NEW REMEDIES

CLINICAL CASES
LESSER WRITINGS
APHORISMS

AND

PRECEPTS

BY

J. T. KENT, A. M., M. D.

Professor Materia Medica, Homoeopath Medical College, St. Louis 1881-8;
Professor Materia Medica and Dean of the Post-Graduate School of Homoeopathy,
Philadelphia, 1890-9; Professor Materia Medica, Hahnemann Medical College and
Hospital, Chicago, 1903-9; Hering Medical College and Hospital, 1909; President
and Trustee Chicago Homoeopathic Hospital, Member American Institute Homoeo-
pathy; Internation al Hahnemannian Association Illinois State Homoeopathic Medi-
cal Society; British *Homoeopathic Society (honorary). Author: Repertory of the
Homoeopathic Materia Medica; What the Doctor Needs to Know, etc.

B. Jain Publishers Pvt. Ltd.
New Delhi (India)

Printed in India

Reprint edition : 2000

Price : Rs. 110.00

Published by:

B. Jain Publishers (P) Ltd.
1921, Street No. 10th Chuna Mandi,
Paharganj, New Delhi-110055 (INDIA)

Printed in India by :
J.J. Offset Printers
7, Wazirpur Printing Press Area,
Ring Road, Wazirpur, Delhi

ISBN 81—7021—070—4

BOOK CODE B-2336

PREFACE

This volume is published at the request of many of Doctor Kent's admirers from all parts of the world. It contains remedies which have never before appeared in book form. They were published in medical journals several years ago and are all verified by Doctor Kent himself.

The various articles appearing are addresses and papers delivered by Doctor Kent at meetings both National and State; to students in classes at college covering a period of many years of his life.

The clinical cases published herewith are only a few of those reported by Doctor Kent and have been carefully selected. All are considered of great value to the student of Homœopathy.

These are only a part of Doctor Kent's writings and were selected from various libraries after considerable effort and are considered the best results of his pen. It is sincerely hoped by the publishers that this book will meet the expectations and be of value to its readers.

W. W. SHERWOOD, M. D.

KENT'S NEW REMEDIES

ALETRIS FARINOSA

This most useful and neglected remedy has been frequently indicated in the complaints of women, especially in those predisposed to hemorrhages; uterine hemorrhages particularly whether it be after an abortion or in connection with menstruation. Copious bleeding from the uterus is characteristic; hemorrhages when the uterus fills with blood until it becomes distended, and its contents are expelled in large clots, followed by copious hemorrhage with or without painful contractions.

A copious menstrual flow followed by watery oozing during the intermenstrual period, now and then dilating into copious gushing flow with black clots; this remedy is useful at the critical period when it is attended with hemorrhage.

The hemorrhages of this medicine are particularly due to a relaxed or debilitated state of the uterus. Weakness of the reproductive organs may be said to be the guiding feature; atony. Weakness of the uterus with repeated abortion or hemorrhages with debility of the individual. Bruised feeling in the region of the ovaries, particularly in the right. Bearing down in the region of the uterus as if the contents of the pelvis would escape. Much worse while walking.

An attack of hemorrhage that came on with great violence in the middle of the night, the patient waking, unable to speak, so exhausted from the flow: was cured by Aletris 45m. This patient lost her urine when coughing, sleeping or walking, and this symptom which has been present many years was entirely cured by Aletris. This involuntary escape of urine was always brought on by catching cold.

Disgust for food; nausea; obstinate indigestion.

The patient has a pale sickly chlorotic face, would like to lie down all day and do nothing but rest. Such de-

5

bilitated patients, when they become pregnant, suffer from vomiting and colic; the stomach seems to be in the same weak condition as the reproductive organs.

Most inveterate constipation.

Until this remedy was known, Kreosote was the most promising remedy for copious frothy eructations with vomiting; this remedy must take the place of Kreosote in the vomiting of pregnant women, when the symptoms agree.

There are violent pains in the rectum and anus. Stool very large and hard, most difficult to expel. Painful constipation.

ALUMINA PHOSPHORICA

The symptoms present aggravations, MORNING, forenoon, AFTERNOON, NIGHT; before midnight, after midnight. Strong desire for open air; open air ameliorates. Marked general anæmia. Single parts go to sleep. Catarrhal conditions generally. Chlorosis. The patient is sensitive to cold and cold generally makes the symptoms worse. He is sensitive to both cold and warm room in a general way; symptoms worse from cold air and from becoming cold; takes cold on slight exposure to cold. Constriction about the body like a band. It is marked for its convulsive action of muscles; its convulsions are clonic; epileptic; hysterical; inclined to fall; with marked stiffness; tonic contraction; convulsive movements. The blood vessels are distended. Symptoms are worse after eating and there is *marked aggravation from physical exertion.* Faint feeling and frequent fainting. General emaciation. Cold drinks and cold food, milk, potatoes and *warm foods* disagree. Formication all over the body. *Lack of vital heat.* A general feeling of heaviness. A lack of physical irritability. Symptoms worse by jarring and stepping. Jerking of muscles and limbs; FEELING OF EXTREME LASSITUDE; desire to lie down. Lying aggravates the breathing but ameliorates the headache; worse after lying long, worse lying on the back. Symptoms worse before, during and after menses; most symptoms are worse from motion, but the pains in the back are better from motion. There is a marked aversion to motion and exertion. There is numbness in the limbs and external parts. Congestion and orgasm of blood. The pains are boring, *bruised*, *burning*, cutting, digging, jerking, *pressing*, sticking and tearing. It is destined to become one of our most useful remedies in paralysis, especially of the lower limbs. It has paralysis of one side, of organs; the paralysis is painless. There is strong internal pulsation. It has fast, weak, irregular pulse. Great internal and external sensitiveness. General amelioration from pressure. The weakness and nervous prostration are as though from sexual excess. Electric shocks are very common and the symptoms are worse after sleep. Standing is a very tiresome position. Tension all over the body. Trembling and twitching. Walking and walking in the open air increase the symptoms, though the open air is grateful to the patient. Great weakness in the morning on waking; from a diarrhoea; from *exertion*; during menses; WALKING; nervous and paralytic weakness. *Extreme weariness.*

Aversion to answering questions and to company; anxiety in the morning on waking; evening; night; of conscience, with fear; about the future; about his health. He is absent-minded and it is impossible to concentrate the mind; confusion of mind in the morning. He is discouraged, discontented, contrary and sure he is going to die. Very excitable and forgetful. Fear in the evening; of death; of disease; that something will happen; of insanity; of misfortune; of people; on waking. It is a remedy to overcome the chronic effects of grief and follows IGNATIA At times there is great hurry, excitement and his mind is full of ideas and this changes to dullness, heedlessness, deficiency of ideas and indifference much like imbecility.

Irresolution is very marked and irritability is extreme. Insane actions, and speech. Aversion to work and laments constantly over his imaginary misfortunes. Spasmodic laughter, maniacal actions, wildly mirthful; moods change rapidly and mental state alternates; loathing of life; extremely obstinate; moments of reserve and absence of all imagination. Mental prostration is a strong feature of this wonderful remedy. Sadness in the morning on waking also in the afternoon; dullness of the senses; very sensitive to noise. Extremely serious at times. Inclination to sit in silence. Starting on falling asleep. It is a very useful remedy after *sexual excesses and prolonged mental efforts*. It is often suited to a mental breakdown at the end of college life. Indisposed to converse with friends; stupefication of mind; disposed to dwell on suicidal thoughts. Talking in sleep. Becomes very timid. Thinking of his symptoms makes them worse. Periods of unconsciousness. Weeping in the morning on waking; during the night; alternating with laughter; involuntary; in sleep. VERTIGO in the *morning*; afternoon, evening; *on closing eyes*; lying amelioriates; with nausea; sitting; stooping; walking. Objects turn in a circle, tendency to fall forward.

This remedy will cure the particulars given below where the generals above strongly predominate.

Coldness of the head; occiput; Rush of blood to head. Constriction of head; forehead. Empty sensation in head. Hair falls out. Heat in head morning and evening; after eating; in forehead. Heaviness of the head in the morning; on stooping. Itching of scalp; forehead. Numbness of scalp. Pain in head, morning in bed; on waking; noon; afternoon; evening; night; ascending; binding up the hair; *after eating* must lie down; before and during menses; moving head; pulsating; sitting; after sleep; from spirituous liquors; stepping heavily; stooping; walking; *warm room*. Pains are better in open air, better lying, better from pressure. Headaches are periodical, every other day. Pain felt deep in brain; pain in the forehead in the morning on waking; afternoon; evening; above the eyes. Pain in *occiput*; *after sleep*, on stooping. PAIN IN THE SIDES OF HEAD; in temples, evening. Pulsating pain in vertex in afternoon. Boring in temples. Bruised feeling in head. Burning in forehead and temples. Bursting, cramping in the head. Cutting in temples. Drawing pains in side of head. Dull pain in the whole head. Pressing pain in head in evening; worse on pressure; in forehead; pressing outward in forehead, over eyes. Pressing in occiput; sides of head, temples, worse night; pressing inward in temples; pressing vertex. Shooting in occiput; vertex; Sore pain in whole head; Stitching pain in head on coughing; in forehead over eyes; sides of head; temples; right side; vertex; stunning pains in head, tearing in forehead; sides of head; temples; vertex. Pulsation in forehead; occiput; sides; temples; vertex. Shocks in head.

Lids stick together during the night. Cracks in the canthi. Yellow, purulent dischrages from eyes. The upper lids are heavy and seem paralyzed. Dryness of the eyes. Inflammation of the conjunctivæ. Itching of the lids and inner canthi. Lachrymation in the open air. Opening lids difficult from dryness, from weakness of lids and from being stuck together with discharge. Pain in eyes from reading. Burning in morning on waking and in *evening*; in the canthi. Pain as though a foreign body in the eye; *pressing*, as though sand in eyes; sore, stitching. Photophobia and quivering of lids. Redness of the eyes. Swollen lids. Twitching of the lids. Styes on the lids. He sees bright colors; halo of colors around the light. *Vision is dim*; exertion of vision causes many symptoms. Flickering and foggy vision. Atrophy of the optic nerve. It has cured blindness from anæmia of the optic nerve.

Purulent discharge from ears. Eruptions on ears. Sensation of flapping in ears; they are hot and red. Itching of the ears and inside. Noises in ears, in morning; evening; with vertigo; buzzing; fluttering; humming; ringing; roaring; whizzing. Roaring in the evening. Pain in ear on blowing nose and swallowing. Boring, burning, stitching, and *tearing in ears.* There is pulsation and a stopped sensation in ears; swelling of the ears. Hearing is acute, later impaired.

Dry coryza alternating with fluent; with cough. Discharge bloody; copious; crusts; excoriating; *greenish*; offensive; purulent; yellow-green; yellow; viscid; thick. It cures most stubborn nasal catarrh. Painful dryness in the nose. The nose bleeds on blowing it. The nose is very red and it itches. One-sided obstruction of the nose. Pain in the nose and root of nose, worse on touch or pressure; soreness in nose; burning in nose; *smell lost*; nose swollen; ulceration in nose; frequent sneezing.

Dry, cracked lips. Sickly, pale, bluish, red; alternating with pallor, red spots. Eruptions on cheeks, chin, forehead and nose; eczema and pimples; pimples on forehead; itching and heat of face. Pain in face worse in open air and from chewing; worse from motion of jaws; drawing, stitching and tearing pains; tearing in bones of face. Sweat on face; swollen face and lips; sensation of white of egg dried on face.

The gums bleed easily and the tongue is coated white. The mouth is very dry and the breath is offensive, even putrid. Pain in gums and palate; sore gums and palate; burning of the mouth. The gums are much swollen and the saliva is abundant. Taste is bitter, insipid, metallic, saltish, sweetish; taste is lost. Burning ulcers in the mouth; pain in teeth in evening, in open air, from masticating, from touch; pain boring, drawing, stitching, tearing.

Constriction of the throat from dryness in evening and on waking. Much hawking to clear the throat of tenacious mucus. Inflammation of the throat. Sensation ot a lump in the throat. Pain in the throat in the morning, on *swallowing*. Burning, pressing, rawness, soreness; worse in morning; stitching on swallowing. Swallowing is difficult. Swollen tonsils.

Appetite increased, even ravenous, without relish of food; hungry even after eating. Appetite wanting. Aversion to his accustomed beer and cigar; to food and meat. Coldness in the stomach. Constriction of stomach. Desires coffee, fruit and sour things. Distension after eating. Emptiness not relieved by eating; without hunger. Eructations in the evening; after milk; bitter; empty; sour; waterbrash; eructations give some relief. He suffers much from heart burn. Fullness and heaviness after eating. Hiccough after eating. He suffers much from indigestion. Nausea, in the morning, evening, night, after eating, during headache. Pain in evening and night; after eating; better after warm drinks; cramping, cutting, drawing, gnawing, pressing, sore, stitching. Retching. Sensation of sinking. Extreme thirst. Thirstless during fever. Vomiting on coughing; after drinking water; bile; blood; food; mucus; watery.

Sensation of coldness and fullness of the abdomen. Flatulent distension. The abdomen feels heavy and constricted. Pain in abdomen morning and afternoon; after eating; before menses; when walking; better from warmth. Cramping, like colic. Pain in the liver. Burning, cutting, nd stitching pains; stitching in liver and sides of abomen; rumbling; sensation of retraction of abdomen; erking in abdominal muscles; sensation of weakness in abdomen.

Constipation with very difficult stools; no desire for stool and fruitless straining; constriction of anus during stool. Diarrhœa morning; afternoon; after breakfast; after eating; during menses. Abscess of the anus. Fistula ani. Flatus very offensive. Formication of anus. Hemorrhoids that bleed and protrude, worse walking.

Itching and moisture of anus. Pain in anus and rectum. Burning during stool. Cutting during stool. Pressing pain. Soreness during stool. Stitching and tenesmus; paralysis of rectum. Stricture. Stool black, bloody, dry, *green, hard, knotty,* large, long and narrow, soft, *thin.*

Frequent ineffectual urging to urinate at night; tenesmus; retention of the urine; paralysis of bladder. Pressure in bladder. Urination difficult; *feeble stream, frequent at night*; involuntary on coughing; must wait long for urine to start; must press a long time before urine flows; an unsatisfied feeling after urination. A feeling of weakness in the bladder. Pain and inflammation of the kidneys. Enlarged prostate gland. Emission of prostatic fluid with stool. Gleety discharge from the urethra. It has cured chronic gonorrhœa with yellow discharge. Burning during flow of urine. Cutting during the flow of urine. Swollen urethra. The urine is acrid, albuminous, burning, cloudy on standing, dark, *pale, copious*; cuticle on the surface; *scanty*; the urinary sediment is red, thick or white.

Erections very troublesome during the night; frequent, painful, violent, later impotency, inflammation of glands; itching of the genitals; soreness of testes; swollen testes; sweat on the genitals.

The woman has aversion to coition; coition without enjoyment. *Leucorrhoea excoriating,* bloody, burning, copious, thin, yellow, before menses, after menses. Menses irregular, too soon or too late; painful, pale, scanty, short; prolapsus uteri, ulceration of the os uteri.

Catarrh of larynx and trachea; dryness of larynx, mucus in larynx, rawness and soreness in larynx and trachea; itching in the larynx, hoarseness in the evening, with coryza worse from talking; the voice is rough, hollow and finally lost. Difficult breathing at night; asthmatic, rattling and wheezing; breathing arrested from coughing; desire for a deep breath.

Cough MORNING, afternoon, evening, night; before midnight; in cold air; asthmatic; dry evening and night; dry evening and loose morning cough; hacking in evening; from irritation in larynx, trachea; loose in morning; paroxysmal; rattling; short; from talking, tormenting; violent. Expectoration in the morning; bloody and copious; difficult; mucus, bloody; putrid; salty; sweetish; viscid; white; yellow.

Anxiety and constriction of the heart. Sensation of heat in chest. Inflammation of bronchia. Itching of skin of chest especially of mammæ. Oppression at night. Pain in chest at night; on coughing; after eating; on inspiring; in sides of chest; aching and burning; pressing; rawness on coughing; soreness on coughing; stitches on inspiring.

Palpitation in morning on waking; evening; anxious; after eating; during menses; on waking; tumultuous. Weak sensation in chest.

The back feels cold. Pimples on the back. Inflammation of the spinal cord. Itching of the back. *Pain in the back*, better by motion; rising from a seat; worse while walking. Pain in cervical region on moving the head. Pain between the scapulæ. Pain in the lumbar region; sacrum; coccyx when touched; spine. Aching in lumbar region during motion and walking; cutting pains in the back. *Sore, bruised* pain in spine; in sacrum. Stitching in back; scapulæ, lumbar region. Tearing in scapulæ; lumbar region. Stiffness of back; cervical region. Weak feeling in lumbar region.

While walking he staggers. Old chilblains came back. Coldness of hands, legs and feet. His corns smart and sting. Hands and fingers cracked. Cramps in the calf. Boils on nates and thighs. Eruptions on legs. Formication on upper limbs and feet. The hands are hot. Heaviness of *upper* and *lower limbs*. Ingrowing toe nail. Itching of limbs evening, worse after scratching; upper limbs and hands; *lower limbs*. Jerking in lower limbs. Numbness of limbs, upper limbs, lower limbs, legs, feet. Pain in limbs at night; in joints; pain in upper limbs when they hang down; in left shoulder; elbow; pain in thighs, legs, feet and soles; aching in legs. Burning in upper limbs; soles. Drawing pain in limbs; arm; forearm; thighs; knees. Sore, bruised limbs; joints; lower limbs; legs. Stitching pain in limbs; upper limbs; arms; elbow; lower limbs; hips; knees; legs; soles; toes. Tearing pain in upper limbs; shoulders; arms; elbow, forearm; hands; fingers; *lower limbs*; hips; *thighs*; *knees*; legs, foot. Paralysis of limbs; *one-sided*; painless; *lower limbs*. Stiffness of lower limbs. Tension of thighs and legs. Tingling upper limbs; hands; fingers, lower limbs; feet; trembling of limbs, hands and knees. Twitching of the muscles of limbs. Weakness of limbs; upper limbs, *lower limbs*; *thighs*; *knees*.

Deep sleep. Dreams anxious; of death; of falling; of robbers; of vexations. Late falling asleep. Restless sleep. Sleepiness in morning; forenoon; evening; after dinner. Sleepless *before midnight*. After sleep he is unrefreshed. *Frequent waking*.

Chill forenoon; noon; afternoon; *evening in bed*; *night*, before midnight. Chilliness after eating; internal chill; coldness predominates. Shaking, quotidian chill; chill or coldness one-sided; warm room does not ameliorate the chill; desire for warmth which does not ameliorate.

Fever afternoon; evening; night without sweat; fever alternates with chill; heat goes from below upwards. Flushes of heat.

Perspiration morning and during night; during least exertion; from *least anxiety*.

Biting and burning. Anæsthesia. The skin is dry burning or cold. Red spots on the skin. Yellow, as if jaundiced. Eruptions biting; boils; blood boils; burning; coppery, become moist with yellow discharge; dry; eczema. Herpes burning, corrosive, itching, scabby, stinging; eruptions itch in a warm room.   Pimples, rash and scabby eruption; smarting, sore, stinging eruptions.   Urticaria, nodules after scratching.   Vesicular eruptions.   *Formication*, Itching a night in bed; biting, burning, crawling, worse after scratching; stinging; worse in warm bed; moisture after scratching.   Pain in skin after scratching. Hyperæsthesia of the skin.   Itching and stinging after scratching.   A feeling of tension in the skin.   Ulcers; offensive; with yellow pus; *indolent*, itching, sensitive, smarting, stinging, unhealthy.   The skin refuses to heal where injured.

ALUMINA SILICATE

This valuable remedy is made from a species of rock known as andalusite and composed of aluminum sixty-three and silica thirty-seven parts.   It was prepared by trituration in the usual way.

It has been proved and used clinically by the author for many years.   It is a deep and long acting remedy and cures chronic complaints of the brain, spinal cord, bowels and the nerves, that have heretofore been most stubborn.

Its complaints are sometimes noticed in the forenoon, but mostly in the afternoon and evening.   Some symptoms come on in the night, even after midnight.

There is a desire for open air which is grateful, but cold air aggravates all complaints; much worse after becoming cold and a marked tendency to take cold.   There is great coldness during pains and all pains are better from warmth and warm applications.   The prover loses flesh, and it has cured patients markedly emaciated and anæmic. There is great weakness and many symptoms are worse going upstairs.   Congestion of brain and cord and spinal nerves, with marked burning and stinging.   It has cured multiple neuritis and locomotor ataxia.   Constriction is a marked general symptom, also constriction of orifices, a sensation as if constricted. It has been of great service in epileptic and epileptiform convulsion; not when the convulsion is on but as a constitutional remedy causing the attacks to diminish and come less frequently, and finally disappear. Stiffness and tonic contractions occur with provers. Distention of all the veins, and fainting spells. The symptoms are worse after eating and he is better fasting or eating very small quantities of food; worse from cold drinks, cold food, milk and very warm foods.

Formication of the skin, extremities along the *course of nerves* and in internal parts. A sensation of fullness throughout the body, with distended veins. Heaviness of the body and all the limbs. Induration of parts inflamed. Inflammation of the nerves, with burning, stinging, crawling and numbness; the brain, spine and abdominal viscera are extremely sensitive to a jar, as in riding in a carriage over rough roads. Jerking and twitching in muscles. The lassitude is so great that she was compelled to keep to the bed; she must lie down, a marked sense of spinal weakness. It cured a woman who had lain in bed many years from weakness. Straining of muscles from lifting, like Rhus tox. Yet some symptoms are worse lying in bed, but lying generally helps and rests the patient. She says, "I am so comfortable while lying." Some symptoms are worse lying on the back. She desires perfect rest, aversion to all motion and worse from all motion. The mucous secretions are increased.   It has cured lupus. Numbness of single parts and of painful parts; numbness with neuritis. There is orgasm of blood, flushes of heat, even great rushes of heat to head from body.

The pains are worse from excitement and motion and better from external warmth and perfect rest. The pains are of all kinds, boring, *burning and stinging.* Constricting, cutting, digging, gnawing, jerking, paralyzing, pinching, *pressing.* The whole body is sore to touch and pressure, *stitching*, TEARING, *ulcerative* pain wandering from place to place.

The pains as well as many other symptoms show a marked periodicity. Pressure sometimes increases and sometimes helps the pains. Pulsation all over the body and in the head and abdomen. The pulse is fast, evening and night. The patient is better resting in bed and worse rising up from bed or chair. Sensitive externally and internally. Complaints all worse standing.

Extreme heat of summer takes her strength. There is swelling in affected parts and of glands. Throughout the body and limbs a feeling of tension. The limbs tremble and she trembles all over. Twitching all over. Complaints felt on waking. Walking is almost impossible; walking fast or any exertion brings out all symptoms; weakness from walking. Wet weather increases the symptoms. Close, warm room causes many symptoms.

It is very useful in nervous debility where there is great mental excitement and aggravations from anger and vexation. Absent minded. *Anxiety*, evening, *night*; anxiety of conscience, anxiety about her health; worse after sleep. One prover felt that she would become insane and urged to have the 30th, which she had taken, antidoted. Wants this and that and never satisfied, she criticises everybody. She desires to be alone, but becomes worse when alone and better in company. She has much difficulty in concentrating the mind. Confusion of mind every morning, worse on waking. Worse from contradiction. Contrary and whimsical.

Several provers were timid and cowardly.

She thinks she is growing smaller and that she will fall if she rises to her feet; she sees visions; there is despair; she is discontented, discouraged and distracted; long periods of dullness of mind; dullness of mind after sleep.

There is marked exaltation of fancy. The mind is in a constant state of fear; wakes up with fear and frightened easily. There is a marked mental weakness, forgetful, indifferent, irresolution, deficiency of ideas, so that it is easy to see the resemblance to imbecility or the borderland of insanity. She laughs much as in hysteria and many mental symptoms are hysterical in character. She is morose and obstinate and the memory is weak. Changeable moods. She makes mistakes in speaking and writing and uses wrong words. There is remorse; religious affections of the mind and great mental weakness bordering on insanity. It is useful in brain-fag after prolonged mental exertion. The mind is anxious and restless at night. There is great *sadness*. One prover said she was never so unhappy in her life, but she felt better after telling it to somebody. Great dullness of the senses. She is very sensitive to noise. She sits a long while without appearing to notice what goes on. She walks in sleep. Starting on falling asleep. She thinks much about suicide, loathes life and desires to die. She sits long, indisposed to talk; she talks in sleep; weeping in sleep. Will power very weak. Aversion to mental as well as physical work.

Vertigo morning and evening; while sitting; stooping; walking; turning the head suddenly; ameliorated while lying. Vertigo while closing the eyes, tendency to fall forward; on turning there is a tendency to fall in the direction turned; vertigo as if intoxicated, with nausea.

Rush of blood to the head, with boiling sensation and coldness of the occiput; constriction of the scalp. especially of the forehead. The head feels empty. Heat and *heaviness* of the head in the evening, especially of the forehead. Much itching and formication of the scalp. There is much pain in the head, *morning, afternoon, evening* and *night*. The headaches are worse from bending the head forward, binding up the hair, after eating; when biting the teeth together, before and during menses, while sitting; after sleep, after stimulants, stepping heavily. stooping. The headaches are better from binding up the head, *from cold applications, cold air, lying,* moving head, pressure standing, and walking. There are intermittent pains day and night. Periodical headaches. Noise causes the headache to become pulsating. She wants the body wrapped up, but wants head in cold air. Sensation of crawling, as though ants in the brain, this sensation travels down the body and leaves at the toes. Pain in the *forehead,* over eyes afternoon and evening. Pain in occiput, temples, vertex and sides of head, worse on the right side. The pains in the head are burning, bursting, cutting, drawing, pressing, shooting, sore as if bruised, stitching and tearing. There is a dull pain in occiput, vertex and temples, worse from pressure and mental work. Pressing in forehead, pressing outward over eyes. Pressing in temples, vertex and occiput. The head is so sore during pain she cannot comb or brush the hair. Stitching pain in *forehead,* sides of head and temples. Many of the headaches were so severe that she was stunned by the pain. Violent, tearing pains in the evening; tearing in forehead in evening; tearing in frontal eminence; tearing pain in temples and vertex. Wandering pains in the head, better during rest and while sitting. Pulsating headache worse from noise; pulsating in forehead and vertex. The brain seems to be sensitive to a noise. When something drops on the floor it seems to drop on her sore head.

The eyelids are stuck together during the night, and in the morning discharge thick mucus; dark rings around the eyes; eyes feel enlarged with dryness; catarrhal inflammation in the open air, with itching. Pain in the eyes; burning in the evening as from smoke; burning in lids and in the canthi; pressing pain in the eyes; soreness and pain as from sand in the eyes; stitching in the eyes. *Photophobia.* Redness of the eyes; styes and swollen lids. The vision is dim, worse at night by artificial light, and exertion of vision. The vision is foggy, weak. Hypermetropia.

Purulent discharge from the ears, with itching in the auditory canal. The ears are hot. Noises in the ears; humming, fluttering, ringing, roaring and whizzing. Pain deep in the ear; boring, stitching and tearing pains in the ear. Stopped sensation with pulsation. Hearing at first acute, later impaired.

The air feels cold in the nose on breathing. Catarrh of the nasal cavity and posterior nares. The discharge is BLOODY, containing crusts, *excoriating, greenish,* hard lumps; offensive, purulent, thick, sometimes watery, yellow, or yellowish-green. Coryza with cough; dry, alternating with fluent, violent coryza; much dryness in the nasal cavity. Epistaxis on blowing the nose; the nose feels full, itching in the nose. The nose is obstructed with thick mucus and crusts. Burning and tearing in the nose; much soreness in nose, root of nose and septum sore to touch; dull pain in nose on breathing transmitted upward to middle of vertex. Smell first acute, then diminished, later lost. Frequent sneezing, with and without coryza. Ulceration in the nose. The nose is greatly swollen.

Pain in the face; pain in malar bones, with pain in temple; pain from temples to malar bones and worse in open air and when chewing. Drawing, stitching and tearing pains in the face. The face is purple.

Apthæ covering the mucous membranes of the whole mouth; the gums bleed and the tongue is coated white. Dryness of the mouth; when a chill or lacerating pain in head comes on the lips stick together. Mucus collects in the mouth, and the odor from the mouth is offensive; pain in gums and teeth from cold air, on biting, and after eating. Sore gums, palate and tongue; stitching and tearing pains in the teeth; *salivation,* swollen gums; the taste is bloody, metallic, sour, or wanting. Food is *tasteless.* Ulceration of gums. Teeth very sensitive. Pain from roots of upper teeth to head, when biting teeth together.

Mild form of inflammation in the throat and tonsils.

Hawks up much mucus; dryness of the throat on waking; sensation of a lump in the throat; tough, tenacious mucus in the throat; pain in the throat on swallowing; burning, rawness and soreness in the throat. Splinter sensation in the throat; stitching pain on swallowing; swallowing is slow and difficult; ulceration of the throat and the tonsils are swollen. Swollen cervical glands.

The appetite is increased, later ravenous, but the first mouthful causes nausea. The appetite is strong, but food is not properly relished; appetite for things not obtainable. Aversion to food, to meat, to coffee; thinks she cannot digest food; an empty feeling, which is not helped by eating. Eructations bitter, empty, sour, of food, after eating tasting like spoiled meat, waterbrash, eructations give relief. Fullness after eating, often only a mouthful. Weight in the stomach after eating; hiccough, heartburn and loathing of food. Nausea morning, evening and night; after eating, during headache. The sight and thought of food causes nausea. Pain in stomach, evening and night, aggravated by eating. Burning extending upwards, *cramping*, pressing, gnawing, cutting stitching; pressing pain after eating, better by eructations. Soreness on pressure. Retchings. Sinking sensation. Sensation of a stone in the stomach. Water tastes as if spoiled. Some thirst, but no thirst during fever. Vomiting or *coughing* after eating and during headache; vomiting of bile, black blood, of food, mucus and water.

Obstructed flatulence in the abdomen, fullness, distension, hardness, heaviness, constriction; distension worse after eating. Pain in abdomen, worse after eating, before menses, during menses, worse walking and better by warm applications. Pain in region of the liver; burning in the abdomen. Cramping, colicy pains begin in the stomach and pass down into bowels, with urging to stool. Cramping all over abdomen, and then must run and pass a watery, fetid, ye"ow stool. Cutting and pressing, stitching pains in left hypochondrium and in the liver; tearing pains in abdomen. Rumbling and tensions.

Constipation, very difficult stool; unsatisfactory, scanty stool; much straining, even soft stool is difficult. Constriction of the anus during stool. Diarrhœa driving out of bed at 5 a. m.; first undigested, then watery, clear, with much flatus, from fruit. Passes much flatus with stool; flatus offensive without stool. Crawling at the anus. Hemorrhage from external piles. Inactivity of the rectum; itching of the anus—worse by scratching; moisture around the anus; pain in anus during stool; burning during stool. Cutting, pressing, soreness and stitching. Tenesmus of the rectum; paralysis of the rectum. Ineffectual urging to stool. The stool is bloody, copious, dark, dry, hard, knotty, large, offensive, scanty, soft, thin, watery, undigested.

Paralytic weakness of the bladder. Retention of urine. Tenesmus while passing urine. Ineffectual urging to urinate. Frequent urging to pass urine, worse at night; urination in feeble stream, frequent during the night; must wait long for urine to flow; unsatisfactory feeling in the bladder after urination; involuntary urination.

Emission of prostatic fluid during stool, the gland is enlarged, sore and painful; prostate gland inflamed.

Discharge of mucus and pus from the urethra; burning when passing urine; cutting during the flow of urine.

Urine copious, later scanty, burning, cloudy and red. Red sediment, specific gravity normal, no sugar, no albumen.

Troublesome erections of the male during the night, which are very strong and painful; the testes are swollen and hard; the glans penis is red and excoriated; the scrotum itches and perspires. Frequent seminal emissions, sexual excitement is strong during the evening and night.

The woman has tormenting itching and crawling; worse after urination, worse after scratching, better by cold applications. Leucorrhea acrid, bloody, copious, purulent, thin, white or yellow; worse before and after menses. Menses in one prover too frequent, in several provers, too late, intermittent, offensive, painful, scanty. Suppressed menses has been cured. Burning pain in the genitals; prolapsus of the uterus; ulceration of the labia.

Irritation of the larynx, mucus in larynx and trachea. It cures catarrh of larynx and trachea. Rawness and soreness in larynx. Must scrape mucus from the larynx very often. Constant tickling in the larynx and trachea. Husky, rough voice. Hoarseness, worse in the morning.

The breathing is arrested by coughing, wheezing, asthmatic breathing; rattling breathing. Difficult breathing from coughing.

Cough in the daytime, morning *evening* and *night*. Asthmatic cough. Dry cough morning and *night*; dry cough with expectoration only in the morning; the cough is worse in cold air. Dry, hacking cough in the *evening*. Much irritation in larynx and trachea from hard coughing. Loud cough in the morning with fever. Lying on the right side causes coughing spells. Racking, paroxysmal cough from tickling in the larynx. Violent coughing spells.

Expectoration daytime, *morning*, evening and night, *acrid*, bloody, copious, offensive, viscid, white or *yellow*.

Orgasm of blood or a feeling of congestion in the chest. Constriction of the chest; oppression, heat and blood spitting; inflammation of bronchial tubes; pain in chest during the night; during cough, in the sides of chest. Burning in chest. Crushing pain in chest; rawness in chest when coughing; sore, bruised chest-walls from coughing. Stitching pain in chest from coughing and inspiring. Weakness felt in the chest and palpitation of the heart.

On exposure to cold air the back is cold as if cold water were poured on it. Many eruptions on the back. Itching of the *cervical* and dorsal regions; pain in the back on motion, rising from a seat, *stooping* or *walking*. Lying perfectly quiet the pain is relieved, but turning or trying to help herself out of a chair causes pain in back near the spine. Pain in cervical region, in dorsal region between the scapulæ, in the sacrum, in the coccyx and in the *whole spine*; aching in the spine, but especially lumbar region and sacrum. Great burning in the spine, burning pain in the cervical region and between the scapulæ. Pricking like needles in the lumbar region on exertion; better during rest. Sore and bruised feeling in the spine, especially the lumbar region; sticking like needles in the lumbar region. Stitching pains in the back, in the cervical region, in the scapulæ and between the scapulæ. Tearing pain in the back. *Stiffness* of the back and of the *cervical* region; extreme weakness of the back compelling her to remain in bed.

Awkwardness of the limbs, more in the lower limbs. A blue painful spot on the hand where she had a wart removed many years ago. The nails became brittle; the hands are constantly chapped; coldness of hands, *legs* and *feet*; hands cold as ice and fingers blue. Cramps in the calf. Emaciation of all the limbs, numerous eruptions on the limbs, notably boils and red rash. *Formication* is extreme. The hands are very hot. Heaviness of *upper limbs*, of *lower limbs, hands and feet*. Violent itching without eruption, upper limbs, hands and fingers, *lower limbs, thighs* and *soles*. Painful itching in arms along the course of nerves. Jerking in all the limbs. Numbness of all the limbs, upper limbs in forenoon, numbness of hands and fingers, numbness of lower limbs, *legs, feet* and heel; numbness of first two toes of right foot while lying on the back. Pain in the limbs from excitement, worse from motion, worse during the night. Pain in the joints; pain in upper limbs, shoulders, elbow, forearm, hand and fingers; pain along the course of nerves. Pain in lower limbs from motion and excitement; pain in thighs, legs and feet, pain along the course of nerves. Pain travels from below upwards, worse on left side; pain goes to cardiac region and then to left temple. Aching pain in legs. Burning pain in limbs; burning pain in arms from *excitement*; burning in the soles. Crushing pain in the bones of legs, and in the muscles. Drawing pain in upper arm and in forearm; drawing pain in thighs, knees and ankles; pricking pain, thinks a knitting needle is thrust deep into muscle of right hip. Sore, bruised limbs, *lower limbs*, legs, tibia, SOLES; stitching pains in upper limbs, shoulder, upper arm, elbow and wrist; stitching pains in hip, knee, calf, sole, toes. Tearing in upper limbs, shoulder, upper arm, elbow, forearm, hands and fingers; tearing pain *lower limbs*, *hip*, thighs, KNEES, LEGS, calf, ankles, feet; tearing pains along the course of nerves. Wandering pains of all kinds in the limbs. Painless paralysis of lower limbs, also pain in the paralyzed parts. Tension in the upper limbs and in the arms when lifting anything; tension in the calf and feet. Swelling of the fingers. Stiffness in the lower limbs. Tingling prickling in all the limbs, upper limbs, hands and fingers, lower limbs and feet. Trembling all over, in limbs, hands and knees. Twitching of limbs, in shoulder, lower limbs, legs, feet. Ulceration about the nails. Weakness in the limbs, *upper limbs*, LOWER LIMBS, *thighs*, *legs*.

He is unable to step up when ascending stairs; it seems to him that he cannot lift his body to the next step.

Sleep is disturbed by visions; dreams anxious, confused, amorous, of death, *nightmare*, pleasant, of quarreling, vexatious. Sleep is restless and broken. Sleepiness in the morning, forenoon and evening, and after dinner. Sleepless before midnight; unrefreshing sleep, waking too early, *frequent waking*. Yawning.

Chilliness in the forenoon, noon, afternoon, evening; chilliness in the evening in bed; chilliness in the open air, after eating, better after warm drink; external coldness; internal coldness. Chilliness on moving in bed. Shaking chill at 5 p. m. One-sided coldness. Chilliness during stool. Desire for warmth which ameliorates the chill.

Heat afternoon, *evening* and *night.* Fever begins between 8 and 10 p. m., with severe crushing pain in both legs; pain goes to heart and left temple. External heat with chilliness. Flushes of heat; heat during sleep.

Perspiration morning, night, with anxiety; perspiration on motion—profuse after waking.

Dryness of the skin, coldness, biting, anæsthesia, yellow spots. *Burning,* cracked. Eruptions, blisters, boils, burning; chapping, DRY eczema. Herpes, dry, itching, stinging. Itching eruptions worse by warmth. Painful eruptions. Nodular urticaria, vesicular eruptions. Marked eruption moist after scratching, smarting after scratching. Stinging and burning eruptions. Suppurating phagedenic eruptions. Nodular urticaria, vesicular eruptions. Marked formication of the skin all over body, itching worse in evening in bed. Biting, burning, crawling; better by keeping perfectly still. Itching better by scratching. Stinging burning in the skin all over, but worse on the back of hands, arms and feet. Moisture of the skin after scratching. Skin extremely sensitive. Much tension in the skin. Ulceration, with itchiñg, soreness and stinging. The skin is slow to heal after injury.

ARSENICUM SULPHURETUM FLAVUM

This is one of our deepest remedies and is to used against psora and syphilis, especially in old broken constitutions. The Encyclopedia and Guiding Symptoms furnish valuable fragmentary provings. This study is based also upon new provings and extensive clinical observations. It is a most useful medicine in old cases of malaria, in great weakness following the abuse of quinine. When eruptions have been suppressed from local treatment, and there is great weakness and lack of reaction.

The symptoms are worse in *morning,* forenoon, *afternoon, evening,* in twilight, NIGHT, *before midnight, after midnight.* It has a marked tendency to form abscesses. Aversion to open air. Aversion to open air alternating with a desire for open air. Extremely sensitive to a draft. Open air makes some symptoms better and some worse. ANÆMIA and PHYSICAL ANXIETY. Weakness and suffocation from going up stairs. Parts feel constricted as with a band. He takes cold from bathing and all symptoms are worse. It is a most useful remedy in combating the symptoms of epithelioma, lupus and scirrhus, even where ulceration is far advanced. The appearance of the face and skin is much like chlorosis. Choreic action of the muscles all over the body. In general the patient is cold, worse from cold air, from becoming cold, from cold, wet weather; takes cold easily. Convulsions, abdomen puffed up; offensive bilious diarrhœa, slimy vomiting. Discharges from all mucous membranes and outlets *very excoriating, offensive, thin and yellow.* Dropsy of the extremities and in abdomen. The symptoms are worse before and AFTER EATING. There is marked emaciation of the body. Slight exertion increases all conditions and symptoms. Faintness from many causes, but *especially after stool.* Worse from cold drinks, sour food, cold food, fat food, fruit and milk. Formication all over the body. The mucous membranes bleeding easily. The body feels heavy and loggy. Sometimes he is too warm and sometimes chilly. Inflamed parts and base of ulcers indurate. Inflammation of organs and glands. Lassitude and lack of reaction. He always desires to lie down. He feels worse lying, worse after lying awhile, worse lying on back, yet he feels better in bed. Symptoms all worse during menstruation. Motion in general ameliorates, yet motion aggravates some sympoms. The patient dreads motion. Old people much broken down, seem to rally under its action. Pains are cutting, BURNING, internal and external, PRESSING, *stitching,* tearing; tearing downward, tearing in muscles. *Thrusting pains*. Periodicity is very marked. Perspiration gives no relief. Complaints after suppressed sweat. Pulsations all over the body. The pulse is fast, irregular, intermittent, small, weak. Running or fast walking increases all symptoms. Extremely sensitive to pain. Shocks felt throughout the body; many symptoms worse on right side of the body. Complaints worse sitting. Symptoms before sleep, on going to sleep and during sleep. Standing aggravates. Stiffness in body and limbs. Dropsical swelling and swelling of glands. Affected parts sore to touch. Trembling of body and limbs. Twitching of muscles. Varicose veins. Many symptoms worse after sleep. Walking ameliorates, walking in open air aggravates; walking fast aggravates. Warmth of bed ameliorates. Extreme weakness, weakness in morning, during menses, after exertion, after eating, from perspiration, after stool, from walking in open air.

Absent minded and he is greatly affected from anger. Aversion to answering questions and when he does answer his mind works slowly. ANXIETY, *morning*, EVENING, EVENING IN BED, *during the night*. Anxiety of conscience, with fear, during fever, about salvation, after a swoon, during stool, on waking. He is very critical with his friends and desires things which are not useful to him. Confusion of mind in the morning on waking. Over-conscientious about small matters. Longs for death. Delirious and raving during the night. His mind is full of delusions. A general feeling of despair. He is discontented and very excitable. His mind is full of *fear at night*; fear of a crowd, of *death,* of evil, of ghosts, of people, of *solitude.* Memory at first active, later he is forgetful. *Easily frightened or startled,* starting on going to sleep and during sleep. It has been useful during fevers when he picks the bed clothing. Hurried feeling and always hasty in actions. Many hysterical symptoms. Impatience, indifference, indolence. He seems to be growing weak-minded. It has been used in insane conditions, in drunkards. *Extremely irritable* during chill; in the morning on waking. Loathing of life. Sometimes he is lamenting and again he is laughing. At times very talkative and again very malicious, almost maniacal like one intoxicated. It has been used in mania-a-potu. Mental work is impossible after eating. Great liveliness, then muttering. Extremely unreasonable and obstinate. Offended without cause and quarrelsome followed by insane fury. Religious affections, remorse. Great mental fatigue. Restlessness evening, *night*, tossing in bed, during fever, during menses. Sadness evening, during heat, during sweat. Extremely sensitive and touchy. Inclined to take all matters seriously. Speech incoherent and wandering. Aversion to being spoken to, indisposed to converse on any subject. Suspicious of all his friends and his family. Periods of stupefication, vanishing of thought. Weeping at night. Weeping in sleep. Extremely timid, bashful, feeling of weakness in head.

Vertigo evening, as if dancing up and down. Inclined to fall to the right. Vertigo with headache. Looking downward, with nausea; walking in the open air.

Whenever the general sympoms given above strongly predominate in any given case, the following particulars will yield to this remedy.

The head is cold during headache, especially the forehead. A feeling of tightness of the forehead and marked hyperæmia of the brain, moist crusts and scales on the scalp. *It has been very useful in eczema.* Pustules on the scalp. Inflamed patches much like erysipelas. Much heat in the head and especially in the forehead. Great weight in forehead morning and evening. Itching of the scalp. The head is painful in the morning on waking. Pain in the afternoon. Pain at 5 p. m. and 4 p. m. Pain in the head evening and *night*. Pain worse in cold air, on coughing, after eating, from exercising, in bright light, moving head, riding in a carriage, in a warm room, shaking the head, after sleep, from stimulants, from stooping, from walking in the open air. Pain comes during chill, during menses, comes periodically, every two weeks. Pain is violent and pulsating. Violent pain deep in the brain, in frontal region and right ear. Pain in forehead worse in right side, better after sleep. Waking often with dull pain above the eyes extending to the top of the head. Pain in the occiput extending to sides of head 7 to 11 a. m. Pain in sides of head. Pain in vertex. Sore, bruised pain in whole head, in forehead. Burning in head. Drawing pain in forehead. Pressing pain in forehead, occiput and temples. Dull pain in right frontal region, which increases in severity and becomes a sharp, pulsating and shooting pain extending to occiput on the right side, worse from motion and stooping, 4 p. m. Stitching pain in the head, in temple, worse on coughing. Tearing pain in occiput. Cold sweat on the forehead; temple worse on coughing. Pulsation in the head. Shocks in the head.

Eyelids stuck together in the morning. Discharges from eyes acrid, bloody, yellow. Dryness of the eyes. Dullness. Eruptions about the eyes. Excoriation of the lids. Glassy look of the eyes. Gum in canthi. Granular lids. Chronic inflammation of eyes, of conjunctiva, cornea, iris, lids. The veins of eyes are injected. Lachrymation. Half open eyes. Opening lids difficult. Pain in eyes evening, on moving eyes, when reading, aching in the eyes. Burning in evening when reading. Burning in margin of lids. Pains are drawing, pressing, sore, bruised, stitching, tearing, paralysis of optic nerve. Photophobia in sunlight. The eyes feel as if protruding. Redness of lids, of veins, spots on the cornea; sunken eyes. Swollen lids. The tears are acrid. Twitching of the lids. Ulceration of the cornea. In the field of vision there are sparks, flickerings and dark colors. Objects look yellow. Foggy vision. Dim vision.

Discharges from ear fetid and offensive. Eruptions on and behind ears. Formication. Heat of ears. Sensation of fullness in ears. Itching of ears and in ears. Noises; buzzing, humming, ringing, soaring, rushing, snapping. Pain in ears in evening. Pain behind ears. Pain in ears; burning, drawing, pressing outward, stitching, tearing. Pulsation in ears. Ears feel stopped. Tingling of ears. Tensive feeling behind right ear on stroking the hair. Hearing impaired.

Cold nose. Fluent coryza. Nasal discharge bloody burning, crusty, excoriating, greenish, offensive, thick, white, yellow. *Dryness in nose.* Bleeding from the nose. The nose is obstructed with thick mucus. Offensive odor from nose. Burning inside of nose. Smell at first acute, later wanting. *Frequent sneezing.* The nose is swollen. Ulceration high up in nose.

It has cured epithelioma of the lip. The face is chlorotic and cold. The lips are cracked. The face is bluish and there are dark circles under the eyes. Earthy, pale or sallow. Jaundiced face. Circumscribed red cheeks. Red spots. Redness of the face. Dryness of the lips. Eruptions, acne, pimples, pustules, rash, scurf, vesicles. It cures eczema when the symptoms agree. The expression is *anxious, sickly,* suffering. Heat and itching of the face. Inflammation of the submaxillary gland. Pain worse in open air and better from warmth; comes on periodically. Pain in the submaxillary gland. Pains of face are BURNING, drawing, *tearing.* Cold sweat on face. Pulsation in right side of face. The face looks sunken. Swelling of the face and *submaxillary gland.* Twitching of the face. Ulceration of the lips.

Copious aphthæ in mouth and on the tongue. Bleeding of the gums. Cracked tongue. The tongue is red or coated brown, white or yellow. Mouth and tongue very dry. Inflammation of the tongue. Much frothy mucus in the mouth. The mucous membrane of the mouth and tongue is inflamed and excoriated, offensive odor from the mouth. Burning mouth and tongue. Copious saliva. Scorbutic gums. Shining tongue. Speech difficult. Taste is bad; better in morning on waking; bloody, insipid, putrid, saltish, sour, sweetish, ulcers in the mouth and on the tongue. The mouth is full of vesicles.

Choking in the throat and constriction of the œsophagus. The right tonsil is enlarged. Dryness, redness and heat in the throat. Inflammation of throat and *tonsils*. Sensation of a lump in throat. Much mucus in throat. Pain in throat in evening on swallowing. Burning, rawness, soreness and stitching. Scraping in the throat, swallowing difficult. The throat is swollen. Ulceration of pharynx. It is a very useful remedy in stubborn syphilitic ulceration of throat with rapid destruction of tissue.

A feeling of anxiety in the stomach. Appetite ravenous, with easy satiety. Appetite wanting for the evening meal. Aversion to fats, to food, to rich food, to meat. Sensation of coldness in stomach. Constriction of stomach. Craves stimulants. Coffee, fruit, sour things, sweets, warm things, warm drinks. The stomach is disordered from milk. A sensation of emptiness. Eructations acrid, bitter, empty; of food, foul, SOUR. Gnawing in the stomach. Fullness in stomach after eating, especially after breakfast. Heartburn. Weight in stomach after eating. Hiccough after eating. Indigestion from all heavy food. Loathing of food. Nausea after cold water, after eating, during headache, during stool. Pain in stomach after eating. Burning, cramping, cutting, pressing and stitching pains. Burning after cold drinks, pressing after eating. Extreme tenderness of the stomach. Pulsation. Retching when coughing. Sensation of a stone in the stomach. Thirst morning, evening and *night*. Burning thirst.

Thirst after chill. Extreme thirst during heat. Unquenchable thirst. Vomiting worse nights; on coughing, after
drinking, after eating, during headache, after milk; vomiting bile, black substance, blood, food, mucus; *sour*, watery
substances.

A feeling of anxiety in the abdomen after stool.
Bluish spots over the abdomen and thighs. Cold abdomen
during chill. Distension after eating. Tympanitic abdomen. Dropsy of peritoneum. It has cured enlarged spleen.
Eruptions on the abdomen. Flatulence, fullness, and *gurgling. Fullness in the hypo-gastric region.* Itching of the
skin. The abdomen feels heavy and the liver is hard.
Pain in the abdomen at night. Pain as though diarrhœa
would come on. Pain in abdomen after coughing; after
eating, during menses, while walking; better by external
warmth. Pain in the liver and in the hypogastrium.
Burning in the bowels. Cramping before and after stool.
Cramping and vomiting. Cutting pain before stool, worse
walking, better by pressure. Great tenderness in the abdomen. Strong pulsations in abdomen. Rumbling in abdomen; worse before stool. It has cured painful and
swollen spleen in old malarial cases. Sensation of tightness in the abdomen. Ulceration of the navel.

Constipation alternating with diarrhœa. Stools hard
and knotty. Difficult. Diarrhœa in the morning after rising, daily at 8 a. m., afternoon, NIGHT, AFTER MIDNIGHT.
Stools acrid, black, pure bile, bloody mucus, offensive,
mushy and yellow, undigested, thin. Diarrhœa after
drinking, after eating, after fruit, during menses. The
diarrhœa is generally painful, but sometimes painless.
Dysentery with bloody mucus, scanty stool. Excoriation
of the anus and around it. The anus is fissured. Flatus
copious and offensive. Hemorrhoids worse during the
night, external, large; worse walking. Itching of the anus.
Moisture that excoriates. Pain in rectum and anus DURING

3

STOOL and after stool, during straining to stool. During urination. *Burning during* and after stool. Cutting during stool. Soreness and stitching pains. Tenesmus with dysentery and after a yellow mushy stool. Paralysis and prolapsus of rectum.

Fullness of the bladder. Inflammation of the bladder. Pain in the bladder. Paralysis of bladder. Retention of urine. Urging to urinate worse at night, constant ineffectual, sudden, must hasten or will lose the urine. Urination dribbling, painful, difficult, involuntary at night, unsatisfactory. Inflammation of kidneys; urine suppressed. Burning in urethra when passing urine. The urine is albuminous, bloody, burning, cloudy on standing, copious or scanty, offensive, with purulent sediment; thick; specific gravity is high. *Specific gravity low.* Gonorrhœa with terrible pains; discharge copious, yellow, constant burning day and night along the entire urethra with restlessness.

Stitching of glans penis and scrotum, perspiration of genitals, drawing pain in left spermatic cord. Seminal emissions. Ulcers on prepuce. Itching of the vulva. *Leucorrhoea; excoriating, bloody,* burning, *copious,* thick, *yellow,* after menses. Menses copious, dark, too frequent, protracted, burning in the vulva.

Catarrh with viscid mucus, Itching in the larynx, causing coughing. Dryness in larynx, causing choking. Soreness, burning and rawness in larynx. Hoarseness. Voice lost.

Asthmatic breathing during the night. Dyspnœa evening and during the night. Dyspnœa worse ascending stairs, after eating, from least exertion, while lying. Respiration is rattling, short, singing, *suffocative,* wheezing.

Cough MORNING, afternoon, *evening in bed,* NIGHT, from cold air, open air, asthmatic, on becoming cold, after eating, *lying.* Dry cough from tickling in the larynx. Hacking cough; loose cough; racking, spasmodic cough;

suffocative cough.   Whooping cough.   Expectoration;
bloody, copious, frothy, offensive mucus; *purulent,* thick,
viscid, *yellow.*

Anxiety of the chest. It has been of great service in
cancerous ulceration of the breast. It is a most useful
remedy in bronchial catarrh. The chest feels cold, sensat-
tion of tightness of the chest. Effusion in the pleura and
pericardium. Eruptions of many kinds on the chest.
Hemorrhage of the lungs. Inflammation of the lungs,
pericardium and pleura. Oppression of the chest on
ascending, when coughing, after eating, when walking.
Pain in the chest when coughing, worse from motion and
from breathing. Pain in the sides of chest and in regions
of heart. Burning in chest. Cutting in chest, worse
from motion; 5 a. m., between fifth and sixth ribs. Cutting *in heart*; worse from respiration. Pressing pain.
Sore bruised chest from coughing. Stitching in chest on
coughing. Stitching in sternum and heart. *Violent palpitation*; worse during the night and from exertion. It is
a most useful remedy in phthisis in all stages, when incurable it is a great palliative. Feeling of weakness in
chest, with weak voice.

The back is constantly cold. Many eruptions on the
back. Pain in back evening and night; during chill and
fever; during menses. Pain in back of neck and *between
the scapulae.* Pain in lumbar region and sacrum. Pain in
coccyx to anus, morning on rising. Aching in lumbar
region. Burning, drawing and tearing in back. Drawing
in lumbar region. Sore, bruised pain in lumbar region. Tenderness of coccyx. Perspiration of the back. Stiffness of
cervical region. Weakness of lumbar region.

Cold hands, legs and *feet.* Cramps in *calf,* feet and
sole. Blueness of fingers and nails *during chill.* Eruptions; boils; *pimples*; *pustules*; vesicles. Desquamation of
limbs. Excoriation between the thighs and nates. Formi-

cation of lower limbs. Heat of feet. Heaviness of lower limbs; *of feet*. Itching of limbs worse after scratching; of lower limbs at 1 p. m., of thighs and toes. Jerking of lower limbs. Numbness of upper and lower limbs; of feet; of heel and outer side of foot. Pain in limbs evening; night; *after midnight*; during chill; rheumatic in cold weather; wandering; relieved by external warmth and warmth of bed; in wet weather. Pain in *joints, bones*. Pain in upper limbs, as though in the bones relieved by warmth; rheumatic, worse toward morning; wandering. *lower limbs*; sciatica; right thigh; knee; leg. Pain in lower third of tibia relieved by motion. Burning hands and feet. Bruised pain in limbs. Stitching pains in limbs. Tearing pain in all limbs; upper limbs; shoulder, arm, elbow, forearm, fingers. Tearing in *thighs, legs and feet*. Paralysis of limbs; hemisplegia; painless; upper limbs; right for three days; lower limbs. Perspiration of hands cold; of *feet offensive and cold*. Restless limbs, legs, feet. Stiffness in knees. Stiffness in all the joints after recovering from the poison. Swelling dropsical and inflammatory; joints; upper limbs; hands; fingers; knees; legs; ankles; feet. Trembling of body and limbs; upper limbs and hands; lower limbs and feet. Twitching of thighs. Ulcers on legs. Weakness of all the limbs; of *joints*; upper limbs; *lower limbs*; knees; legs; ankles; feet.

Deep sleep, even comatose. Dreams; amorous; anxious; of death; of the dead; frightful; of misfortune; nightmare; vexatious; vivid. Falling asleep late. *Restless sleep*. SLEEPLESSNESS *afternoon and evening*. Sleeplessness before midnight; after midnight; after 3 a. m. If he wakens cannot get to sleep again. Unrefreshing sleep. Waking easily and frequently.

Morning on waking; FORENOON, noon, *afternoon*, evening in bed; *night*, midnight. Chill in open air; in cold air; walking in cold air. Chill alternating with sweat. Chill ascending the body; the back. Chilliness with sweat. Creeping chills in the evening. Chill after drinking cold water; after eating; worse from motion. External and internal coldness. Congestive chill. Chill followed by sweat. Quartan, quotidian and tertian chill. SHAKING chill afternoon and evening. Trembling with the chill. Warm room does not relieve the coldness nor the chill, but is grateful. Specific times of chill: 1 a. m., 10 a. m., 1 p. m., 2 p. m., 4 p. m., 5 p. m., 6 p. m., 7 p. m., 8 p. m., 12 p. m.

Morning, afternoon and *evening* heat. Evening fever with chilliness. Fever *during night with* chilliness. Fever after midnight. Fever alternates with chill and with perspiration. Burning fever afternoon, evening and *night.* Fever without chill at night. Fever and chill intermingled. Continued fever worse during the night. Long lasting *dry heat.* External heat with chilliness. Flushes of heat. It has done excellent service in hectic fever. It should become one of the best remedies in intermittent fever. It has fever with sweat and without sweat. It is suitable in remittent fevers as its fevers are afternoon, evening and night and there is a remission in the morning and forenoon. During the fever he wants to be uncovered. It is a strong remedy in zymotic fevers.

It has morning sweat and again during the night Sweat from the least excitement or anxiety; from the warmth of the bed; on coughing; while eating; from least exertion; on motion; *during sleep* and *after waking.* The sweat is cold, clammy, debilitating, offensive, sour. Profuse night sweat. Sweat of single parts. His symptoms are not relieved while sweating. *If he becomes cooled while perspiring he suffers much.*

Burning of the skin after scratching. Burning in spots. Marked coldness of skin of body and limbs. Discoloration of skin; blotches; blue spots; liver spots; pale, red spots; white spots; periodical dry burning skin. Eruptions; blisters; bloody after scratching; boils; burning; carbuncles; desquamating; *dry*; ECZEMA; fetid; herpes itching; moist with corrosive yellow discharge; painful petechia; painful pimples; *psoriasis*; PUSTULES; rash; SCABBY *after scratching*; bran-like scales; stinging; *suppurating*; URTICARIA that is nodular and worse after scratching; vascular, worse after scratching, with yellow fluid. All eruptions *worse after scratching* and the itching without eruption is also *worse after scratching*. Inflammation of the skin like erysipelas. Excoriation of the skin. Formication, inactivity and marked *induration*. Itching, burning, crawling and stinging, worse after scratching. Moisture *after scratching*. Pain in the skin after scratching. Purpura hemorrhagica. The skin is very sensitive to touch. Sticking, stinging and swelling of skin in places and spots. Ulcers bleeding; *burning*; CANCEROUS; crusty; DEEP; indolent; inflamed; *painful*; *phagedenic*; pulsating; RED; STINGING; stinging margins; SUPPURATING. Ulcers discharging corrosive, offensive, thin, watery, yellow pus.

AURUM ARSENICUM

The symptoms of this remedy present themselves in morning, in forenoon, afternoon, evening during the night, after midnight. The symptoms are worse in the open air, worse in cold air. He desires open air. Worse on ascending. Asleep-feeling in single parts. A sensation of a band around parts. It is a most useful remedy in cancerous affections; in epithelioma; in caries of bone; worse in cold, wet weather. It is a useful remedy in many kinds of convulsions; clonic spasms with consciousness; epileptiform; hysterical. Dropsy of the extremities and of cavities. The symptoms are worse during and after eating. The body emaciates, complaints come on after slight exertion and after cold drinks. Formication all over the body.

The body and limbs feel heavy. Induration is a common
feature; in glands; cancerous induration. Inflammation
and congestion in many parts; in mucous membranes;
bones; glands; periosteum; serous membranes. Marked
physical irritability. Desire to lie down, but lying brings
on great restlessness and many symptoms are worse lying.
Worse after lying awhile. Lying in warm bed ameliorates
many symptons. Motion aggravates in general. He
is restless and desires to move. The mucous membranes are much affected. Numbness of many parts; in
suffering parts. Orgasm of blood. There are pains of all
kinds in all parts of the body; pains in bones and glands;
boring; bruised; burning; cutting; pressing in internal
parts; stitching; tearing. Painless paralysis. It is useful
in broken down as well as in plethoric people. Strong internal pulsation. The pulse is fast, irregular, small, weak.
Any exertion or hurry like running is impossible. General
sensitiveness; sensitive to pain. The symptoms resemble
persons much debilitated by sexual excesses and vices.
The symptoms are predominantly right sided. Symptoms
come on going to sleep and during sleep. He is better in
summer and worse in winter. The glands are swollen. It
is one of our most useful remedies in advanced stages of
syphilis; in nervous syphilis. General aggravation from
touch. Trembling in all parts. Ulceration of glands with
marked induration; in cancerous conditions. Symptoms
appear after sleep; worse from uncovering the body; while
walking. Worse walking in open air; walking fast; walking in the wind. Marked general weakness; in the morning; from mental exertion; from physical exertion; weariness. Worse in windy weather and in winter.

Absent minded. Easily angered and complaints from
anger; anger with silent grief; from contradiction. He
suffers from anguish. Anxiety day and night; of conscience; with fear; about salvation. Inclined to criticise
and find fault with everybody. Confusion of mind in the

morning. Over conscientious. Contrary. Desires death.
Delirious at night. Delusions: about animals; thinks he
has done wrong; illusions of fancy. Despair: during chill;
with pain; periodical; of recovery, religious. Excitable
and discontented. Excitement during chill. Symptoms
are worse from mental exertion. Exaltation of fancy.
Fear; evening and night; in a crowd; of death; of evil; of
people, when alone. Forgetful and easily frightened. He
suffers from grief and lasting complaints come on after
grief. Always excited and in a hurry. Hysterical disposition and conduct; disorderly methods and perverted desires. Neglects the household and children. It is a many
sided remedy. Ideas abundant, clear minded. Imbecility,
impatience, indolent, even marked aversion to work or in-
dustrious and loves activity. Insanity of fanatics; of
drunkards; religious. Irresolution. Extreme irritability;
alternating with cheerfulness; during chill; when spoken
to. Lamenting, loquacity and laughter. Loathing of life.
Malicious. Mania. Memory active; weak. Obstinate and
easily offended. Mental prostration. Quarrelsome. Remorse. Reproaches himself for having done wrong. Reproaches others for imaginary injury. Insane reserve.
Restlessness, night; anxious. Sadness in the evening;
from suppressed menses; during perspiration. Oversensitive; to noise; to voices. Mental symptoms from sexual
excesses and from secret vice. Shrieking; prolonged periods of silence. Wandering speech. Aversion to being
spoken to. Suicidal disposition, during perspiration;
wants to jump out of window. Indisposed to talk. The
symptoms are worse when he thinks of them. Timid.
One moment he is tranquil, the next he is violent. Weary
of life. Weeping; during chill, in hysteria, in sleep. Vertigo during headache; while walking in open air.

Hyperæmia, fullness and heat of head from mental exertion. Eruptions on the scalp; crusts; pimples;. The
hair falls out. Heaviness in the head in the morning on

rising. Hydrocephalus. Itching of the scalp. Pain in the head; morning; afternoon; evening; in cold air; in cold weather; rheumatic; from binding up the hair; on coughing; hammering; hysterical; lying; from mental exertion; from motion; nervous; periodical; pulsating; on rising from lying; after sleep; in windy weather; heat ameliorates. Pain in forehead. Pain in one side; either side or in both sides. Pain in temples; in temple and forehead. Bruised pain in head. Burning pain in head; in forehead; in vertex. Drawing pain in head. Pressing pain in head; in forehead; in occiput; in temples. Stitching pain in head. Tearing pain in head; in forehead; in occiput. Pulsation in head; in forehead; on sides of head. Uncovering head brings on complaints.

Discharge of mucus and pus from eyes and the lids are stuck together in the morning with yellow pus. Granular lids. The lashes fall out. The eyes feel hot. Inflammation of eyes; catarrhal; scrofulous; of the cornea; of the iris; from syphilis. Lachrymation. Unable to open the eyes. Pain in the eyes; morning; night; from light; when reading; warmth ameliorates; aching; burning; pressing; core; as from sand; stitching; tearing. Paralysis of the optic nerve. Photophobia. Protrusion. Pulsation. Pupils contracted. Redness of the eyes; of lids; staring. A stye near the inner canthus. Swollen lids. Ulceration of the cornea. Vision blurred; bright colors before the eyes; dim; foggy; hemiopia, upper half lost; sparks; vision lost.

Mastoid caries. Discharge from the ear; fetid; offensive; purulent; thick; yellow. Sensation of flapping in ears. Itching in ears. Noises in ears; buzzing; crackling; humming; ringing; roaring; rushing. Pain in ear; behind ear; inside ear; burning, stitching. Hearing acute at first; for noise; later impaired; finally lost.

Caries of the bones of nose in old cases of syphilis. It is a most useful remedy in old stubborn catarrhs. The nose is red. He has frequent attacks of coryza, fluent or dry. Discharge from nose: bloody; crusts; offensive; fetid; greenish; purulent; suppressed; thick; watery; yellow. The nose is obstructed and there is itching and bleeding. It is a useful remedy in ozæna. Pain in the nose; in the bones; boring; burning; sore inside; ulcerative pain. Smell at first acute, later lost. Frequent sneezing. The nose is swollen. Ulceration in nose.

Epithelioma of face and lips. Lupus. Cracked lips; discoloration: bluish; bluish like; earthy; pale; red spots; eruptions: nose; acne rosacea face and forehead; comedones; coppery eruptions; pimples face and forehead; pustules; scurfy eruptions. Suffering expression. Erysipelas. The face is hot. Inflammation of the parotid gland. Pain in face; in parotid gland; in submaxillary gland; burning lips; drawing pain in face; stitching; tearing. Perspiration of face; cold. Swelling of the face; lips; parotid; submaxillary; ulcer on lip.

Apthæ in the mouth. The gums bleed easily. Cracked tongue. Brown tongue, red tongue, dry tongue. Heat in the tongue, mucus in the mouth. Odor from the mouth offensive; putrid. Burning tongue, soreness of gums. Speech difficult. Swollen gums; tongue. Taste: bitter; insipid; metallic; putrid; sour; sweetish; wanting. Ulcers in mouth syphilis; on gum; tongue; vesicles in mouth. Caries, sensation of elongation and loosening of teeth. Grinding of teeth in the night. Pain in teeth; night; when masticating; on touch; tearing.

Inflammation in throat. Lump in throat, mucus in throat. Pain in throat on swallowing; burning; stitching; scraping and swelling. Swallowing difficult.

Appetite is ravenous. Aversion to food; to meat; desires alcoholic stimulants; bread; coffee; cold drinks; milk; distension, emptiness and bitter eructations. Nausea with headache. Hiccough. Pain in stomach; violent; burning;

cutting, pressing; stitching. Extreme thirst. Vomiting
bile.

Atrophy of the liver. Suppurating bubo in groin.
Distension of abdomen. Enlarged liver. Fullness and
great flatulence. Hardening of the liver. It has cured
numerous liver conditions and complaints. Itching of the
skin of the abdomen. Pain in abdomen; night; colic; on
coughing; after eating; during menses; warmth ameliorates; in right hypochondrium; in inguinal region; cramping; cutting in right hypochondrium; soreness in abdomen;
in hypogastrium. Stitching pain in hypochondria; in hypogastrium. Rumbling in abdomen. Swelling of mesenteric glands; inguinal glands.

Constipation; alternating with diarrhœa. Diarrhœa in
morning; night. Offensive flatus. Bleeding from anus.
External piles. Moisture at the anus. Pain in the anus;
during stool. Burning pain in anus with diarrhœa; during
and after stool. Soreness and stitching pains. Urging in
the rectum and prolapsus ani. Stool: copious; green;
green mucus; hard; knotty; large; offensive; thin.

Retention of urine. Urging constant; ineffectual.
Urination dribbling; dysuria; involuntary at night; seldom;
unsatisfactory. Suppression of urine. Inflammation in
urethra with burning. Urine albuminous; bloody; burning; cloudy on standing; red; copious; offensive; scanty;
mucous sediment; sand; thick; watery. Inflammation of
glans penis; testes; sore pain in testes. Perspiration of
genitals. Swollen testes. Ulcers on the penis; chancres.

It is a very useful remedy in cancer of the uterus.
The desire is increased. Eruptions on the vulva. Inflammation of ovaries and uterus. Itching of the vulva. Leucorrhœa; acrid; copious; thick; white; yellow. Menses absent; copious; too frequent; scanty; suppressed. Pain in
ovaries and uterus. Burning in the vulva. Prolapsus of
uterus.

Mucus in larynx and trachea. Hoarseness. Respiration is rapid. Asthmatic at night; difficult at night, on ascending, while lying and while walking; irregular; short; suffocative.

Cough: morning; night; in cold air; dry at night; short; spasmodic at night. Expectoration; morning; evening; bloody; mucus; offensive; purulent; tasting sweetish; tough; yellow.

It is a most useful remedy in heart affections. Angina Pectoris. Anxiety in chest; in the heart. Constriction of chest; of heart. Fluttering of heart. Heat in chest. Oppression of chest, from rapid motion; when lying; while walking; of the heart. Pain in chest; on coughing; on inspiration; in sides of chest on inspiration; in heart; burning in chest; pressing in chest; in sternum; in heart. Stitching pains in chest on inspiring; in sides; in sternum; in heart. Palpitation: at night; anxious; on least exertion; during menses; on motion; tumultuous; on walking; trembling of the heart, weak heart.

Coldness in the back. Pain in the back on inspiration; in lumbar region; sacrum; spine; pressing pain in lumbar region; sore in lumbar region; stitching in lumbar region. Weakness in lumbar region.

Chilblains on the feet and toes. Cold hands; icy cold; legs, feet, during headache. Blueness of nails. Heaviness of upper limbs; of feet. Itching of limbs; palms; lower limbs; feet. Numbness of limbs; during rest; upper limbs; lower limbs. Pain in limbs; at night; during chill; in joints; gouty, rheumatic, wandering; in upper limbs; shoulders, rheumatic; forearm; knees; heel; aching in legs; burning in toes. Drawing pains in limbs; upper arm, knees; feet. Gnawing pain in legs. Stitching pain in limbs; in shoulders; in wrist; knee; foot. Tearing pain in limbs; joints; upper limbs; upper arms; elbow; wrist; fingers; thigh; soles. Painless paralysis of limbs. Sensation of paralysis in fingers. Restlessness of limbs; of lower limbs. Stiffness of the joints; of lower limbs; of knee. Swelling of the joints; dropsical swelling of limbs, forearm, and hand, lower limbs, legs and feet. Ulceration of nails. Weakness of joints; of upper limbs; lower limbs; knees.

Deep or comatose sleep. Dreams amorous; anxious; of dead people; of death; frightful; vivid; restless sleep; sleepiness in afternoon. Sleeplessness before midnight; after midnight, after waking. Unrefreshed after sleep. Waking too early; waking frequently.

Coldness in evening. At night in bed. Chilliness when undressing. Shaking chill. Fever at night. Burning hot in blood-vessels; intense heat; aversion to uncovering. Perspiration in morning; in night; profuse; aversion to uncovering.

Burning skin. At times marked coldness of skin. Discoloration; blue; liver spots; spots yellow. Eruptions: blisters; boils; burning eczema; herpes; painful, pimples; psoriasis; red; scabby; scaly; bran like; smarting; syphilitic; urticaria; vesicular; erysipelas. Formication, itching; sensitive; sore feeling in skin. Dropsical swelling of skin. Tension in skin. Ulcers; bluish, burning; cancerous; deep; discharging. Green, ichorous, offensive, yellow pus; fistulous; foul; indurated; painful; sensitive; suppurating; syphilitic. Warts that are syphilitic.

AURUM IODATUM

The symptoms are prominent in morning, afternoon, evening and night. *Strong desire for open air and feels better in open air.* Asleep feeling in single parts. A sensation of a band around parts. It is very useful in cancerous affections and in caries of bones. The patient feels better when cool and worse when in warm air. Congestion of blood to glands and organs. Dropsy in cavities and limbs. Exertion increases all complaints. Induration is characteristic and especially in glands. Inflammation of organs; bones; glands; serous membranes. *Lying aggravates,* especially lying in a warm bed. Motion increases the suffering. Numbness in many parts, especially of painful parts. *Orgasm of blood.* Pain in bones; in glands; bruised feeling internally; internal burning; pressing internally and externally; stitching pains, tearing pains. internal pulsation. Pulse is fast. It is one of our great heart remedies. Running brings on many symptoms. The symptoms are strong and *right-sided.* Sitting increases the suffering. Swollen, painful glands. It is a most useful remedy in syphilis. Trembling. Walking fast aggravates. Slow walking ameliorates. Warmth in general aggravates; warm air; becoming warm in open air; warm bed; warm room; warm wraps. Weakness in morning.

Anxiety day and night. Spells of unusual cheerfulness. Aversion to company. Want of self confidence. Confusion of mind in the morning. Over-conscientious about small matters. Despair of her salvation and of recovery. *Excitement. Worse from exertion of mind.* Fear of evil and of people. Feels hurried and seems hysterical. Fretful and impatient. Dread of all work. Indolence. Insanity with enlarged heart, orgasm of blood, red face, full veins, bloated appearance. Irresolution, irritability and mania. Mirthful without cause. Moods alternate and changeable. Mental prostration. Extreme sadness; restlessness, sensitive to noise. Timid, weeping and dizziness.

Heat, heaviness and rush of blood to head. Itching of scalp. Pain in the head in the morning; better in cold air and by cold applications; in forehead on left side; one-sided. Pressing pain in head; in forehead; occiput; temples; vertex. Stitching pains in head. Tearing in head; in temples. Pulsation in forehead.

Inflammation: conjunctiva; catarrhal; scrofulous; syphilis; iritis. Lachrymation. Pain in eyes, pressing, stitching. Protrusion of eyes. Redness of eyes and swollen. Bright colors before the eyes. Dim vision, diplopia; foggy vision; sparks.

Purulent fetid discharge from ears. Noises in ears; buzzing; humming; ringing; roaring. Stitching pain in ears. Hearing acute for noise. Impaired.

Post-nasal catarrh. The nose is red. Fluent or dry coryza. Discharge from nose; bloody; greenish; hard chunks; *offensive*; PURULENT; *thick*; *yellow*. Dryness in in nose. Epistaxis. *Obstruction in the nose*. Pain in the nose, boring pain. Smell lost. Much sneezing. The nose is swollen. ULCERATION in NOSE.

The face is pale. Sometimes red. Eruptions on face and nose; pimples. Pain in the face. Pain in submaxillary glands; in lymphatic glands.

Aphthæ in mouth, and bleeding gums. Redness of gums. Brown tongue. Dryness of tongue. Putrid odor from mouth. Burning pain in tongue. Salivation, swollen gums. Taste putrid, sour, sweetish. Ulceration of gums. Drawing, tearing pain in teeth, and the teeth feel too long.

Much mucus in the throat and burning pain. Swallowing is difficult. The throat is swollen and ulcerated. It has cured goitre. It has cured enlarged thyroid with fast pulse and protruding eyes. The goitre is right-sided like *Lycopodium*.

The appetite is INCREASED; RAVENOUS. Aversion to food. Desires alcoholic stimulants. Distension of the stomach. A sensation of emptiness in the stomach. Eructations which ameliorate. Hiccough and nausea. Pain in the stomach; burning; cutting; pressing; stitching. *Thirst*: burning; *extreme*. Vomiting bile.

It is a very useful remedy in a variety of liver affections. The liver is enlarged but it is of great service in atrophy of the liver. Obstructed flatulence. Pain in the abdomen. Colic; after eating; during menses; in the right hypochondrium; in inguinal region; burning in the liver; cramping; cutting in right side; drawing; pressing in right hypochondrium. Rumbling in abdomen. TABES MESEN-TERICA.

Constipation alternating with diarrhœa. Difficult stool; inactivity of the rectum. Morning diarrhœa. Much flatus. External piles. Burning in the rectum. Stool copious; offensive; hard; knotty. Retention of urine. Urination dribbling, frequent. Urine is *albuminous*; cloudy; *copious*; offensive.

Atrophy of the testes. Erections troublesome at night; later impotency. Hydrocele. *Induration of testes. Pain in testes*; ACHING. Perspiration of the genitals. Sexual desire increased. *Swollen testes.*

In the female the desire is also increased. INDURA-TION OF THE OVARIES; UTERUS; cervix uteri. Inflammation of *ovaries and uterus. Leucorrhoea*, acrid; copious, *thick*; YELLOW. Menses absent; copious; late; suppressed. Pain in ovaries and uterus. Prolapsus uteri. *Sterility.*

Hoarseness. Respiration is fast; asthmatic; difficult at night with cardiac affections and when ascending; irregular; short; suffocating.

Cough: dry; short; spasmodic. Expectoration in the morning. Bloody with cardiac affections; difficult; mucus; offensive; tough; yellow.

Anxiety in region of heart. Congestion to chest. CONSTRICTION OF CHEST; *of heart.* Heat in chest. *Hypertrophy of heart.* Inflammation of heart; endocardium. Milk suppressed. Cardiac murmurs. Oppression of chest; OF HEART. Pain in chest; during cough; sides of chest; in heart; burning in chest; cutting pain in chest; stitching pain in chest. Palpitation of heart; *at night*; *anxious*; *on least exertion*; on motion; TUMULTUOUS; when walking. Swelling of axillary glands without any tendency to suppurate.

Pain in sacrum; stitching pain in lumbar region.

Cold hands with hot head. Cold legs and feet. Heaviness of feet. Hip joint disease Itching limbs. Lower limbs. Pain in limbs; *joints*; gouty rheumatic; elbow; hip; drawing pain in knee; stitching in shoulder and wrist; tearing pain in limbs; upper limbs; fingers; finger joints; joints of thumb. Dropsical swelling of limbs; hands; legs; feet; weakness of limbs upper; lower; knees.

Dreams: amorous; *anxious*; distressing; frightful; vivid. Restless sleep; *sleepiness*. Waking too early.

Chill in warm bed. Shaking chill. Perspiration morning and night; profuse.

Skin burning. Coldness of skin. Eczema of neck, chest and forearms. Herpetic eruptions. Itching and burning. Ulcers: cancerous; discharging; yellow pus: sensitive.

AURUM SULPHURICUM

The symptoms of this remedy appear in the MORNING, forenoon, afternoon, *evening*, and DURING THE NIGHT. DESIRE FOR OPEN AIR. The open air aggravates many symptoms. Ascending brings on many symptoms. Asleep feeling in single parts; a sensation of a band around parts. Cancerous affections; ULCERS. Worse from cold in general; from cold air; from becoming cold; after becoming cold. Congestion of blood. Hysterical convulsions. Dropsical tendency. Worse during and after eating and from exertion. Formication. Fullness of the veins and a feeling of distension; lack of vital heat. Induration of glands and other parts. Inflammation of internal organs; of bones; of glands; of serous membranes. Desire to lie down, but lying aggravates some symptoms; worse lying in bed. A most useful remedy in cases abused by mercury. Motion intensifies most symptoms. Mucous secretions much increased. Violent orgasm of blood in

4

chest and head. Pain in bones and glands; aching, *boring*, cutting, *pressing*, stitching, tearing pains in many parts; bearing downward in bones and muscles; paralysis of organs. It is most useful in red-faced, full-blooded people. Pulsation in internal parts; the pulse is *small*, FAST, *irregular and weak*. Marked aggravation follows hurried actions, like running. Oversensitive to pain, in glands. Complaints are predominantly right-sided. Sitting erect aggravates some symptoms; standing aggravates many symptoms. Swelling of affected parts; of the glands.

A feeling of tension all over the body; symptoms are worse *from touch*. Trembling in body and limbs. Walking ameliorates; walking fast aggravates; walking in open air aggravates. Warm bed increases some symptoms, in some cases worse from both heat and cold; worse in warm room and from warm wraps. Marked general weakness; weariness. Complaints worse in winter.

Absent minded; irascible, even violent; ANXIETY; of conscience; with fear; about salvation. Very critical with all her friends; morbidly cheerful and gay; *aversion to company*. She has lost all confidence in herself. Confusion in the morning, worse from mental exertion; very timid, even cowardly. Loathing of life and *desires death*. Delusions about animals. *Despair of recovery* and salvation; EXCITEMENT and discontentment; exerion of mind makes all the mental symptoms worse. Marked increase in her imaginative powers. Fear on going into a crowd; of death; of evil; of people; of robbers; very forgetful and easily frightened. It is a very useful remedy for chronic complaints that date back to grief. Hysterical and in a hurried state of mind; at first mental activity, later dullness; imbecility. He is becoming weak-minded and indolent; will not work, becomes like a tramp. These states change to excitement and a mania for work. It should become an excellent remedy for insanity, irresolution and *extreme irritability*; moaning and lamenting. Maniacal conduct and loquacity, weakness of memory; insane mirth; moods constantly changing; morose, obstinate and easily offended; MENTAL PROSTRATION; quarrelsome. Great restlessness, worse during the night. Extreme sadness in the morning but worse in the EVENING and during perspiration. Generally oversensitive. Desire to sit and brood. Averse to being spoken to; SUICIDAL THOUGHTS occupy his mind; suspicious; indisposed to talk; weeping, worse at night; alternating with laughter.

Vertigo in the open air; with headache; must lie down; when standing; when stooping; walking in open air.

Fullness of head; constant hyperæmia of brain. *The hair falls out.* Heat in head; burning scalp. Heaviness in moving or rising; in occiput; hydrocephalus, itching of scalp worse at night. Nodding of head like paralysis agitans. Pain in head; morning in bed, afternoon; evening; better in open air, worse from binding up the hair; from coughing; worse lying; from motion; from strong odors; from warm room; after sleep; from straining the eyes; from talking; in windy, stormy weather. Aching pain in forehead, worse from motion, in occiput; in occiput and forehead; in sides of head; in temples; in temples and forehead. Boring in head; in forehead; in vertex. Drawing pain in head; lancinating pain in occiput. Pressing pain in head; *in forehead*; in occiput; in temples; in vertex. Stitching pains in head; in forehead; in sides of head. TEARING PAIN IN HEAD; in forehead; in occiput; in sides of head; in temples. Pulsating in head on coughing and on motion; in sides of head.

The eyelids stick together in the morning; discharge of yellow mucus from the eyes; heat in eyes. Inflammation of eyes; catarrhal; SCROFULOUS; *syphilis*; of chancroid, with ulceration of cornea; of iris. Itching of lids; of canthi. Much and easy lachrymation; OPACITY OF THE

CORNEA. Pain in the eyes; from motion; when reading; aching, burning in the eyes and canthi; *cutting, pressing*; as from sand; stitching. *Paralysis of the optic nerve.* Photophobia, protrusion and *pulsation* in eyes. The pupils are contracted. *Redness of eyes*; of *lids*. *Scrofulous affections of eyes.* Spots on the cornea; stye near outer canthus; swollen lids. Floating black specks in the field of vision; DIM VISION; *diplopic*. All the eye symptoms are worse from any exertion of vision. FOGGY VISION. Hemiopia; can see only the lower half of objects. Vision lost from paralysis of the optic nerves; vision smoky; sparks; stars.

Discharge from the ear; fetid; offensive; purulent; sequelæ after *suppressed eruption*; the ears are red; dryness in ears; scanty wax; stitching of the ears; noises; buzzing; crackling; fluttering; *humming*; *ringing*; *roaring*; rushing sounds. Pain inside the ear; stitching in and behind ears; tearing in ears. The ears burn. Hearing acute; for noise; *impaired*; *lost*.

Catarrh of nose; discharge *bloody*; dry crusts, worse on on right side; greenish; HARD; OFFENSIVE; PURULENT; THICK; YELLOW. The nose is red and swollen; most marked at tip. Coryza fluent and dry; dryness in nose; epistaxis on blowing nose; itching of skin of nose and inside. The nose is obstructed; offensive odor from nose; œzena. Pain in nose at night; in bones of nose; on touch; burning; soreness; ulcerative pain, right side; polypus in nose. Nose very sensitive to touch. Smell acute, later lost. **Frequent sneezing.** *Swollen nose.* ULCERATION in NOSE.

Epithelioma of lip; cracked lips. **Discoloration of face,** earthy, pale, red, red spots. Eruptions on face; **forehead;** *nose*; acne rosacea; comedones; crusty, crusty on nose; pimples on face and forehead; pustules; scurf. **Pain in** face; right side; worse in cold air; in parotid gland; in *submaxillary gland*; *burning pain in lip*; drawing in face;

stitching, tearing; tearing in cheek bones and lower jaw. Perspiration of face; cold. Swelling of the face, cheeks, glands in general; lips; *parotid gland*; submaxillary gland; ulceration of lip.

Apathæ in mouth and on tongue; Bleeding gums. The tongue is cracked. The mouth feels hot. Offensive, even putrid odor from mouth. Speech is difficult. The gums are swollen. Taste: bitter, insipid, metallic, putrid, sour, sweetish, lost. Ulcers on gums and tongue. Vesicles in the mouth. Caries of teeth. Sensation of elongation of teeth. Grinding teeth in sleep. The teeth become loose. Pain in the teeth, worse from touch; drawing, stitching, *tearing*.

Inflammation of throat and *tonsils*, with elongation of uvula. Sensation of a lump in throat; much mucus forms in the throat. Pain in throat on swallowing; burning, stitching, scraping. Suppuration of tonsils; swallowing difficult. Swelling of throat and *tonsils*; swelling of thyroid gland. Ulceration throat, tonsils, uvula, *syphilitic*.

The appetite is ravenous. Aversion to food, to meat. Desires stimulants, coffee, cold drinks, milk. Distention of stomach. Digestion very slow; a sensation of emptiness. Eructations watery, bitter, tasting of food, ameliorate. Fullness in the stomach; flushes of heat. HICCOUGH. Nausea after eating; during headache. Pain in the stomach; burning, cutting, *pressing*, stitching. Thirst burning; extreme. Vomiting bile.

Atrophy of the liver; *enlargement of liver*. Abdomen distended with gas; with serum. Bubo in groin. Flatulence obstructed. Fullness and heaviness. Pain in abdomen: night, after midnight, *from colic*; on coughing; after eating; during menses; in hypochondria; in inguinal region as though a hernia would appear; burning in right hypochondrium; cramping, cutting, pressing pain in abdomen; in hypochondria; in hypogastrium. Rumbling in abdomen; swelling of *inguinal glands*.

Condylomata of anus. *Constipation*; *alternating with diarrhoea*; *difficult stool*; inactivity of rectum, during menses. Diarrhœa; morning, night, with burning in anus. Fistula in ano. Flatus passed from rectum; *offensive*, which ameliorates. Bleeding piles; external piles. Itching in anus. Moisture at anus. Pain in anus during stool; burning in anus with diarrhœa; soreness at anus; stitching pain in anus; prolapsus ani. Urging in rectum. Stool: gray, green-mucus, thin mucus, *hard*, KNOTTY, LARGE.

The bladder symptoms are very numerous and important. Pressing in the bladder. Retention of urine. Urging to urinate constant; ineffectual. Urination dribbling, difficult, *frequent, involuntary at night*; unsatisfactory. Suppression of urine. Prostatic discharge. Burning in urethra when passing urine; stitching and tearing in the urethra. Urine: *albuminous, bloody*, burning, cloudy on standing, copious, offensive; sand in the urine; SCANTY; mucus sediment; thick, yellow.

Condylomata of the glans penis. Impotency. Hydrocele in boys. Induration of the testes. Inflammation of glans penis; of testes; of epididymis. Itching of the scrotum. Pain in the TESTES; ACHING IN TESTES; drawing pain in testes; lancination in penis; PRESSING IN TESTES. PERSPIRATION OF GENITALS; *scrotum*. *Seminal emissions*. Sexual desire increased, with relaxed penis. Swelling of testes; especially the right. *Chancres on penis*; in syphilitic cases that have had much mercury; cancer of uterus. Sexual desire increased in women. Inflammation of the uerus. Itching of the vulva. Leucorrhœa: worse in the morning, acrid, *copious, thick*, transparent, *white*, YELLOW. Menses absent; copious; irregular; first menses delayed in girls; too frequent; late; scanty; suppressed. Pain in ovaries, in uterus; bruised; bearing down in uterus, especially during menses; burning in genitals and vagina.

Lancination in vulva. PROLAPSUS UTERI. The vulva is swollen.

Mucus in the larynx and trachea; hoarseness. **Respiration is rapid, asthmatic: dyspnœa at *night*; on ascending, while lying, while walking; respiration is irregular, short and suffocative, worse at night.**

Cough in the morning; nightly paroxyms; worse in cold air; short, dry, hard, racking; short, spasmodic. Expectoration in morning and evening; bloody, difficult; scanty, greenish, offensive, *purulent*, yellow.

Congestion of chest with anxiety; spasmodic constriction of chest. Cracked nipples. Fluttering of the heart. Heat in chest. Milk disappearing or is suppressed. Oppression of chest worse at night. Pain in chest; on coughing; on inspiration; in sides of chest on deep inspiration; aching in heart; burning in chest, cutting in chest and in heart; pressing in chest, sides and sternum; soreness in chest; stitching pain in chest; on inspiring; in sides of chest on inspiring or deep breathing; in sternum; in heart; in nipples. Palpitation at night; on *ascending*; anxious; from least excitement; on slight exertion; during menses; on motion; tumultuous; visible; when walking. Swollen mammæ; swollen *auxiliary glands*. Trembling of the heart.

The back is cold; heat in lumbar region; itching of the back. Pain in the back in the morning; on breathing; in dorsal region; lumbar region, worse while sitting; in sacrum, in spine; aching in sacrum; bruised in lumbar region; drawing in cervical region; pressing in back and in lumbar region; stitching in lumbar region. *Stiffness in back*, weakness in lumbar region.

Gouty nodosites in the finger joints; caries of bone. COLD HANDS, LEGS AND FEET. Cracked skin of hands, Blueness of finger nails. The feet feel heavy. *Hip joint disease.* Itching of the upper and lower limbs. Numbness of the limbs while lying and on waking; lower limbs. Pain in limbs while lying and on waking; lower limbs. Pain in joints; in shoulder, upper arm, elbow, forearm, *hip*; bruised pain in all the limbs; drawing in all the limbs, but especially in knees and feet; stitching in shoulder, wrist, feet, and toes; tearing in the limbs, joints, upper limbs, upper arm, *fingers*, FINGER JOINTS, thighs, toes. Painless paralysis of limbs. Staggering gait. Stiffness of knees. Dropsical swelling of legs and *feet*. Tension of thighs; weakness of limbs; of joints, upper limbs, lower limbs, knees.

Comatose sleep. Dreams: amorous, anxious, of assassins, of dead people, of death, *distressing, frightful*, of thieves; pleasant, VIVID. Sleep is very restless; sleepiness afternoon; after dinner. Sleepless before midnight; after midnight. Waking easily.

Coldness in evening in bed; chilliness; shaking chill. Fever of a mild nondescript type. Perspiration in the morning; during the night; profuse.

Burning of the skin, cold skin. Eruptions; blisters; boils; burning; eczema; *herpes*; pustules; scabby; urticaria; vesicles. Erysipelas; excrescences. Formication. Itching, itching burning, itching creeping, itching stinging. Sensitive skin. Sore feeling in the skin. *Ulcers*: burning, *cancerous, deep*, offensive, discharging yellow pus; fistulous, sensitive, suppurating, *syphilitic*. It has cured *syphilitic warts*.

BARIUM IODATUM

Complaints come on in the morning; afternoon; evening; night; after midnight; strong desire for open air; better in open air; better in cold air. Takes cold easily; worse in cold, wet weather. Congestion of many parts. Convulsive action of muscles. Feels worse before eating and when fasting; worse after eating; some symptoms are better after eating. Emaciation. Exertion aggravates most symptoms. Fainting spells. Formication all over body. General sensation of fullness. Easy hemorrhage. Induration in many parts; in glands. Inflammation or congestion in internal organs; in glands. Lassitude; continued lying rests him. Lying on the back aggravates. Lying in bed increases some symptoms. Worse before and during menses. Motion increases the symptoms. Pain in bones and glands. Pressing, sore, stitching pains. Tearing in many parts; downward; in muscles. It suits the complaints of plethoric people. Pressure aggravates many symptoms. Pulsation all over body. Pulse fast; full; hard; small. Very sensitive to pain; glands sensitive. Swelling and inflammation of affected parts and of glands. Tension all over body. Touch aggravates. Trembling and twitching. Walking aggravates all symptoms. Worse from warmth in general; in a warm room; on becoming warm. Weakness; during menses, nervous; while walking.

Anger, anxiety and aversion to company. Concentration of mind difficult. Confusion of mind. Timidity even cowardly. Delusion; thinks he sees dead people. Illusions of fancy. Marked dullness of mind. Fear of evil and of people. Memory weak; very forgetful. She feels hurried and hysterical. Impatience. Irresolution; indolence; indifference. Talkative and irritable. Mental weakness marked. Alternation of moods. Marked restlessness. Sadness and weeping. Over-sensitive to noise. Desire to sit and brood over events. Vertigo while lying, stooping; walking.

The head feels cold. Heat and hyperæmia of head evening and night. Heaviness of head. Pain in head; morning on rising; forenoon; afternoon; better or worse in open air; worse binding up the hair; from noise; while walking; warm room. Pain in forehead; right side; evening; above eyes; occiput, side of head; temples. Bruised pain in head. Pressing pain in head; in forehead; over eyes; in occiput; temples; vertex. Shooting in occiput; stitching in head; occiput; sides of head; temples. Stunning pains. Tearing in vertex. Perspiration of scalp. Pulsation in forehead and temples.

Inflammation of conjunctiva. Tubercular iritis. Itching of eyes. Opacity of the cornea. Pain in eyes worse from light; aching; burning; pressing; as from sand; tender feeling. Photophobia; protrusion; pupils dilated. Redness of eyes and lids. Swollen lids. Vision dim; diplopia; flickering; foggy; sparks; weak.

Discharge of pus from ear. Sensation of flapping in ears. Noises in ears; when chewing; buzzing; fluttering; ringing; roaring. Tearing pain in ears. Stopped feeling in ears. Hearing acute for noise; impaired.

Catarrh of nose; discharge bloody; copious; hard mucus; thick; yellow; post nasal. Redness of nose. Dryness in nose. Fluent coryza with cough. Epistaxis on blowing nose. Obstruction of nose at night. Pain in nose; in root of nose. Frequent sneezing. The nose is swollen and red.

Coldness of face. The face is congested and red; the lips are blue; face sometimes pale and sometimes circumambient redness. Face looks drawn and shrunken. Emaciated. Eruption on face and nose; boils and pimples. Pain in face; in submaxillary gland. Swelling of glands of lower jaw; parotid gland; submaxillary gland.

Bleeding gums, cracked tongue. The gums are detached from the teeth and the teeth become loose. Dry mouth in morning; dry tongue. Mucus in mouth which is offensive, even putrid. Burning tongue; sore gums. Salivation. Swollen gums. Taste bad; bitter; sour. Drawing and tearing in teeth.

Throat dry and constricted. The tonsils are enlarged. Inflammation with marked swelling of tonsils. Membranous exudation in throat. Pain in throat on empty swallowing; burning. Swallowing difficult. Swollen and indurated glands of neck.

Appetite diminished; increased, even ravenous with emaciation; without relish of food; wanting, aversion to food. Emptiness. Eructations: empty; sour; waterbrash; ameliorate. Fullness and heartburn. Flashes of heat in stomach. Heaviness after eating. Indigestion with hiccough. Nausea and loathing of food. Inflammation of stomach. Pain in stomach after eating; cramping; gnawing; pressing; soreness; stitching. Retching. Feeling of tension in stomach. Thirst extreme; unquenchable. Vomiting bile; watery.

Distension of abdomen; enlarged mesenteric glands. Flatulence; rumbling. Pain in abdomen; after eating; before and during menses; in hypochondria; inguinal region; umbilical region; cramping; cutting; drawing; pressing in hypogastrium; stitching in hypochondria and sides of abdomen. Distension of abdomen.

Constipation; difficult stool; inactivity of rectum; insufficient stool; hard, knotty stool. Diarrhœa with yellow, watery stools, much flatus, external piles. Itching anus. Pain in rectum; burning after stool; tenesmus. Ineffectual urging to stool.

Retention of urine; constant; frequent. Urination frequent at night; involuntary. Enlarged prostate gland. Urine copious.

Induration of testes. Erections wanting. Seminal emissions. In the female the desire is increased. Leucorrhœa bloody; before menses. Menses copious; frequent; painful; short; suppressed.

Mucus in the trachea. Voice: hoarse; lost; rough, weak. Respiration fast; asthmatic; difficult at night and on ascending; rattling; short; suffocative.

Cough morning; evening; asthmatic; dry in morning; from irritation in larynx or trachea; rattling; spasmodic; suffocative; as talking; from tickling in larynx and trachea. Expectoration in morning and evening; difficult; mucus; purulent; salty; viscid; yellow.

Catarrh of chest. Constriction of chest. Inflammation bronchial tubes; of lungs. Oppression of chest. Pain in chest; stitching in chest and in mammæ. Palpitation of heart; night; tumultuous. Paralysis of lungs. Swollen axillary glands.

Pain in sacrum; stitching pain in back and in lumbar region.

Cold hands, legs and feet. Hot hands. Heaviness of limbs. Itching limbs. Numbness of arms and fingers. Pain in joints; gouty; in hip; thigh; knees. Stitching in knees; tearing in knees and legs. Perspiration of hands; palms; feet. Weariness of knees.

Dreams: amorous, anxious; vivid.

BARIUM SULPHURICUM

The symptoms of this remedy appear in the *morning*; *forenoon*; afternoon; evening; *night*; after midnight. Desire for open air which ameliorates; the mental symptoms are better in the open air. There is a marked physical anxiety. Many symptoms show themselves or are worse on *exertion and ascending stairs*. Single parts become numb and prickle. Generally worse from bathing; in a close room; from cold; from cold air; from becoming cold; symptoms are worse after becoming cold; takes cold easily; there is a lack of vital heat; worse in cold, wet weather. Constriction of many parts. Clonic spasms and epileptic convulsions. The blood vessels are distended. Symptoms come on during and after eating; worse after eating to satiety. Emaciation; faintness and the muscles become flabby. Formication and a sensation of fullness. Induration of glands. Heaviness and lassitude. Inflammation of glands. Lack of reaction. Jerking in muscles. Desire to lie down. Symptoms come on before and during menses. Aversion to motion. Most symptoms are worse from motion. The patient feels worse from motion. Orgasm of blood in body. Pain in the bones; in glands; boring; burning; gnawing; jerking; pressing; stitching; tearing. Tearing in glands; tearing downwards. Paralysis, *one-sided*; of organs; painless; pressure aggravates the pain and many symptoms. Pulsation all over the body. Pulse feeble on motion. Rising up aggravates. Sensitiveness in external parts; to pain. Electric shocks felt in the body. It is a one-sided remedy; mostly *right-sided*. Sitting erect and standing cause some symptoms. Stiffness of muscles and joints. Swelling of glands. Tension felt all over body. Trembling in body and limbs. Walking brings on many symptoms. Walking in open air ameliorates. Weakness after eating; during menses; while walking.

Anxiety in the evening in bed; during the night; before midnight; with fear; WITH FEVER; about the future. Desires things which are not needed and soon put aside. She is very critical. Aversion to company. Concentration of mind impossible. Confusion in the morning; in the evening; better in the open air. Fear in the evening; in a crowd; of death; of evil; of people. Forgetful especially of words. Easily frightened. Always in a hurry and becomes hysterical after grief. Mentally weak like imbecility. Impatience, indifference, indolence and *loss of will power*. Irritability is very marked, but worse in the evening. Memory weak. Moaning and lamenting. *Suspicious* and dread of conversation. Bashful. Talks in sleep. *Fainting spells*; *unconscious*. Weeping, worse at night. Aversion to mental work. Vertigo; objects turn in a circle; when standing; when walking.

The head is sometimes cold, again there is marked hyperæmia with cold feet. Constriction of forehead and occiput. Empty feeling in the head. Eruptions on the scalp; crusts; moist; pimples. Formication of the scalp and the hair falls out. Heaviness of the head in the evening; of the forehead; of the occiput. ITCHING OF THE

SCALP. A feeling of looseness of the brain. A sensation of motions in the head. Pain in the head in the morning in bed; in the forenoon; in the afternoon; *in the evening*; better in the open air; worse from coughing; after eating; from becoming heated; from a jar; when lying; moving head and eyes; from pressure; shaking the head; after sleep; from sneezing; *when stooping*; in the summer; from heat of the sun; violent; when walking; worse in a warm room; better while walking in open air. Pain in forehead; in the evening; worse on the right side; above the eyes; in the occiput; in the SIDES OF THE HEAD; in the temples; boring in forehead and temples; bursting in head and forehead; drawing in forehead, sides of head and temples; dull pain in head; jerking pain in head. Pressing pain in head; as though in a vise; *in forehead,* outward; over eyes; occiput; side of head; temples; vertex. Shooting pain in head; in vertex. Sore-bruised pain in head. *Stitching* pains in head; in *forehead*; in frontal eminence; in temples; in vertex. Stunning pains in head. Tearing pains in occiput. Perspiration on scalp. Pulsation in temples. Electric shocks in head.

The eyelids are stuck together in the morning. It has cured cataract. Dryness of eyes. Inflammation of the conjunctiva, of the lids. Itching and lachrymation. It has cured opacity of the cornea. Pain in eyes on exertion of vision; WORSE FROM LIGHT; aching; burning on using eyes; burning in canthi, pressing; pain as from sand; tearing. Paralysis of optic nerve. *Photophobia.* Protrusion of eyes. It has cured exophthalmic goitre. Pupils dilated and insensible to light. Redness of eyes. Swollen lids. Black spots; specks and flies before the eyes. *Dim vision. Exertion of vision aggravates. Foggy vision.* Sparks before the eyes. Weak vision.

Bloody discharge from ear. *Eruption behind ears.*

Formication of ears. *Itching in ear.* Noises in ears; *buzzing*; cracking; crackling; fluttering; reverberations; *ringing*; ROARING. Pain in right ear; behind ear; drawing behind and in ear; *stitching in ear*; tearing pain in ear. Pulsation in ear. Twitching of ears. HEARING IMPAIRED.

Constant inclination to blow the nose. Fluent coryza with cough. Catarrh of the nose with discharge bloody; copious; crusts; hard lumps; offensive; thick; yellow. DRYNESS IN THE NOSE. Epistaxis on blowing the nose. The nose is often obstructed. Smell is acute. Much sneezing. The nose is swollen.

The face is cold. Convulsive twitching of face. The lips are dry and cracked. The face is pale or red. Eruptions on the face; forehead; nose; acne; boils; crusty; eczema; herpes; pimples. The face is red and hot. Pain in face; in *submaxillary gland.* Drawing pains in face. Swelling of face; *parotid gland*; SUBMAXILLARY gland; PAINFUL.

Bleeding gums. Cracked tongue. The gums are detached from the teeth. The tongue is coated white. Dry mouth and tongue in the morning. Mucus in the mouth. Offensive, even putrid odor from mouth. The tongue burns. Salivation. Speech difficult. Swollen gums. Taste is bad, bitter or sour. Burning vesicles in mouth and on tongue. Pain in teeth worse from cold things; cold drinks; after eating; from warm things; boring; drawing; stitching; tearing. Constriction in throat. Dryness in the throat. Enlarged tonsils. Hawking mucus from throat. Chronic inflammation of throat and tonsils. Liquids are forced into nose. Sensation of a lump in throat. The membrane of throat is covered with exudate and throat is full of viscid mucus. Pain in throat on *empty swallowing*; burning, stitching on swallowing. Roughness in throat. Spasms of the esophagus on swallowing. Swelling and suppuration of tonsils. Swallowing difficult of solids. Induration of cervical glands. Pain in external throat. Swollen cervical glands. Tension in neck.

Appetite is variable; diminished; *ravenous*; easy satiety; *wanting*. Aversion to food. Sensation of coldness in stomach. Craves sweets. A sensation of *emptiness*. Eructations; after eating; bitter; empty; sour; watery; WATERBRASH. Fullness in stomach even after eating so little. Heaviness after eating. Heat felt in stomach. Heartburn. Hiccough. Weak and slow digestion. Loathing of food. Nausea in the morning. Pain in stomach; after eating; cramping; gnawing; PRESSING AFTER EATING; tenderness; stitching; severe retching. Tightness. Thirst in the evening; unquenchable. *Vomiting*; bile, mucus, *sour*, watery. The abdomen is distended with flatulence and feels full. The abdomen is large and hard; the mesenteric glands are enlarged. Pain in abdomen in the morning, after eating; during menses; on motion; on pressure; after stool; in inguinal region; cramping; cutting; before stool; stitching in inguinal region and sides of abdomen; tearing; rumbling and tension. Constipation; inactivity of rectum; difficult stool; unsatisfactory stool; *hard, knotty stool*. Diarrhœa; worse at night from taking cold; yellow watery stools. Offensive flatus. Crawling and itching in rectum and anus. Bleeding from anus; from piles. *External piles*. Involuntary stool. *Constant moisture at anus*. Pain during and after stool; pressure; soreness; stitching; tenesmus. Constant or frequent ineffectual urging to stool. Ascarides in the stool.

Retention of urine. Urging to urinate; constant; *frequent*; sudden, must hasten to urinate or lose it. Dysurea. Urination frequent at night. Involuntary during the night. Urine copious at night. Discharge from urethra gleety; purulent. In the male there is no sexual desire and erections are wanting. Induration of testes. Sweat on the scrotum. *Seminal emissions.*

In the female desire is also absent. *Leucorrhoea*; smarting; *copious*; before the menses. Menses *scanty*; frequent; protracted; suppressed. Burning of the vulva. Catarrh of the trachea with copious mucus. Voice: hoarseness; lost, rough; weak.

Respiration: accelerated; asthmatic; difficult at night and on ascending; *rattling*; suffocation.

Cough: morning after rising; evening; night; in cold air; in open air; in damp cold air; asthmatic; dry morning and evening; from irritation in larynx and trachea; rattling; spasmodic; suffocative; worse talking; from tickling in larnyx and trachea; tormenting; whooping cough. Expectoration morning and evening; difficult; mucus; purulent; scanty; viscid; yellow.

Catarrh of chest with marked constriction and oppression. Pustules on the chest. A feeling of fullness in the chest. Chronic inflammation of the bronchial tubes. Itching of chest; of mammæ. Pain in the chest in evening. Soreness in the walls of chest. Pressing and stitching pains in chest. *Palpitation*; night; anxious tumultuous. Swollen axillary glands.

Feeling of weight in the back. Itching of the back. Pain in the back; before and during menses; while sitting; in cervical region; in lumbar region in evening and before and during menses; in the sacrum; aching in back and especially in lumbar region; burning in spine and in lumbar region; drawing pain in lumbar region; stitching in back, in cervical and lumbar regions. Pulsation in lumbar region. Stiffness in the back; in cervical regions. Tension in back; in cervical region; lumbar region; sacrum. Weakness in lumbar region.

Cold hands and feet. The corns sting and burn and are sore and painful. Cracked hands and fingers. Cramps

5

in the calf. The hands are very dry. Painful eruptions on the limbs; pimples. The hands are hot. Heaviness of upper and lower limbs. Itching limbs; upper; lower, thighs. Jerking of the lower limbs. Numbness upper limbs; hands; fingers. Pain in limbs; joints; upper limbs; shoulder; hands; hip; thigh; knee; leg; bruised limbs and joints; drawing in upper limbs, LOWER LIMBS; thighs and legs; stitching in knees; tearing pain in all the limbs; forearm; wrist; lower limbs; thighs; KNEES; legs; feet. Painless paralysis of upper limbs. Perspiration of hands, palms; offensive sweat of feet; suppressed foot sweat. Tension of thighs. Ulcers on legs; weakness of lower limbs.

Deep sleep. Dreams; anxious; frightful; of misfortune; vivid. Falling asleep late. *Restless sleep*. Sleepiness in afternoon; evening; after dinner. Sleeplessness before midnight with sleepiness.

Chill in the morning; forenoon; noon; afternoon; evening; night; chilliness in the open air; in the least draft; coldness in bed; external coldness; daily spells of coldness; shaking chill; one-sided chill; generally left-sided; coldness relieved in a warm room. Fever evening and night; alternating with chilliness; burning heat; flushes of heat. Perspiration after midnight; cold; while eating; offensive; on single parts; during sleep; on waking.

Burning skin at times; otherwise coldness; cracked skin. Pale skin; red spots. Dry burning skin. Eruptions; burning, with yellow moisture; DRY; herpes; ringworm; itching; painful; eating; pimples; rash; scabby; worse after scratching place bare; after scratching; smarting; stinging; suppurating; tubercles; nodular; urticaria; vesicular; vesicles after scratching. Excoriation of the skin. *Formication*. Itching at night; itching; burning; *itching crawling*; unchanged by scratching; *itching stinging*; *in a warm bed*. Moisture of the skin after scratching. The skin is very sensitive. Stitching in the skin after scratching. Stinging in the skin. Tension. Small wounds slow to heal and often fester. WARTS; small stinging.

CALCAREA IODATA

The symptoms appear or are worse in the morning; afternoon; *evening* NIGHT; *after midnight*. It has produced abscesses. Strong desire for open air; open air excites and also ameliorates symptoms. The tendency is towards anæmia. There is general physical anxiety; asleep feeling in single parts; choreic movements. Becoming cold ameliorates many symptoms, but there is a tendency to take cold; cold weather aggravates. It is a most useful remedy in tuberculosis. It has cured convulsions; clonic; epileptiform; with falling. Convulsive movements. Many symptoms come on before eating and are better after eating; some symptoms are worse before and after eating. There is marked loss of flesh. Exertion is impossible. There are fainting spells, fainting in a warm room. Fasting brings on many symptoms. Feeling of fullness internally. Internal hemorrhage. It is a most useful remedy in induration, especially following inflammation. Great lassitude; lying ameliorates, but lying long in bed aggravates, as the patient is worse from the warm bed. There is surging of blood in the body; pains are numerous but mild and flitting, burning, cutting, jerking, pinching, pressing, stitching, tearing; there is more weakness than pain. He perspires easily and becomes chilled during sweat. Pulsation all over. Many of the symptoms are right-sided. Swelling of affected parts and glands; swelling that suppurates. *Trembling* and *twitching*. The symptoms as well as the patient are worse from warmth, warm air, warm bed, warm room, warm wraps. GREAT GENERAL WEAKNESS; in the morning; during menses.

He becomes very angry over small matters. Frequent spells of anxiety; anxious over trifles. Aversion to company; confusion of mind; delusions; sees dead people. Despair; discontented; discouraged. Dullness of mind. Worse from mental exertion. Fear of insanity; of misfortune; of people. Impatience; indifference; indolence; irresolution. Irritability; during headache. Symptoms like insanity and mania. Mirthful. Mental prostration. Restless and anxious. EXTREME SADNESS. Dullness of the senses; starting in sleep; *weeping*. Vertigo in the morning on rising; while walking; with headache.

The head feels cold. There are congestion, heat and heaviness of the head; especially during menses. Crusty eruptions on the scalp. The hair falls out. It has cured Hydrocephalus. Itching of the scalp. Pain in the head; in the morning, binding up the hair makes the pain worse; with coryza and catarrh; compelled to lie down; before the menses; moving the head; noise; riding against a cold wind; stooping; talking; walking; warm room; wrapping up the head. Pain in the forehead above the eyes; in the *occiput*; pain in occiput before menses; sides of head but mostly in the right; temples, vertex. Pressing pain in forehead, occiput, sides of head, temples and *vertex*. Sharp pain in right temple. Shooting in head; in the occiput. Sore, bruised pain in head. Stitching pains in head, in the occiput, in sides of head, in temples, in vertex; stunning pains in the head; tearing pains in the head, in the temples. Perspiration on the scalp; on the forehead. Pulsation in the head; forehead; temples.

Dullness of the eyes; inflammation of the conjunctiva; scrofulous inflammation of the eyes. Lachrymation. Pain in the eyes; burning in the eyes. The ball of the eye is tender to touch. Protrusion of the eyes, exophthalmus. *Pupils dilated.* Redness of the eyes; of the lids; sunken eyes; swollen lids; twitching lids. **Weak eyes. Vision** foggy, dim. Colors before the eyes; sparks.

Catarrh of the eustachian tubes; discharge from the ears. The ears are hot. Noises in the ears; buzzing, humming, ringing, roaring. Pain in the ear; pressing, tearing. Hearing acute; later impaired.

Catarrh of the nose, also of the posterior nares; redness of the nose. Coryza FLUENT and dry. Discharges from the nose; excoriating; fetid; greenish; purulent; thick; watery; yellow. Dryness in the nose. Epistaxis. The nose is obstructed and smell is lost; much *sneezing.* The nose is swollen.

The face is cold and sunken and the muscles twitch. The face is discolored, earthy *pale,* red, *yellow.* Scaly eruptions on the face. Pain in the face. Swollen submaxillary gland.

Aphthæ in the mouth; the gums bleed easily; the tongue is fissured; dryness of the tongue. Offensive odor from the mouth. Pain in the gums; teeth, and tongue burns. Salivation. Swollen gums and tongue. Taste astringent, bad, bitter, sour, sweetish. Ulceration in the mouth.

Dryness and constriction of the throat; enlarged tonsils, honeycombed with small crypts; viscid mucus in the throat. Pain in the throat on swallowing; pressing pain. External throat swollen; many hard glands. It has cured GOITRE, even exophthalmic goitre.

Appetite INCREASED, ravenous or *wanting;* aversion to food. Desires stimulants. Eructations empty; sour; waterbrash; heartburn. Fullness in the stomach; flushes of heat in the stomach. Hiccough. Nausea at night and after eating. Pain in the stomach after eating; burning, cramping, cutting, *pressing,* SORE, stitching. *Pulsating* in the stomach. Thirst extreme, unquenchable. Vomiting on coughing, after eating, bile, blood, food.

Distension of the abdomen, tympanitic. Enlarged ab-

domen, mesenteric glands, spleen. Flatulence; obstructed.
Hardness of the liver, mesenteric glands. Pain in abdomen; during menses, in hypochrondria, in liver; burning,
cramping, *cutting*, pressing in the hypogastrium. Pulsation in abdomen. Rumbling.

Constipation; inactivity of the rectum; difficult stool;
hard stool. Diarrhœa; evening, after eating. Exhausting;
stool bloody, copious, watery, white, yellow; passing of
copious flatus. Hemorrhoid. *Itching* of the anus; burning
after stool; tenesmus after stool; ineffectual urging to
stool.

Retention or suppression of urine; much urging at
night; frequent urination during the night; involuntary
urination. Frequent paroxysms if busy; stinging pain in
neck of bladder with frequent urging to urinate. It has
been useful in Addison's disease. The urine is acrid, albuminous, cloudy, dark, pale, red, copious, with offensive
odor and cuticle on the surface.

Erections wanting; seminal emissions; sexual passion
increased without erections. Pain in the testes; induration
of testes; swollen testes.

Sexual desire increased in the woman; congestion of
the uterus. *Leucorrhoea* acrid, bloody, copious, yellow.
Menses absent, *copious*, frequent, irregular, painful, suppressed. Metrorrhagia. Pain in ovaries and uterus. Sterility. Tumors on ovaries. Pain in both ovaries before
menses.

Catarrh of the larynx and trachea; constriction, croup.
Inflammation of the larynx; mucus in the air passages;
pain in the larynx; phthisis of larynx; tickling in the
larynx. HOARSENESS.

Accelerated respiration, asthmatic, difficult at night
and on ascending steps; rattling, short. Suffocation.

Cough morning; evening, after midnight, asthmatic,
DRY; from irritation in the larynx and trachea, short,

spasmodic; from tickling in the larynx. Expectoration: morning; bloody, greenish, mucus, offensive, purulent, viscid, yellow. Violent, hard cough after pneumonia.

Anxiety in chest and heart; catarrh of the bronchial tubes; constriction of the heart. Induration of the mammæ. Inflammation of the bronchial tubes, of the pleura; oppression of the chest; pain in the chest on coughing; in the heart; burning, cutting, pressing, rawness; stitching on coughing; stitching in mammæ. Palpitation of the heart, warm during the night. PHTHISIS. *Trembling in the heart.* It has cured nodular tumors in mammæ, tender to touch, painful on moving the arm.

Pain in the sacrum; soreness in the spine; stitching pain in back and lumbar region.

Enlarged points of the fingers; coldness of the upper limbs, hands, legs, feet; cramps in the feet; heat of the hands; heaviness of the limbs; of the feet; itching of the limbs; numbness of the hands, fingers, lower limbs, legs; pain in the limbs, in the joints; in gouty joints; in the thighs, in the knees. Stitching pain in the shoulders, in the knees. Tearing in the joints, in the upper limbs, in the elbow, in the knees; perspiration of the hands, of the palms, of the FEET; stiffness in the limbs; swelling of the hands, legs, knees, feet; œdematous; trembling of upper limbs, of the hands, lower limbs; twitching of the upper limbs, thighs, legs; weakness of the upper limbs, of the knees.

Dreams amorous, anxious, of dead people; nightmare vivid. Restless sleep; sleepiness in the evening; sleeplessness; waking too early.

Chill, external, internal; *shaking chill*; tertian; warmth does not ameliorate.

Fever in the afternoon; fever alternating with chill; *flushes of heat*; hectic fever.

Perspiration in the morning; during the night; in bed cold; on SLIGHT EXERTION; on motion; profuse.

Burning of the skin; coldness. Red and yellow spots. Dry skin; eruptions, boils, herpes, rash, scaly. Erysipelas.

CALCAREA SILICATA

The silicate of lime is a very deep-acting remedy. The symptoms come on during all parts of the day and night—*morning*, forenoon, afternoon, EVENING, NIGHT, *after midnight*. It acts profoundly upon the skin, mucous membranes, bones and glands. Abscesses, catarrhal discharges, ulcers, are marked with *thick, greenish-yellow pus*. Thick, greenish-yellow expectoration. Aversion to the open air. Extreme sensitiveness to drafts. One prover felt better in open air; very sensitive to wine and alcoholic stimulants. Marked paleness as in anæmia. Weakness and out of breath ascending stairs, like *calcarea*. Aversion to bathing and worse from bathing; especially cold bathing makes worse, in a prover who had always enjoyed cold bathing. Complaints worse after breakfast. It has cured epithelioma and lupus. From what is known of both calcarea and silica it ought to be a remedy in caries where the symptoms agree. Change of weather, from warm to cold, makes all symptoms worse. Many symptoms are worse after coition. Worse from cold in general, cold air, becoming cold and after becoming cold; worse in cold, wet weather. Takes cold in cold weather; seems to be constantly taking cold; many internal congestions. Contraction of orifices, a convulsive tendency. It greatly mitigates the constitutional condition in patients suffering from epilepsy, making the fits lighter and farther apart. The veins are greatly distended and a sensation of fullness in many parts. The symptoms are worse during and *after eating*. Emaciation is marked and especially in children who have inherited phthisis. Weakness, night sweats and seminal emission. The least exertion prostrates and increases many symptoms. Faintness creeps over her. The muscles become flabby. He is more comfortable on low diet or when fasting; cold food, cold milk and cold drinks make many complaints worse. The mucous membranes bleed easily. Hemorrhage from throat, nose, larynx and chest. He is cold all the time; marked lack of vital heat. One chilly prover became warm after the proving, curative action. Great aggravation from being overheated. The body feels heavy and the organs drag down. Inflammation in external and internal parts; in *bones* and *glands*. Extremely sensitive to a jar in all internal parts. Lassitude day and night, but worse evening and night; must lie down all the time.

The muscles, tendons and joints are weak and easily strained. The weakness is much like arsenicum and china, or as though from loss of fluids. He is most comfortable when lying in bed on the back; lying helps most symptoms; after lying a while he seems very well, but as soon as he walks about all the lassitude returns and he must lie down. Many symptoms come at the menstrual period—before, during and after. All symptoms are worse from motion. Mucous secretions increased and greenish-yellow. Numbness of single parts, of parts lain on and of painful parts. The weakness suggests it in complaints following onanism. The blood seems to rush from body to head with great flushes of heat.

The pains are boring, burning, CUTTING, jerking, pressing, bruised, *stitching, tearing*. Burning in internal parts. The function of organs and glands much impaired and slow. Slow digestion, slow action of bowels and liver. Periodicity is marked in many symptoms. When perspiring a slight draft or cold air will suppress the sweat and he becomes lame and the symptoms in general are worse. Pulsation all over the body—internal and external.

Sensitive all over, sensitive to pain; sore internally. The bones are sore to touch. Its symptoms are like those that have come on from sexual excesses. The weakness and many other symptoms are worse standing. Stiffness in body, back and limbs when cold, after exertion and after sweating. It has swelling from dropsy and from inflammation; swelling of affected parts, of *glands* with hardness. Touch aggravates many parts and he dreads being touched. Trembling all over and in limbs, much twitching of muscles. It is most useful in restraining malignant ulceration in the mammary gland. Symptoms worse from uncovering. Walking fast and walking in cold air makes him worse. Great weakness, especially in the morning on waking, after least exertion, from mental exertion, walking in open air. Great nervous weakness. *He is always so weary.* Wet weather brings out all his sufferings. It seems that he can hardly get through the winter, so much are his symptoms increased, and he is correspondingly improved in the summer.

He is absent-minded and excitable and easily angered and his symptoms are worse after anger. Symptoms worse when alone. Anxiety in evening in bed and during the night about her health, worse during menses and on waking in the morning. Wants many things and soon tires of them; desires the unobtainable; nothing suits and he is very critical. Inability to concentrate the mind on what he is reading or listening to. He has lost all confidence in himself. *Confusion* of mind in the morning on waking and in the evening, after eating, after *mental exertion* and while sitting. Consolation irritates him; contrary and timid, even cowardly. She sits long in one place and locks into space and does not answer when spoken to. Passive delirium; talks and acts like one insane; talking to imaginary people who have long been dead. Talks nonsense and foolish things; talks coherently, but about impossible things. Answers questions correctly and goes off into muttering. Wants to go out of the window. Thinks her husband, long dead, is in the next room, and grieves because they will not let her go to him; her living son she calls by the name of one long dead. Mutters foolish things and sees dead people. She wanders all night in her room without sleep. She seems to see and converse with dead friends, with her dead son and her dead husband; wants to get dinner for her dead husband. She imagines her husband will starve if she does not find him. Many delusions about dead people; sees dead people and corpses; she sees dogs and images nights. Horrible visions; sees disagreeable persons when half awake. Illusions of fancy; she hears voices and answers the voices of the dead. Discontent and *despair*; discouraged about her disease and thinks it proving an incurable disease. Dullness of mind; imaginary fears and vexations after mental exertion. Emotional and easily moved to laughter or tears; exaltation of fancy. Exertion of mind aggravates all mental and many physical symptoms. Great fear at night; fear of brain lesion with headache in the morning; fear about family matters also about financial matters; fear or dread of work or any exertion. Complaints from fear. He is so forgetful that he cannot recall the sentence just spoken. *Easily frightened*, all the time in a hurry. Many hysterical manifestations, and at night his ideas are abundant, but in daytime deficient. Many of the mental symptoms and his appearance are like one approaching imbecility. He is very impatient with everything and everybody. "Utterly ambitionless," no desire for physical or mental work and aversion to exercise. Irresolution. Marked irritability in the morning and evening, after coition, from consolation, during headache, about trifles. Lamenting and wailing. Las-

civious. Loathing of life. Memory very weak. Mistakes
in speaking; misplaces words. Changeable mood, morose,
generally better when occupied; during the proving mild
and yielding. Extreme prostration of mind; restless and
anxious during the night; sadness in the morning and during the day; sadness during heat. *Mental depression* without cause. Dullness of the senses; very sensitive to noise
and to mild rebuke from a friend. The mental symptoms
are worse from sexual excesses. Shrieking during sleep.
Easily startled. Starting during sleep. Stupefaction and
disposition to suicide; indisposed to talk or to be talked to,
and inclined to sit in silence. Timid and bashful. She is
unconscious and her conduct is automatic; weary of life.
Weeping at night, in sleep; almost impossible to keep
from bursting into sobs from imaginary fears and worries;
sits and weeps by the hour; the will is almost lost; great
aversion to mental work.

Vertigo, morning on rising, after rising, in evening,
tendency to fall backward during headache. *Vertigo,* looking upwards, while lying, from mental exertion, with
nausea, on rising from stooping, while sitting, on stooping,
while walking in the open air.

Coldness of the head, especially of occiput, and on vertex; congestion of the head at night, and when coughing;
constriction of the forehead; eruptions on the scalp; crusts,
eczema, pustules; the head inclines to fall forward; marked
sensation of fullness in the head. There is bristling of the
hair; the hair falls out. Heat in the whole head, worse in
forehead, in the evening. Heaviness in the head in the
morning; heaviness in forehead. *Hydrocephalus.* Itching
scalp; itching occiput. Sensation as if the brain was in
motion.

The head pains are severe and in all parts of the head.
Worse *morning,* but felt also afternoon and evening, lasting all night; worse from *cold air* and A DRAFT; ascending

steps; binding up the hair, in women; after coition; becoming cold, from taking cold; from cold, damp weather; with coryza; after eating; also worse from becoming overheated, and during heat with hammering; *worse from a jar*; *from light*; must lie down; worse before and during menses; *from mental exertion*; worse from moving about the room, from moving the head, *from noise*. The pain comes in paroxysms. It cures periodical headaches that come every day or only once each week; pulsating headaches. Pain is worse *after sleep*, from stimulants, stooping and stepping heavily, and from taking cold. Headache from *eye strain*. Head pains from touch, walking, wine, writing. The pains extend to occiput and nape of the neck. Aching deep in the brain, with pulsation on motion. Hard pain in forehead in the morning; steady dull heavy pain, better after eating and occupation; worse from mental exertion, *motion*, and walking and writing; better from perfect rest. Headache morning on waking; worse lying, worse rising from bed, better by occupation, better standing and walking. Severe headache in the forehead; pain over the eyes, pulsating; worse walking, worse from motion, better from lying, heat and pressure. Hard pain in occiput, and sides of the head, worse in right side. Severe pain in temples and vertex; burning pain in head; bursting pain in head, mostly in vertex; cutting in head; drawing pain in forehead and occiput; dull pain in whole head in the morning. Jerking with the pain like a jerking pain. Pressing pains in forehead; *occiput*, sides of occiput, *temples* and *vertex*. Pressing-out pain in forehead. Shooting pains in whole head. Shooting in occiput. Scalp is sore to touch and whole brain is sensitive to motion and jar, as if bruised. Stitching pains in forehead, occiput, sides of head and temples. The pain is so violent that *he feels stunned*; tearing in the *forehead* and frontal eminence, *occiput* and temples. Perspiration of the whole scalp; perspiration of *forehead*. Pulsating in forehead and whole head. Shaking or undulating sensation in brain. Twitching of muscles of head.

The eyelids are agglutinated with pus. It has cured *cataract*. Discharges from the eye of thick, greenish-yellow mucus and pus. Heaviness of the lids. Inflammation of the conjunctiva with thick discharges, also of lids. Injected, dark veins. Itching of the eyes. Lachrymation in open air, lachrymation of right eye with coryza. It has cured opacity of the cornea. Very severe pain in the eyes, worse from light, before and during a storm, with redness. The pains are burning, cutting, pressing, as though sand in the eyes; sore, bruised, stitching, and *tearing*. Paralysis of the optic nerve; *photophobia*; pulsation in the eyes and the pupils are contracted; marked redness in eyes, especially inner canthi, of lids, of veins; spots on the cornea; swollen lids; twitching of the lids. It has cured ulceration of the cornea. The eyes look weak.

Colors before the eyes, spots, floating spots, dark colors. Dazzling. Cannot see to read with the usual glasses. He thought he was going blind. Hypermetropia. Exertion of vision causes headaches and many nervous symptoms; flickering and foggy visions before the eyes; dimness of vision; sparks before the eyes.

From the ear there is an offensive, *purulent, thick* yellow and greenish-yellow discharge; watery offensive discharge; bloody, watery discharge. Flapping in the ears. The ears are hot. Itching deep in ears. Noises in ears, cracking in ears when chewing. Fluttering in ears. Humming, ringing, roaring and whizzing in ears; violent drawing, jerking, stitching, tearing pain in ears. There is pulsation with and without pain; swelling inside with stopped feeling; increased wax in ears; twitching in the ears. Hearing first acute, later *impaired*.

It causes vicious catarrh of nose and posterior *nares*, extending to frontal sinuses in tubercular constitutions, chronic coryza with cough; *coryza* with discharges fluent in open air, but patient feels better himself. It has cured many cases of hay fever. Copious discharges in morning after rising; albuminous and shiny in the daytime. Crusts blown out of nose. Hard crusts, excoriating, greenish, *offensive, purulent, thick* and *yellow or yellowish green*; copious, bloody, thin or watery discharges. Extreme dryness inside of nose. Epistaxis, bright red blood, on blowing nose; itching inside of nose; obstruction at night and in morning on rising. It is a most useful remedy in *ozoena*. Much pain high up in nose, in root of nose; soreness inside of nose; stitching pains in nose; polypus in nose has been cured by this remedy. Sense of smell at first acute, later diminished and finally lost. Sneezing, ulceration in nose; swelling of the nose.

The face is very pale, an earthly color; lips bluish and cracked; red face during headache; circumscribed red cheeks; dryness of the lips. Eruptions of the face, cheeks, chin, forehead, lips, on the nose, and around the mouth. *Acne,* boils, comedones, *eczema,* herpes pimples; scurfy eruptions on the face; the face is hot and red. Inflammation and suppuration of the parotid gland. Pain in face from cold, better by *warmth*. The pains of the face are boring, drawing, stitching and tearing. Perspiration of the face and scalp. Swelling of glands; swelling of the parotid and *submaxillary* glands.

Mucous membranes of mouth covered with aphthæ and the gums bleed; the tongue is coated white; the mouth is very dry, but at times copious mucus; offensive, even putrid odor from the mouth. The tongue is very sore, saliva is copious and speech is difficult. Swollen gums and tongue; bad taste, alkaline, bitter in the morning, metallic, putrid, sour. Taste is sometimes wanting. Ulceration of mucous membrane, lower lip, on left side; stinging, smarting, splinter-like pain, spreading, painful to pressure, lardacious, inflamed edges; small ulcer appeared on right side. The teeth become loose and feel as though too long; caries of the teeth. Pain in the teeth at night. The teeth are very sore when masticating; pain worse from cold air, from anything cold in the mouth; while eating, after sleep, better from external warmth and warm things in the mouth. The pains are boring, digging, drawing, *jerking*, piercing, pressing, *stitching* and tearing.

Inflammation of the throat, pharynx and tonsils with dryness and redness; constant effort to clear the throat, worse in the morning. Tenacious mucus in the throat; lump in the throat. Much pain in the throat on becoming cold, on coughing, on swallowing. Sore pain and burning; splinter-like pain on swallowing. Stitching pain on swallowing; swallowing is difficult. Tonsils and uvula swollen; ulceration in the throat. Pain and swelling in cervical glands. Induration in the glands of the neck. It has cured goitre.

A feeling of anxiety in the stomach. The appetite is at first increased, then ravenous, and finally wanting, with aversion to food, especially to meat and milk. Some provers desire sour things and milk. Sensation of coldness in the stomach; sensation of emptiness not relieved by eating; sinking sensation in the pit of the stomach; eructations in the morning, after eating; bitter, empty, tasting like food eaten; *sour*. *Waterbrash*. *Heartburn*. Hiccough. Fullness in stomach after eating; loathing of food. Nausea in the *morning*, afternoon, evening, night; while eating, after eating, better after empty eructations, during headache, while walking. Pain in stomach, evening and night; after cold drinks, on coughing, after eating, while walking in the open air. The pains are burning, cramping, *cutting, pressing, bruised* and stitching; pressing pains in evening after eating, like a weight. Pulsation in the stomach; sensation of a stone in the stomach;

marked sensation of tension. Thirst afternoon and *night*; *burning thirst*; *extreme thirst*. Vomiting morning and night; on coughing, after drinking, after eating, during headache, after milk; vomiting bile, bitter substance, black *blood*, *food*, mucus, watery substances.

Distension of the abdomen after eating; dropsy of the abdomen, enlarged liver. Flatulence with much rumbling and fullness. The abdomen is very hard, the liver is hard. Inflammation of the peritoneum. Sensation of movements in the abdomen from flatus. Pain morning and *night*; pain before menses; pain in right hypochondrium; pain in liver and in the inguinal region. The pains are burning, *cramping*, cutting, *pressing*, stitching, tearing, twisting, stitching pains in sides of abdomen and in liver. Marked tension in abdomen; tympanitic abdomen.

Extreme constipation, with inactivity of the rectum; *difficult* stool, paralyzed feeling in rectum; constriction of anus; constipation, with dry stool, *hard*, knotty, *large* and soft, *light colored*, with much straining. Diarrhœa painless, with stool copious, lienteric, *offensive,* even putrid, sour, pasty, thin and watery. Dysentery; with bloody, scanty stools. Copious, offensive flatus. It has cured fistula in anus. Itching and crawling of anus. Hemorrhoids protrude during stool, sore to touch, worse when walking. Bleeding from rectum and anus with stool; itching after stool. Moisture about the anus, pain during and after stool, burning during and after stool. Pains are pressing, stitching and *tearing*; marked soreness of anus. Paralyzed feeling in rectum. Stricture of the rectum not allowing feces to pass larger than a pencil, was cured. Tenesmus. Much urging to stool, urging during stool; ineffectual urging.

Tenesmus of bladder and retention of urine, pressing pain in the bladder, catarrh of the bladder with much mucus in the urine; urging to urinate at night, worse moving

6

about, better lying. Sudden urging, ineffectual urging. Frequent urination during the night; involuntary urination during night in sleep; unsatisfactory urination. The urine is scanty.

The prostate gland is enlarged and tender; emission of prostatic fluid when straining to pass stool.

Urethral discharge purulent, greenish, yellow; cutting and burning urination. It has cured stricture of the urethra. The urine is copious, later scanty, red, cloudy, burning, containing mucus, with sediment purulent and sandy It has cured diabetes mellitus.

Erection at night without thought or dreams; eruptions on the genitals of the male, on the prepuce. It has cured hydrocele and induration of testes. Marked redness of glans penis; itching of glans penis and scrotum; stitching pain in penis. Foul sweat on the male genitals. Sweat on the scrotum. *Seminal emissions.* Sexual passion increased, sexual desire strong without erections. Swollen testes.

In the female the desire is increased; eruptions on the vulva with much itching. Heaviness of the uterus and prolapsus. Leucorrhœa excoriating, bloody, *copious*, before and after menses, milky, white or purulent and yellow or yellowish-green. Menstrual flow acrid, bright red, copious, too soon, protracted, or scanty; menstrual flow absent or suppressed, painful and irregular. Flow of blood between the menstrual periods; pain in the uterus, aching, burning, labor-like and tearing; soreness in the genitals; ulceration of labia, vagina and os uteri.

Chronic irritation of the air passages, larynx and trachea; catarrh of the larynx and trachea, with copious yellow-green mucus; rawness in larynx and trachea; phthisis of the larynx. He constantly scrapes the larynx. Tickling in the larynx and trachea. Respiration fast, *asthmatic*, deep; difficult during cough and when lying, rattlng, short, sighing and suffocative.

It is one of our greatest cough remedies in phthisical subjects. The cough comes at *night*, but also morning after rising, and in evening in bed. Cough from cold air, from cold damp air, asthmatic, from cold drinks. It has a dry cough at night, with much expectoration in the morning; cough during fever; hacking, hoarse cough; cough from irritation of larynx and trachea; hoarse cough, especially in the morning; paroxysmal, spasmodic cough in the evening racking the whole body. Cough worse lying, talking; virulent cough after waking in the morning. Expectoration in the *morning, bloody, greenish-yellow, copious*, offensive, *purulent*, thick, viscid—sometimes white. It has cured abscesses of lungs and axilla. It has restrained cancerous ulceration of mammæ. It has cured desperate cases of catarrh of the bronchial tubes, constriction of chest, eruption of chest and excoriation of the nipples. Hemorrhage of the lungs. Chronic inflammation of bronchial tubes and lungs. Oppression of the chest. The milk is suppressed or absent. Pain in both lungs. Pain in chest during cough, on inspiration, on deep breathing. Pain in the sides of chest. The pains in the chest are burning, *pressing*, soreness, stitching and rawness in chest. Stitching pains on inspiring, in sides of chest, and in the mammary glands. Palpitation of the heart *at night*, after eating, from *exertion*, and even from slight motion. Perspiration all over the chest. *Phthisical conditions*. Extreme weakness of chest.

The back feels cold and there is a sensation of coldness in back of neck and sacrum. Eruption in the cervical region, pimples and pustules. Itching of the back. *Much pain in the back*, especially *at night*. Pain in back *during menses*, on motion, rising from sitting and while sitting. Pain in the cervical region, scapula and in the spine between the scapula; pain in lumbar region when *rising from a seat*; pain in coccyx. Hard aching in the back, in lumbar region when rising from a seat, and in the sacrum. Drawing pain in the lumbar region, pressing pain in the lumbar region. The spine is sore to touch in many places. Stitching pains in the cervical region, scapulæ, lumbar region and sacrum. Tearing pains in the cervical region. Perspiration on the back, worse on the back of the neck. *Stiffness of the back, especially of the cervical region*; *stiff neck*. Tension in the cervical region. *Weakness of the back.* Weakness of the lumbar region.

It is a remedy for gouty nodosites of the fingers, awkwardness of the limbs, caries of the bone, chapped hands; chronic jerking of muscles; coldness of all the limbs, hands, palms, lower limbs, LEGS, FEET, *evening and night*. Contractions of tendons of hands and fingers. Many corns, painful *sore* and *stinging*. *Cracked hands* and *fingers*. Cramps in hands, lower limbs, *calf, feet, soles, toes*. Eruptions, vescicles, boils on the upper limbs, vescicles on the upper limbs and fingers; eruptions on lower limbs, itching, pimples. Boils on the thighs; felons on the fingers. Heat of hands, palms, of the feet. Heaviness of all the limbs, especially of *legs and feet*. It has been of great service in hip joint disease; inflammation of all the joints. Intense itching of all the limbs, thighs and legs. The nails have ceased to grow for two years; the nails are hard and brittle. Numbness of all the limbs; upper limbs numb when lying on them; numbness of *hands* and *fingers*; numbness of lower limbs, legs and feet when sitting. Rheumatic and gouty pains in limbs, *joints* and *bones*, evening and night. Pain in upper limbs at night, worse from cold, motion and taking hold of anything; pain in shoulders, upper arm, elbow, forearm, fingers and finger joints; pain in the lower limbs; pain in the sciatic nerve; violent pains in the hip joint; pain in the hip joint as if an abscess were forming; pain in thigh, knee, calf, foot and toes. Aching in all the limbs, with stiffness in cold, damp weather; aching in the shoulder, worse from motion. Burning feet and soles. Drawing pain in upper arm, forearm, wrist and hand; drawing pain in the knee and leg. Sore, bruised pains in upper limbs and thighs. Sensation as if sprained in wrist and ankle. Stitching pains in the *joints*. Stitching pains in the shoulders, upper arm, elbow, wrist and fingers. Stitching pains in hips, knees, calf, ankle, foot, sole, heel, toes, especially the *great toe*. Tearing pain in shoulder, upper arm, elbow, forearm, wrist, hand, fingers and finger-joints; tearing pain in thighs, knee, *leg*, calf, *foot*, soles, toes, and especially the great toe.

Sensation of paralysis in upper limbs and in the hands; paralysis in lower limbs. Cold sweat on all the limbs; cold sweat of *palms*, of hands; cold sweat of *feet*; *offensive cold sweat of feet*. Stiffness of all the limbs, *joints*, *hands*, and *fingers*; stiffness of lower limbs, knees. Swelling of hands, *knees*, legs, *ankles*, feet. Tingling of the fingers; trembling of the upper limbs, of the hands, of the lower limbs; twitching of the upper limbs, thighs and legs. Ulceration of *lower limbs, legs*. Varicose veins. Warts on the hands; on the dorsum of the thumb; on the ball of the thumb; large, hard seed warts. Weakness of all the limbs, and especially the *joints*. Weakness of thighs, *knees, legs*, calf and feet.

Dreams of anger, *anxious*, of business, confused, amorous, of the dead, of death, of disease, fantastic, fire, *frightful, horrible*, murder, nightmare, vivid, vexatious, visionary; dreams of sick people and caring for sick people; a hideous old woman's face appeared in her dreams. Sleep is restless; sleepiness in the morning, forenoon and *evening*, after dinner, *after eating*; sleeplessness *before mid-*

night; sleeplessness with sleepiness; sleepless from much thinking; after once waking cannot sleep again; unrefreshing sleep. Waking early and frequent. Yawning.

Chill in morning, forenoon and evening, in the open air, in the cold air, even in bed, after eating, external and internal, shaking chill; chill with trembling, from uncovering, warm room does not relieve, desires warmth, but it does not relieve; chilliness during stool. Fever forenoon and afternoon, but marked fever in *evening and night*; fever alternating with chill; dry heat at night in bed; external heat with chilliness; flushes of heat. It is useful in hectic fevers. Mild fever *evening* and night. Heat with moist skin. Perspiration in the morning and latter part of the night; perspiration with great anxiety. Cold sweat mostly on the extremities; sweat from coughing, during and after eating, from exertion, from mental exertion; sweat from motion, from walking. *Profuse* hot sweat. Sweat of single parts; sweat during and after sleep; offensive, sour sweat, uncovering while sweating brings on many symptoms. If the perspiration becomes suppressed from uncovering, or from a draft, he suffers much.

Burning of the skin after scratching; the skin is cold to touch; the skin of hands and fingers cracked; the skin is discolored; bluish, liver spots, pale, red, red spots,*white spots,* yellow. Dry, burning skin and inability to perspire. Eruptions are biting, *burning, itching*, painful, *phagedenic*, stinging. Boils and chapping and desquamating. *Eczema* and herpes. *Dry, itching, crusting*, stinging herpes, eruptions discharge a white, pus-like substance. There are pimples, *pustules*, and red rashes; eruptions *scabby* and *scaly* after scratching. Suppurating eruptions, nodular urticaria after scratching. *Vesicles* in many places. Erysipelas with swelling, worse from scratching. Excrescences form upon the skin; formication and goose-flesh.

Indurations. Intertrigo. Itching with and without eruptions, itching, biting, burning, crawling and stinging, worse
after scratching. The itching is ameliorated by radiated
heat It has cured lupus. The skin becomes moist after
scratching. The skin is very sensitive, sore feeling, and
sore, raw places on the skin; sticking and stinging after
scratching. Ulceration of the skin and ulcers bluish, burning, cancerous, *crusty, deep, corrosive,* offensive with yellow pus, *fistulous, foul, indolent, indurated,* stinging, and
unhealthy. Warts painful, *hard,* inflamed, stinging, suppurating and withered. It has cured wens and other cys-
tic growths.

CALENDULA

The proving of Calendula is so nearly worthless that
we cannot expect at present to use it as a guide to the internal administration of the remedy. There are only a
few things that I have ever been able to get out of it. In
injuries Calendula cannot be ignored, in cuts with lacera-
tion, surface or open injuries. Dilute Calendula used locally will keep the wound odorless, will reduce the amount
of pus, and favor granulation in the very best possible
manner, and thus it assists the surgeon in healing up surface wounds. Calendula is all the dressing you will need
for open wounds and severe lacerations. It takes away
the local pain and suffering. You may easily see we are
not now dealing with a condition that exists because of a
state within the economy, but because of something that
is without. There is nothing that will cause these external
injuries to heal so beautifully as the Marigold. Some will
say it is not homœopathic, but these are the individuals
who "strain at a gnat and swallow a camel." If there
are constitutional symptoms suspend all medicated dressing entirely and pay your whole attention to the constitutional symptoms. Sometimes there are no constitutional

symptoms to prescribe on, but when they are present resort locally to cleanliness and nothing else. Do not supress symptoms that you will need to guide you to a remedy.

CAULOPHYLLUM

Weakness in the reproductive system of the woman. From weakness she is sterile, or she aborts in the early months of gestation. During parturition the contractions of the uterus are too feeble to expel the contents, and they are only tormenting. Labor-like pains during menstruation with drawing pains in the thighs and legs, and even the feet and toes. Uterine hemorrhage from inertia of the uterus. Relaxation of muscles and ligaments. Heaviness, and even prolapsus. Subinvolution. Excoriating leucorrhea. Menses too soon, or too late. She is sensitive to cold and wants warm clothing, quite unlike Pulsatilla. She is hysterical, like Ignatia. She is fretful and apprehensive. She is rheumatic, like Cimicifuga, only the small joints are likely to be affected. Later she suffers from after pains, and they are felt in the inguinal region. Rheumatic stiffness of the back, and very sensitive spine. She is sleepless, restless, and withal very excitable. This remedy has cured chorea at puberty when menstruation was late.

CENCHRIS-CONTORTRIX PROVING
(Copperhead)

Bulletin No. 24 of National Museum gives check list of North American reptilia Ancistrodon Contortrix. Dr. Albert Günther, who furnished the article for The Encyclopedia Britannica, calls the "Copperhead" Cenchris-Contortrix, and considers it very similar to the Trigonocephalus family, but smaller in size, generally found near the water-courses, closely related to the Chenchris Piscivarus, which is the water-snake or crater-moccasin.

The Cenchris family belongs to the temperate parts of North America, and its venom is of a deadly nature.

PROVERS

No. 1.   Mrs. K., 6th potency, one dose only.

No. 2.   Dr. Mary S., 6th potency, one dose only.

No. 3.   Dr. Eliza M., 6th potency, one dose only.

No. 4.   J. A. T., 6th potency, one dose only.

No. 5.   Dr. Mary S., 2nd proving, 10m.

No. 6.   Dr. Eliza M., 2d proving, 10m, one dose.

No. 7.   Geo. W. S., 6th and 30th potencies.

MIND—Loss of memory. Feeling of intoxication. Anxiety, with a feeling that she will die *suddenly*[1] (8th day, lasting many days). The horrors of the dreams of the previous night seemed to follow her[1] (8th day). She could not banish the horrors of her dreams[1] (9th day). Instantly after lying down at night she was seized with a horrible, sickening anxiety, all over the body, but most at the heart and through the chest, exclaiming, "I shall die! I shall die!" This soon passed into profound sleep, which was not interrupted until morning, but full of horrible dreams. Afternoon and evening thinks her family plotting to place her in an insane asylum (this lasted four afternoons and ended fourteenth day of proving). Suspicious of everybody. Melancholy (old symptoms worse). No inclination to attend to her usual duties, which are pleasant.[3] Angry when disturbed.[3] Not able to rest in bed, must walk the floor to ease mind.[3] Wants to be alone[3] (4th day). Nervous and irritable[3] (14th day). Catch myself staring into space and forget what people are saying to me, or that there is any one in the room.[2] (4th day). Inability to concentrate mind[2] (4th day, 6th and 10m.). Absent minded[2] (two provers, 5th, 6th and 10m.). *Dreamy, absent minded, took wrong car without realizing where was going.* Misdirected letters[2] (13th day, 6th and 10m.). Very gloomy and discouraged[3] (7th day). So absent minded and stupid that I tremble and shiver, and my teeth chatter for some time before I begin to realize that I feel cold[5] (3rd day). Foreboding, gloomy without cause, frequent sighing[2] (21st day, 6th and 10m.). Crying and very frequent sighing, as if very sad[2] (many days, 6th and 10m.). Lack of de-

termination and snap, have to use all my reserve mental
force to make myself get up and go out[5] (many days).
Painful procrastination, indecision.[5] Time passes too slowly, seems to drag along. I am longing to go, yet I cannot
tear myself out of my chair and move along. When at
last I do pick up enough determination to go, I go very
suddenly.[5] Feel hard and uncharitable[5] (8th day). Selfish, envious, easily slighted. Transient attacks of anger
6 P. M.[5] (9th day, 6 P. M. and 8:30 P. M. 14th day, and
6:30 P. M. 17th). Longing for the woods so intense I
wandered out to the park alone[5] (2d day). Great depression and gloomy foreboding followed by great hilarity[5]
(9th day). Alternation of opposite moods and desires[5]
(9th day).

SENSORIUM—Sensation of intoxication in evening[3] (2d
day). Sensation of intoxication came on at 4 P. M., lasting
3 hours, feeling as if I would fall; unable to walk in a
direct line; go from side to side of pavement[3] (2d day).
Same symptoms 4 P. M. 3d day. Same symptom 4 P. M.
to 7 P. M. 4th day, and came every day for 4 weeks). Vertigo, coming and going, with no inclination to attend to her
usual duties that are very pleasant; nervous and tired all
the time[3] (6th day). Vertigo. Angry when disturbed.[3]
(6th day). Compelled to lie all afternoon. So dizzy[3] (9th
day). Vertigo very bad from 4 P. M. to 7 P. M.[3] (2d to
10 and 11th day). When riding in the car, she rode by
the place she intended to get off at.[3] Her mind is all a
blank for ten minutes, but people did not observe anything
wrong with her appearance. Dreamy feeling[2] (6th day).
Fainting spells.

INNER HEAD—Sensation of fullness about the head[1]
(18th day). Dull, aching pain in the forehead, which
finally extended to the occiput, leaving forehead[1] (1st day),
Feeling as if all the blood in the body rushed to the head[1]
(8th day). Violent headache in both temples in forenoon;

could not stand any warmth in the room; lips dry and parched[1] (13th day). Headache in both temples on rising, passing off after breakfast[3] (4th day). Headache in temples; passes off after eating.[3] Headache, not defined, with disgust for food.[3] Aching in the frontal sinuses, nose, and throat, as though she had taken a severe cold, but no discharge of mucus[2] (4th day). Dull ache in the occiput[2] (4th day). Dull aching in the frontal eminence[2] (4th and 8th days). Dull ache in left frontal eminence[5] (7th day). Hard, aching pain commenced in left frontal eminence and spread down left side to teeth, then spread to right frontal eminence, then to teeth on right side[5] (16th day). Hard pain over left eye[5] (9th day). Dull frontal headache during menstruation[2] (23d day). Dull throbbing in vertex[2] (18th, 19th and 20th days).

OUTER HEAD—Sore feeling in the scalp after the headache passed away[1] (2d day). Itching of scalp, better by scratching[2] (1st and 6th day—6th and 10m.). Transient sensation of prickling in the scalp, like a gentle current of electricity[5] (4th day. One large, dry, scabby pimple on scalp, long and narrow, oval shaped[5] (12th day).

SIGHT AND EYES—Eyes ache, and there is dimness of vision.[3] Lachrymation from left eye; left eyelid red on edges[2] (7th day). Twitching in left eyelid[2] (17th day). Dull ache in eyes, with sense of weakness[5] (16th day). Itching of eyes; begins in left eye and extends to right[1] (17th day). Margins of eyelids red, especially at night[5] (many days).

HEARING AND EARS—Itching of ears at night[3] (an old symptom not had for a year; 5th day). Itching of ears during the day[3] (7th day). Burning of left ear[2] (1st and 7th days; many days—6th and 10m.). Dull pain in and around the left ear[5] (6th day).

SMELL AND NOSE—Sickening odor in the nose (1st day). Copious flow of mucus, thin and watery.[2] Copious flow of mucus. Coryza. Cold nose[2] (several days). Cold nose[2] (6th day, evening 7 P. M.). Aching in throat and nose, tickling sensation in nose, as though discharge would flow, but very little discharge when blowing it[2] (5th and 6th days). Aching in left side of nose as though in the bones, with dull headache[2] (7th day). Sneezing occasionally and eyes filled with water[2] (6th and 8th days). Sneezing in morning when waking[2] (7th day—6th and 10m.; many days). Sneezing violently on awaking in the morning[2] (6th and 8th days). Tingling from left nostril to left eye (lachrymal canal). Slight discharge of water from left eye, sensation of weakness in the eye[2] (6th day. Nose burning sensation inside as though full of pepper[2] (7th day). Nostrils sore, worse left side[2] (7th day). Discharge of yellow mucus, sometimes tinged with blood[2] (7th and 9th days). Discharge of mucus from nose, varying from cream to amber color, specked with blood[2] (8th day). Cannot breathe through the nose[2] (8th day—6th and 10m.; many days). Impossible to breathe through the nose[2] (9th, 10th, 11th days). Scabs in the nose, lasting many days[2] (10th day—6th and 10m.). Dry mucus in nose, cannot breathe through it[2] (13th day). Slight tingling in left nostril[5] (4th day).

FACE—Flushes of heat about the face and head[1] (1st day). Bloating of face, as if intoxicated[1] (9th day). Bloating above and below eyes[1] (9th day). *Besotted countenance.* Mottled skin; purple, deep, dark red face. Dry parched lips in evening, with fever that began at 3 P. M.[1] (10th day). Swelling above eyes, below brow[1] (like Kali c.—12th day). She can see the water bag that fills the upper lid[1] (12th day). Baggy swelling under eyes[5] (many days). Face pale all through the proving.[3] Flushing and burning of face[2] (1st day). Great burning of the face, worse at night[2] (6th and 7th day). Cheeks began to get red and hot about 2 P. M.; keep growing hotter and redder until she goes to sleep at 10 P. M.; became dark red like erysipelas[2] (9th day). Woe-begone expression of face[2] (12th day). Burning face, 2 P. M.[2] (16th day). Burning begins in left cheek and ear, spreads to right cheek 6:30 P. M.[5] (2d day). Blue circles under eyes[5] (all through the proving). Face sallow.[5] Very small red pimples in little clusters, between the eyes and on the upper lip[5] (15th day). Same tiny pimples on end of nose[5] (16th day). Formication on left cheek, like crawling of a fly, also on septum of nose[7] (8th day).

LOWER FACE—Lips cracked and hot. Face chapped, dreads washing it[2] (18th day—6th and 10m.).

TEETH AND GUMS—Aching through jaws after lying down at night, lasting until after midnight[1] (12th day). Teeth ache from hot or cold drinks[5] (12th day). Teeth feel edgy, can feel that I have teeth[5] (12th day). Dull ache in right upper teeth when eating[5] (19th day).

TASTE, SPEECH AND TONGUE—Dry tongue. Bitter taste in mouth on waking in the morning. Taste of copper in the mouth[2] (14th day). Dry tongue[7] (4th day—30th potency).

MOUTH—Dry mouth in evening.[1] Increase of saliva[2] (7th and 8th days). Profuse saliva[2] (8th day). Profuse saliva, running out of mouth on pillow in sleep[7] (4th day—30th potency).

PALATE AND THROAT—Constantly hawking up thick, tough, stringy mucus, difficult to raise[1 5] (1st day). Throat full of mucus, thick and yellow, slightly tinged with blood from posterior nares, in the morning on waking[2] (6th day). During morning, twice discharged glossy, thick mucus from throat, looking like gelatine with bluish tinge, not tough, easily broken up[2] (6th day). Sore throat; painful, empty swallowing, but water swallowed without pain. Sore all over throat, after an hour it located on left side in tonsil, and muscles of left side of neck, was gone next morning[1] (11th day). Throat feels scraped, warm drinks are grateful[2] (4th, 22d, 26th days—6th and 10m.). Right side of throat red and swollen[2] (6th and 7th days). Throat full of mucus, yellow, with specks of blood in it[2] (8th day). Throat feels strained from the exertion of hawking[2] (6th day). Slight pricking in the throat on empty swallowing, but no pain on swallowing liquid or solid food[2] 6th day). Rawness of the throat with increase of saliva, which she swallows[2] (7th day). Throat full of mucus, yellow, with blood vessels plainly outlined on uvula, fauces and pharynx[2] (7th day). Right side of throat (pharynx), behind the posterior pillars of fauces, swollen and dark red, with sticking pains[2] (7th day). Throat feels sore and full, have to swallow often in order to breathe[2] (8th day). Aching in right side of throat[2] (8th day). Constantly swallowing[2] (9th day). The mucus is difficult to raise, loses her breath, and strangles in trying to raise it[2] (9th day). Eustachian tubes filled with mucus[2] (9th day). Had to hawk a half hour before I could get the mucus out of the throat so I could go to sleep; *mucus thick, tough* and yellow[2] (9th day). Throat painful on empty swallowing, but not when swallowing solids or liquids[2] (11th day).

APPETITE, THIRST, DESIRES AND AVERSIONS—Intense thirst for cold water in the evening. Every evening during proving.[1] Intense thirst in evening, with dry mouth.[1] Dislike for everything put before her to eat, and finds fault with everything[3] (5th day). No appetite for anything at breakfast[3] (7th day). Craves salt bacon (7th day). Disgust for food at breakfast[3] (9th day). No appetite.[7]

HICCOUGH, BELCHING, NAUSEA AND VOMITING—Eructations of tasteless gas a short time after eating[2] (3d and 6th days). Vomiting of white gruel-like substance, with mucus and undigested food[5] (2d day).   Nausea > by ice; water makes sick[6] (2d day).

STOMACH—Transient throbbing in the stomach[5] (6th day).   Acute cramping sensation in stomach, > by belching.

HYPOCHONDRIA—Pain in the attachment of the diaphragm, right side[2] (3d day).   Cough felt at the attachments of the diaphragm.[2]   Aching all around the waist, at the attachments of the diaphragm.[2]   Felt as though a cord were tied around the hip.[2]   Pain in the attachment of diaphragm when laughing[5] (9th day).   Hard ache in the attachment of diaphragm, both sides, < by breathing deeply[5] (11th day).   Feeling of a bottle of water in left hypochondrium, shaking up and down with motion of carriage[7] (13th day).

ABDOMEN—Dull pain in two spots directly over pubic arch, 10 A. M., passing off after two hours[3] (2d and 3d days).   Feeling as though that part of abdomen below umbilicus was not sufficiently expanded, on waking in the morning (2d day).   *Bands around the waist unbearable most of the time during the three weeks of proving.*[2]   Dull pains in lower abdomen[2] (2d day, 12th day—6th and 10m.).   Dull pain in abdomen when coughing[2] (14th day).   Transient aching in a spot just above the umbilicus[5] (11th day).   Sensation of a hard lump in left side of abdomen.   Bloating or abdomen after small amount of food, with diarrhœa.[7]   Great deal of rumbling in the bowels, left side[7] (11th day).   During breakfast, sharp, cutting pain in the left hypochondrium, from above downward; pain deep, took breath away, lasting but short time[7] (2d day—30 potency).

STOOL, ANUS AND RECTUM—Itching and soreness of the anus[1] (13th day).   Soreness of anus[5] (20th day).   Hemorrhoids that itch and are sore[1] (13th day).   Urging to stool, which passes away before the closet can be reached[2] (3d day). Unsuccessful urging to stool, strain until rectum feels as though prolapsed, but have no stool[5] (3d day). Waked in morning with itching of anus[5] (13th day). Diarrhœa with tenesmus[5] (35th day). On waking in the morning, had to hasten to the closet; stool watery, dark with a black sediment like coffee grounds; stool intermits, have to sit a long time, passing small quantities every minute or two[6] (2d and 40th days). Stool looks like bran porridge and of same consistency[7] (10th day). Stool gushing and frequent, watery, with a dark sediment at first without pain; after several hours great pain before stool[6] (20th, 21st and 22d days). Flatus at termination of stool. Painless and involuntary stool when passing flatus. Soiled the bed twice in sleep[7] (10th day). Had several diarrhœic stools at night, copious, gray in color, not debilitating. Several copious stools during the day with spluttering flatus, with bloating of abdomen after the smallest amount of food. Desire to be in a warm room, with above symptom[7] (14th day). Several stools, not so frequent; weak to-day, good deal of rumbling in left side of abdomen. Stools profuse, each seems as if it would empty the bowel, but soon full again. Sensation of intestines filled with water. (Crot. tig.) Stool frothy, foamy, air bubbles like yeast[7] (16th day).

URINARY ORGANS—Loses her urine when coughing.[3] Desire to urinate at night, just after getting in bed; must get up and press a long time before a few drops pass[5] (many days). When doing mental work, frequent desire to urinate, pass large quantities of colorless urine[6] (several days).

MALE SEXUAL ORGANS—Violent sexual desire.[4] No sexual desire (unusual) since began the proving[7] (10th day).

FEMALE SEXUAL ORGANS—Yellow leucorrhœa; never had any leucorrhœa before[1] (11th day). White leucorrhœa, only while at stool, during the whole proving.[6] Sexual desire strong, in a widow who had long been free from such sensations. Pain in right ovary[3]. Herpetic eruption on labia majora.[3] Dull aching in the small of the back and sacral region, at night during menses[2] (23d day). Soreness in coccyx and gluteal muscles, and aching in abdomen at night, during menses[2] (23d day). Menstrual flow very profuse, bright red, with dark clots (23d day). Menses two weeks late[5] (old symptom, 13th day). During menses, aching in small of back, when sitting up, must lie down. Easily moved to tears. Throbbing about umbilicus[5] (13th day). Sharp shooting pain in left ovary, upon motion[5] (3d day). Pain in left ovary during menses[5] (10th and 38th days). Cramping pains in uterus at each menstrual period, for four months.[6] Laborlike pains in uterus during menses.

VOICE AND LARYNX—Slight hoarseness, worse at night[2] (26th to 30th days—6th and 10m.). Hoarseness[2] (8th day).

RESPIRATION—Suffocating feeling after lying down in the evening[1] (7th day). Dyspnœa as if dying from anxiety[1] (7th day). Stops breathing on going to sleep[1] (8th day). She was prevented from sleeping by thinking of dreams of the previous night[1] (8th day). After lying down, a suffocating feeling came over her, with anxiety[2] in the chest as if she would die, worse on first lying down. She must lie with head drawn back, as she chokes so[1] (9th day). Dyspnœa on lying down and the thought of sleep brings on great anxiety[1] (12th day). She says: "There is no use lying down, that suffocation will come!" (12th day). Frequent sighing[2] (8th day). Impossible to breathe through the nose and very hard to breathe through the mouth, because of mucus in the throat[2] (9th day). Can hardly find breath enough to talk, have to stop and gasp in the midst of a word or short sentence[2] (9th day). Great

7

difficulty of breathing at night, she had to gasp and struggle for breath[2] (9th day).

COUGH AND EXPECTORATION—Dry, hacking cough, coming on at 3 P. M., continuing through the evening.[3] Irritation to cough, felt in pit of stomach[3]. Soreness in abdomen when coughing.[3] Cough comes on when walking fast or walking up stairs.[3] Coughs only when in the house.[3] Cough at night after retiring[2] (7th day). Cough caused a feeling of helplessness[2] (7th day). Concussive cough, causi: g watering on left eye[2] (7th day). Only cough twice, but felt quite concerned about it; a hopeless feeling comes over her at each cough[2] (7th day). Dark, bloody expectoration; also bright red blood seems to come from throat[2] (12th day). Cough seems to come from the diaphragm, causing violent contraction there. At other times it causes contraction of the umbilicus.[2] Expectoration frothy white, all shades of yellow in morning[2] (14th day). Loose cough in morning, with frothy sputa.[2] Concussive cough at night[2] (18th and 19th days). Dry, short cough at 4 P. M., with constant irritation to cough, lasting until 10 P. M. Cough very hard, dry, frequent[2] (14th day). Concussive, forcible, dry cough, shaking chest walls, cannot be repressed, lasting many days[2] (16th day). Expectoration of white mucus of a metallic taste[2] (18th day). Cough only in evening[2] (20th day). Hoarse, paroxysmal cough, with whitish expectoration[2] (21st day).

LUNGS—Transient hard ache in lower lobes of lungs; am afraid to draw a long breath on account of the pain[5] (9th day).

HEART AND CHEST—Anxiety about the heart in evening after lying down[1] (7th day). Anxiety about the heart with palpitation[1] (8th day). Anxiety in the chest, as if she would die, worse on lying down; must lie with head drawn back, as she chokes so[1] (9th day). Feeling as though the whole chest was distended and the heart very sore[1] (9th day). Feeling as if the heart was distended, or swelled to fill the chest[1] (many days). Anxiety in the region of the heart all night[1] (9th day). Extreme realization of the heart[1] (strongest 12th day, lasting many days). Pulse 120 in the evening[1]. Pulse 105 in the evening[1]. At 3 P. M. sensation of fluttering of heart followed by feeling that heart fell down into abdomen; then pulse became feeble, with heat lasting until after midnight[1] (10th day). At 11 P. M. sudden, sharp stitching pain in the heart, followed by dull pain, which gradually subsided[2] (1st day). Throbbing or fluttering under left scapula[2] (2d). Sudden, sharp stitches in apex of heart, worse evening[2] (3d day). Pain through the attachments of the diaphragm, just below apex of heart. Pain in same region on right side of chest; hard aching, worse from deep inspiration[2] (3d day). Sharp stitches in the heart[2] (4th day, lasting through the proving—four weeks). Dull pain in region of heart at 10 P. M. (7th day). Drawing pain in right side of chest, below mammary gland, on lying down at night (three nights); makes him put the hand on the pain; > by lying on that side and < lying on left side.[4] Sharp stitches in right side of chest[2] (7th day). Dull pain in apex of heart, transient[5] 2d, 4th, 9th and 17th days). Hard ache in heart at 10:30 P. M.[5] (10th day). Sharp, darting pain under right breast[5] (13th and 16th days).

OUTER CHEST—Hard dull aching across the chest, extending to axilla on both sides, < on pressure; moving the hand to opposite shoulder causes pain in muscles of chest[2] (6th day). Transient sense of pressure over the lower sternum[5] (12th day).

NECK AND BACK—During the day, constriction about the neck, clothing disturbed her, choking feeling[1] (8th day). Sore aching feeling below the left scapula, rubbing >[1] (lasting many days). Transient lame stitch in back of neck[2] (4th day). Transient aching feeling in sacrum[3]

(5th day). Throbbing under the scapulæ, dull aching in small of back[2] (13th day). Transient dull aching in back of neck[2] (18th day). Dull aching in small of back[2] (21st day). Throbbing in buttocks[2] 21st day). Soreness in coccyx and gluteal muscles when sitting[2] (21st day). Awoke with throbbing in vulva and in anus, followed by a dull aching in sacral region, relieved by walking about (12th day). Throbbing carotids when lying down[5] (12th day). Awoke at night with pain in region of left kidney, worse lying on left side, better by turning on right side and drawing up limbs[7] (3d day).

UPPER LIMBS—Transient aching in middle of right forearm, on the radius[2] (3d day). Heat in palms in evening[2] (3d day). Hands get chapped easily.[2] Hands vary, one minute hot and dry, then cold, then sweating in palms[5] (3d day). Dull ache in metacarpal bone of thumb[5] (4th day). Dull ache in cushion of right and left thumbs[5] (12th day). Dull ache in left palm[5] (21st day). Itching of left palm[5] (17th day). Cold air makes the hands look red and as though the little red points of blood would ooze out. In the house hands merely look rough[5] (20th day).

LOWER LIMBS—Feet painful in morning[3] (7th day). Sharp itching in 3d toe[3] (old symptom, 5th day). Awoke with dull aching in four lesser toes of right foot, acute pain when stepping or moving foot, gradually subsided after bathing in hot water[2] (19th day). Want to put feet up; unconsciously cross the limbs[5] (throughout proving). Profuse foot-sweat, can almost wring the stockings, not acrid nor offensive[5] (12th day). Corn burns and twinges, cannot bear my usual shoe; < in wet weather[5] (21st and several days following).

LIMBS IN GENERAL—Hands and feet get numb early during proving.[2] Small varicose veins.[5]

NERVES—Extremely restless during night, compelled

to move constantly[1] (Rhus—11th day). Not able to rest in bed, must walk the floor to ease mind and yet has no mental trouble[3] (6th day). Restless after stools[7] (11th day). Hysterical fainting at 7:30 P. M.[3] (an old symptom —11th day). Fainting from nervousness[6] (30th day).

SLEEP AND DREAMS—Unusually sound sleep during entire night[1] (7th day). The night was full of horrible dreams of drunken people, dead people, naked people, robbers, indecent conduct of men and women[1] (7th day). While sleeping in afternoon the breathing ceased and she awoke suffocating[1] (8th day). Sleepless until 3 A. M.[1] (9th day). Wakeful with horrible anxiety and feeling that she must die[1] (many nights). Wakeful until 3 A. M. with anxiety. Sleepless until 1 A. M. (10th day). Sleepless before midnight[1] (11th day). Restless all night, could not lie in one place long enough to go to sleep[1] (12th day). Dreams of wandering in the field with cattle, with fear of being hurt[3] (3d day). Dreams of male animals following her in the field to injure her[3] (6th day). Wakeful until midnight.[3] Dreams of seeing animals copulating (two provers). *Dreams of rape* (confirmed). Late falling to sleep; voluptuous dreams[3] (8th day). Wakeful night with dreams of animals; voluptuous dreams[3] (9th day). Dreams of male and female terrapin. Wakeful, after these dreams of animals[3] (13th day). Dreams of wandering; of naked people; of wild animals pursuing her[3] (14th day). Vivid dreams first night.[2] Vivid, horrible dreams; of dissecting living and dead people; of going up and down ditches; being in peril of engines; woke feeling as though that part of abdomen, the umbilicus, was not sufficiently expanded (constriction)[2] (2d day). Dreams confused[2] (3d day). Sleepy at dark[2] (4th day). Dreams, horrible; of the dead; seeing dead infants[2] (5th day). Very sleepy at 9 A. M., can hardly hold eyes open while people are talking to me[2] (6th and

7th days). Dreams vivid and pleasant[2] (13th day).
Dreams vivid and fantastic[2] (6th day). Dreams vivid[5]
(6th, 7th, 8th days). Dreamed had all the upper incisors
pulled out[7] (8th day). Dreamed all night of snakes, they
were coiled ready to strike, was bitten on left hand by one
and hand swelled and pulse went up to 160 per minute[7]
(9th day). Cold when in bed; not when had my clothes
on[7] (10th day). Coldness of body, especially nates, early
in bed, 8:30[7] (10th day). Sleepy at 11 A. M., took nap.
Biting sensation in left temple on waking[7] (3d day—30th
potency). Sleep all night on left side without moving.
Dreams of plotting to fire the town or any building[7] (4th
day—30th potency). Tongue dry; saliva running upon the
pillow during sleep (unusual). Body always cold in bed
since began the proving[7] (5th day—30th potency).

TIME—Suffocating feeling after lying down in the
evening[1] (7th day). At 3 P. M., most symptoms; chill,
fever, thirst, dry mouth, constriction of neck. Most
symptoms better in the morning. Tired at 10 A. M., wants
to lie down. During breakfast, cutting pain in left hypochondrium. At 11 A. M. sleepy, took a nap.

CHILL, FEVER AND PERSPIRATION—Chill at 3 P. M., icy
cold hands and feet.[1] Flushes of heat to face and head
(1st day). Fever at 3 P. M., lasting until midnight.[1]
Fever, afternoon and evening. At 3 P. M., dry mouth
and lips, mouth feels parched, intense thirst, pulse 105,
choking and sensation as if chest was filling up, causing
constriction and difficult breathing[1] (10th day). Considerable chilliness[3] (10th day). Chilly all morning[3] (12th
day). Very chilly, shiverings pass over body every few
minutes, absent 9 to 10 P. M.[2] (5th day). The body feels
flushed, but the contact of cold things is disagreeable,
causing chills[2] (7th day). Chilly at night[2] (8th day).
Feels flushed all over the body[2] (9th day). Face and

hands feverish in afternoon[2] (12th day). At 10 P. M., cold chills in the back and chest, face and hands still burning[2] (12th day). Felt very cold for about a half hour, could not get warm even when wrapped up warmly[2] (12th day). Went to bed at 11 P. M., still feeling feverish[2] (12th day). Awoke at 5 A. M., still feeling flushed with fever[2] 13th day). At 10 P. M., hands hot and dry, nose cold[2] (14th day). Inclined to be chilly all day and more so at night, must keep wrapped warmly, even when feeling feverish[2] (14th day). Chilly at 11 A. M.[2] (16th day). Chilly, shaking and trembling with cold at night in bed[2] (16th day). Shivering in bed, during evening and night, though (10 P. M.) loaded with blankets[2] (17th day). Sensitive to draft of air.[2] Heat and chilly sensations alternate from 6 to 10 P. M.[5] (8th and 9th days). Chilly, yet face is burning[5] (10th day). Chilly, yet heat gives me a dull headache and makes me feel smothered[5] (12th day). Fever, beginning left side of face and spreading over body about 4 P. M.[6] (2d, 3d, 4th, 16th, 17th days). Chill from 9 to 11 A. M., worse from least motion, even moving finger[6] (2d, 3d, 4th, 16th, 17th days).

SENSATIONS—Sensation of warmth over region of liver[5] (many days). Sense of fluttering and beating, or throbbing in a small spot on the outer side of right thigh, near its middle, commenced at 5 P. M. At 6 and 7 P. M., same sensation under right breast, alternates with that sensation in the thigh. This beating sensation is next felt in left hypochondrium, then in stomach pit, then in right ankle[5] (18th day). Throbbing in left calf[5] (19th day). Throbbing under right breast[5] (21st day). Heat over region of liver extends to heart region[5] (19th day). Cramping sensation[7] (1st day—30th potency). Sensation as though back were going to have a crick, while sitting on feet, < on left side, had to hold back with hands, soon

passed off[7] (3d day—30th potency). Biting sensation, as
of a fly[7] (3d day—30th potency).

TISSUES—*Abscesses.* Hard pain in left iliac bone[5]
(1st day).

TOUCH, MOTION AND MODALITIES—Immediately after
lying down: suffocation; anxiety; palpitation; sinking;
sensation of dying. Horrible anxiety comes over her on
lying down at night, also on lying down in afternoon.
Must lie with head drawn back, she chokes so. Compelled
to move constantly, which seems to quiet for a moment;
compelled to change position from restlessness. Sensitive
to clothing about the body and neck. Symptoms > from
heat, < evening and night. *Restless.* Stomach symptoms
> by belching. Catching sensation in back, < by holding
with hands.

SKIN—Spot on the right calf became red, then copper-
colored; it seemed deep in the skin.[3] Some old scars from
a burn, which became blue and deep red during the proving, have again become white.[2] Itching all over the body;
flying over the body[2] (10th, 13th days).

GENERALITIES—Feeling of general anxiety throughout
the body.[1] Feeling as if the entire body was enlarged to
bursting.[1] All symptoms come on when lying down at
night.[1] Tired at 10 A. M., wants to lie down. Weak, sick
feeling all day[3] (11th day). Has lost much flesh, emaciation spreading from above downward, about the neck and
face, then mammæ, then thighs and legs. Most of symptoms come after 3 P. M.[1] Weary.[2] (4th day). A dog
was bitten and an abscess forms upon his neck, which has
reopened three times; when it is about to open, he scratches
it violently until it opens and discharges a yellow watery
fluid. Tight clothing unbearable[2] (throughout the proving). Throbbing in entire body[2] (21st day). So tired,
the weight of my clothing is burdensome[5] (4th, 5th, 6th

days). Bloated feeling, lasting all day[7] (13th day). Lost from 10 to 20 lbs. during proving.[7]

RELATIONSHIP—Chamomilla antidoted its uterine hæmorrhage. Cenchris antidotes Pulsatilla. Amm. c. > general symptoms.

CULEX MUSCA

When this remedy is needed your patient will present to you a picture of something on fire; he burns like something he would like to mention, and perhaps does mention the place; the itching and burning are present every where in this remedy; he rubs and scratches wherever the eruption appears.

The mental symptoms are just what you would expect would follow the physical symptoms of Culex; impatience, a willingness to quarrel, anxiety and fear of death; poor memory and a disinclination for all work; he is so busy scratching to relieve the itching and so busy walking to relieve the restlessness, that any interruption makes him impatient and ready to quarrel.

The dull frontal headache begins on waking at five a. m. and passes away after lying awake for a while; during the forenoon there is pain, fullness and pressure in the forehead with heat of the face, getting worse by spells until afternoon when it extends to the outer part of the right orbital ridge and extending through to the occiput is accompanied by nausea which lasts until evening. Some of the head pains go from the cerebellum to the forehead or right temple; the boring pains in the temples come on several times a day; the pain comes and goes across the forehead just above the eyes; a rending pain back of the eyeballs. The headache is made worst by the least motion followed by intense vertigo which comes on in the afternoon and is located in a spot over the right eye. Itching and stinging of the scalp.

In the right eye there is a feeling of fullness extending to the parotid gland, from there to the sub lingual and finally involves the right side of the face and head. The margins of the lids are sore and crusted over; the inflammation of the lids is worse in the morning with a discharge of sticky fluid; the eyeballs are inflamed and there is stye-like ulceration. Rending pains in the eyeballs; he could not keep his eyes open yet it pained to keep them shut; the eyes feel tired.

The ears come in for their share of trouble with swelling of the parotid glands and soreness on pressure; pain as if he were going to have mumps; sharp pains in both ears followed by watery discharge of the same sticky character that is present in the saliva.

From the nose there is a watery discharge with bloody scabs on the inside; small scabs come from the nose which may be dry or moist and bloody; usually mixed with a copious discharge which may be greenish or light colored and the head feels stuffed; the itching, stinging and tickling are always present; he rubs and scratches because his nose itches inside and outside and the more he rubs it the more it burns so he stops for a while until he is driven to rub and scratch again only to be compelled to stop while there is a little skin left on his nose. On top of his nose is a shining redness like a rum blossom; the nose is swollen and the eruption on it contains a clear colorless fluid; as the swelling goes down it is followed by itching and to rub it only increases the desire for more rubbing.

There is pain in the posterior nares with green scabs with bleeding after removal of the scabs. Epistaxis morning and night on blowing the nose. The redness is like erysipelas; shining, red, and sore to touch; it is more marked on the right side in the beginning and then extends to both sides of the nose and to the face. An ineffectual desire to sneeze.

Pain over the right malar bone going to the left the next day and here you will see one of the characteristic red spots the size of a twenty-five cent piece feeling as if red pepper had been rubbed in; from the malar bone will be shooting pains to the temple and forehead in the evening, made worse by setting the jaws together. The sub maxillary gland is swollen and tender on pressure. The eruption on the face and between the eyes contains a colorless fluid; there will also be swelling and puffiness under the eyes; in keeping with this remedy we find the heat and redness of the whole right side of the face with a sore bruised feeling.

Constant wetting of the lips; a symptom common to many remedies perhaps from nervousness but in this patient it ameliorated the dryness and the ever present burning; the saliva is of such a character that it leaves the lips sticky; this bad tasting whitish saliva leaves a bad taste in the mouth in the morning on waking; a sickish taste as if he had been drinking warm mineral water. The tongue is coated white and is dry, swollen, thick on waking; there is also numbness of the tongue. Periodical attacks of salivation for months; at night the pillow is wet and in the daytime the saliva accumulates and causes continued swallowing. If you prescribe a remedy on one symptom this patient would probably be given Merc. The entire edge of the tongue is covered with a double row of small painful vesicles. This remedy cured a case of numbness of the tongue with ulceration at the tip following scarlet fever.

On rising in the morning in addition to the other troubles, he must spend much time hawking up from the pharynx dark green scabs and strings of tough mucus tinged with dark blood and coughing from the trachea green scabs corresponding to the green discharge from the nose.

There is burning and dryness of the throat with soreness in throat and in the posterior nares on swallowing solids or fluids. The right side of the throat is always sore.

The appetite is increased but the food does not digest; it sours in the stomach; his appetite is quite likely to be ravenous and he must have his dinner on the minute or he feels faint; he is especially hungry and faint in the morning and cannot wait for the breakfast to be prepared; with this sour condition of the stomach you would expect nausea and it is often present day and night; sometimes even the thought of food will bring on nausea with gagging and retching and inability to vomit; with the disordered stomach are sickening pains and eructation of much offensive gas.

Thirst for cold water which causes burning in the stomach with urging to stool, followed by loose and dark brown offensive stool, much tenesmus lasting several days and gradually subsiding into painless diarrhoea.

On the abdomen are blotches the size of a twenty-five cent piece, itching, burning, with little pimples on the blotches; this is the form of the eruption wherever it is present.

A dull pain in the right side in the region of the kidney extending up the back to the occiput.

Cramps in the abdomen during stool with rumbling and the passing of much offensive flatus; these colicky pains come on about ten a.m. and last from one to three hours. The usual desire for morning stool is absent; the stool is scanty, lumpy, and expelled with effort; the first part of the stool is hard and scratches the anus; it is followed by a soft stool; after stool he has the sensation that he has not finished so he sits and strains until blood comes. (Merc.)

Itching and burning of the anus; it is scalding hot and raw as from a bite; burning of the glans penis and there is a strong smelling discharge from the glans; the itching of the scrotum comes from spots like bee stings; these spots are of the usual circumscribed character that swell and burn and itch; rubbing only aggravates the itching, stinging, burning.

The Majora has the same itching, burning that runs all through the remedy. The itching of the vulva is so intense that she feels as if she could tear it to pieces; this symptom returned at intervals for years and was cured by Culex.

Menses come too soon with a profuse dark clotted flow; violent pains in the uterus compelling her to go to bed.

Hoarseness so that he could scarcely speak a word; usually there is great hoarseness in the morning.

Deep sighing breathing with constant desire for a deep breath; the breath is foul and it seemed as if he could smell it himself.

A distressing cough caused by burning in the chest; a whistling strangling choking cough with red face and water running from the eyes or it may be a dry hacking cough, present day and night; the cough is mostly in the morning with the feeling as if he would vomit; with the cough there is pain low down in the back; there is coughed up a small amount of yellowish white expectoration; sometimes there is one constant racking cough lasting fifteen minutes ending in a long loud inspiration with blue face and protruding eyes followed by great languor and sweat. There is constant desire to sneeze and cough alternately with a discharge of quantities of mucus from the throat which does not relieve the inclination to cough.

In the apex of the right lung there is soreness which is aggravated by deep breathing or raising the right arm, and occasional dull pain in the lower part of the right lung; a painful condition when you consider the desire for deep breathing which is present with oppression and anxiety in the chest; other symptoms give him much trouble; a sensation of fullness in the right lung, soreness on stooping, leaning forward, raising the right shoulder, and with it all there is the sensation of a rubber band around the right lung; not all the pains are dull, there are sudden cutting pains running up and down lasting a minute; there is rawness, a bruised feeling in the right chest; drawing, clawing pains in the right lung going to the left lung and staying there; these pains lasting several hours each day; with these conditions you would expect soreness on stooping, leaning forward, or raising the right shoulder.

Culex Musca has very few heart symptoms which is fortunate considering the many lung symptoms; there are occasional cutting pains that are neither severe nor long lasting; there are pains in the right pectoral muscles and the right side of the neck is swollen.

The hands and fingers are hot and burning, as if frozen, with severe pain; the burning of the palms and on the thumb is as if the hand had been rubbed against nettles; itching, burning, as if he must tear the flesh for relief while the back of the hands felt cold and benumbed.

Rose red, colored, burning eruption on the arm aggravated by heat; the arms and hands are numb and prickling; there is the everlasting itching that is present all through this remedy; the eruption with its colorful fluid, burning after scratching and with it the desire to tear the skin off. There is coldness of the right hand while the left hand is warm.

The lower limbs feel heavy with an uneasy restlessness that is made better by the open air; his feet are tired all day long yet he must drag himself into the open air for relief; he wishes that he knew some place where he could put his poor, tired, heavy limbs that would give him rest. On the thigh there is the blotch the size of a twenty-five cent piece, with little pimples on it, that itches and burns like a flea bite. There is aching of the legs from the knee down; there is no position that will make the pain less so he must get up out of his chair and take a walk in the open air; there is little comfort to his feet while walking as the soles are tender and there is intense itching on the tops of the feet.

Of course his sleep is restless with much tossing about in sleep; the heat of the bed causes him to waken frequently; he must rise early in the morning to move around for relief; he is unrefreshed by sleep which has been restless, and full of dreams of quarrels, fights, and of the dead.

There are hot flushes as if a chill would follow, followed by warm perspiration which is strong smelling and sticky; this stickiness is also noticed in the saliva.

His skin torments him almost beyond endurance, itching, burning, heat, all combine to make him miserable; the skin feels better while scratching but worse after scratching; there is no comfort at home or abroad, in bed or out of it and a place of amusement is not to be thought of; he scratches which makes more trouble yet he must scratch to relieve that terrible, constant itching; you may truthfully say that this remedy has many outward manifestations.

This may be summed up as a right sided remedy with the strange feeling of having been poisoned; there are sharp stinging pains all over the body like needles; lightning like; darting here and there, aggravated by light pressure and ameliorated by hard pressure.

Head, nose, and limb symptoms seem to grow worse until seven p. m. and are ameliorated about eight p. m.; in an hour or two they are gone; the symptoms seem most severe from six to seven p. m.

All symptoms, pain, itching, burning, are worse in a warm room and better in the open air, although he is so tired and weak that he can scarcely move, cannot walk straight, with soreness and aching all over the body, yet he is so nervous that he finds it impossible to keep still; there is almost constant motion of the hands and feet.

FERRUM ARSENICUM

Complaints in general are aggravated in the morning, on waking; afternoon; evening; night, before midnight, after midnight. Aversion to the open air; aggravation in the open air. General physical anxiety. Chlorosis. Anæmia. Chorea in anæmic subjects. In a general way cold air aggravates, and the patient is very sensitive to cold; aggravation from becoming cold, in a cold room. Takes cold easily. In low vitality from malaria, and inherited phthisis. Epileptiform convulsions; tonic spasms. Blood vessels distended. Internal and external dropsy. Many complaints come on, or are worse after eating. Emaciation. She faints easily. Must select the most digestible foods. Butter disorders his whole system. Cold drinks aggravate, fat food aggravates, sour things aggravate, vinegar aggravates. Sensation of fullness. Subject to hemorrhages. Inflamed parts indurate. Inflammation of glands and organs. Increased physical irritability. Sensitive to jar. Jerking in muscles. Languid and must lie down. After hemorrhage or loss of fluids. Lying aggravates many symptoms. The longer he lies the more restless he becomes; must get up and walk about. Motion aggravates inflamed parts, but ameliorates the patient. Desires to move. Catarrhal conditions. Numbness of hands and feet, and painful parts. Surging of blood in the body and head. Aching in the bones. Drawing, pressing paralytic pains. Sore; bruised; stitching; tearing pains. Periodical complaints. Perspiration gives no relief of symptoms. Plethoric subjects. General pulsation, pulsation in parts, and pulsating pains. This is a deep acting antipsoric. Most complaints grow worse during rest. It is useful in malaria cases when much quinine has been taken. Relaxation of the whole muscular system, with a sensation of heaviness or weight in the whole body. Physical exertion or running aggravates, but moderate motion ameliorates. Sensitive to pain. Sitting still aggravates. On first sitting down, amelioration. Some complaints come on during sleep, or on waking. Standing still long aggravates. Much swelling of affected parts. Dropsical swelling. Swelling of glands. Trembling. Varicose veins. Walking long causes. weakness. Walking slowly about ameliorates. Walking in the cold air aggravates. Walking fast aggravates. Great general weakness; evening; from malarial influences, or loss of fluids; paralytic weakness, from exertion or walking. Complaints worse in cold weather or winter. Complaints aggravated in cold wind.

Irascible from contradiction. Anxiety at night. Anxiety as if guilty of a crime, with fear, during fever. Mirthful. Concentration difficult. Confusion of mind in the morning on waking; in the evening. Conscientious about trifles. Thinks of death. Discontented. Distraction. Excitable. Fear of a crowd, of death, of some mischief, of people. Forgetful. Hysterical. Indifference. Irresolution. Irritability. Laughing and mirthfulness. Alternating moods, and change of mental symptoms. Obstinate. Quarrelsome. Religious affections of the mind; remorse. RESTLESSNESS at night, driving out of bed. Tossing about the bed, during heat. Extreme sadness, in the evening, when alone. Oversensitive to noise. Serious mood. Stupefaction of mind. Indisposed to talk. It disturbs him to hear people talk. He is sensitive to their voices. Tranquility. Unconscious. Weeping.

Vertigo; tendency to fall, during headache, looking downward, with nausea, on rising up. When walking he staggers, with obscuration of vision.

Sensation of coldness of scalp. Hyperæmia of the brain. Tension of the scalp. Sensation of emptiness in the head. Fullness in the head. The hair falls out. Heat in the head, with cold feet. Flushes of heat in the head. Heaviness of the head, of the forehead. Itching of the scalp. Violent headache; morning, afternoon, evening; aggravated in cold air, ameliorated in open air. Catarrhal headaches. Pain in head during chill. Cold applications ameliorate. Headaches with coryza. Pain when coughing; after eating. HAMMERING HEADACHES. Headache before and during menses; motion of head. Paroxysmal pains. Periodical headaches. Pulsating pains. Riding in

8

a carriage aggravates. Shaking the head aggravates. Sitting aggravates.

Pain in the forehead; worse right side; evening; above the eyes; occiput. Sides of head; right; temples; right side. Temple and forehead. Vertex. Boring in temples. Bursting, Drawing. Pressing outward. Pressing in forehead; temples. Vertex. Soreness. Stitching in temples. Tearing pains. Pulsating in head; forehead, occiput, temples, vertex. Shocks in the brain.

Lids stick together at night. Discharge of mucus from the eyes. Eyes lusterless. Inflammation of the eyes; scrofulous. Bood vessels injected. Lachrymation. Difficult to open lids. Pain in the eyes; aching, burning; as if sand. Paralysis of optic nerve. Protrusion of eyes. Redness of eyes; of lids. Looks sunken about the eyes. Eyes swollen; lids swollen. Sclerotics yellow. Dim vision.

Discharge from ear, offensive. Itching. Noises in ears; humming, ringing, roaring, singing. Pain in ear. Stitching. Hearing impaired.

Chronic catarrh. Coryza. Discharge bloody; crusts; excoriating; greenish; purulent; watery. Nosebleed. Sneezing.

Dark circles around eyes. Pale, sickly, earthly, waxy face. Greenish. Sickly, suffering expression. Lips pale. Red face during chill. Sallow; jaundiced. Dryness of lips. Heat of face. Flushes of heat. Hippocratic countenance. Pain in face. Perspiration of face. Swelling of face.

Bleeding mouth and gums. White tongue. Dryness. Numbness of tongue. Burning tongue. Increased saliva. Gangrenous sore mouth. Swollen gums. Taste bitter, insipid, putrid, sweetish.

Constriction and choking in throat. Throat feels hot. Lump in throat. Pain in throat on swallowing. Burning, rawness, soreness. Swallowing difficult.

Anxiety in stomach. Appetite increased, or ravenous; yet he does not relish his food. Appetite wanting. Aversion to food; to meat. Constriction. Craves bread, sour things. Distended stomach. Eructations after eating; abortive, bitter, empty; of food; foul; sour. Waterbrash. fullness. Heartburn. Heat. Nausea, before eating, after eating, during pregnancy. Pain, after cold drinks, after eating. Burning; cramping; pressing after eating. Soreness. Pulsating. Thirst extreme. Also thirstless in chronic troubles.

Vomiting, morning, night, after drinking, coughing, after eating; with headache; during fever; during pregnancy. Blood, FOOD sour.

Constriction of abdominal muscles. Distension of abdomen from flatus. Ascites. Flatulence. Fullness. Gurgling. Hardness of abdomen. Sensation of heat in abdomen. Weight in abdomen. Inflammation of bowels. Itching of skin of abdomen. Congestive, sluggish and swollen liver. Pain in abdomen at night, on coughing, after eating, during menses. Paroxysmal pains. Warmth ameliorates. Pain in hypochondria, in hypogastrium, in the liver, sides of abdomen. Cramping before stool, from flatus. Soreness; hypogastrium. Liver. Nervous uneasiness in abdomen. Rumbling. Spleen enlarged. Swollen liver and spleen. Tension of abdomen.

Constipation. Constriction. DIARRHŒA; morning afternoon, NIGHT, AFTER MIDNIGHT; colliquitive; during dentition AFTER DRINKING, after cold water. after eating; aggravated by motion. Painless. Flatus. Hemorrhage from anus. Hemorrhoids, external. large. Involuntary stool. itching of anus. Moisture at the anus Pain during stool. urning during and after stool. Stitching. Tenesmus during stool. Paralysis of rectum Prolapsus during stool. rging to stool; ineffectual; after stool. Stool excoriating, oody, brown, frequent, hard, UNDIGESTED, mucus, watery, own watery.

Pain in the bladder. Tenesmus. Constant urging. Involuntary urination at night

Pain in the kidneys.

Burning in urethra during urination.

Urine albuminous, bloody, burning; cloudy on standing; dark, red, copious, scanty; mucous sediment.

Seminal emissions.

Inflammation of female genitals, Uterus. Itching genitals. Leucorrhea, EXCORIATING, thin, white. Amenorrhea. Menses bright red, copious, dark, too soon, painful, pale, protracted, scanty, suppressed. Uterine hemorrhage. Pain in uterus. Burning in labia. Prolapsus uteri

Catarrh of larynx and trachea. Mucus in larynx and trachea. Burning in air passages. Roughness in air passages. Hoarseness. Voice lost. Respiration arrested on coughing; asthmatic; difficult, evening, night, during cough, lying; rattling; short; suffocative. Subject to asthma after midnight.

Cough morning on rising, evening in bed, lying down, at night, before midnight; cold air, open air, walking in open air; asthmatic; deep breathing aggravates; after drinking. Dry cough in the evening. Cough after eating. Exhausting cough. Cough during fever; from irritation in trachea. Loose cough; lying aggravates; cough in bed, motion aggravates; on rising; must sit up. Spasmodic cough. Talking aggravates the cough. Tickling cough. Tickling in larynx and trachea. Whooping cough.

Expectoration in daytime, morning, night; bloody, blood streaked, copious, difficult; greenish mucus; offensive, purulent; nausiosis; putrid, sweetish, thick, viscid, whitish, yellow.

Anxiety of chest in heart symptoms. Catarrh of chest. Constriction of chest; constriction of heart. Fullness of chest. HEMORRHAGE OF LUNGS. Heat in chest. Inflammation of lungs. Cardiac and anæmic murmurs. OPPRESSION OF CHEST in the evening. Pain in the chest, during cough; in sides of chest; sternum. Soreness in chest on coughing. Stitching on coughing. Palpitation at night with anxiety. Spasms of chest.

Coldness of back. Pain in the back at night, during menses, during stool. Pain in cervical region, between shoulders, in lumbar region. Aching in back. Bruised pain in lumbar region. Tearing in back. Pulsating in back. Stiff neck.

Cold extremities, hands and feet. Contraction of fingers and toes. Cramps in hands, thighs, calves, feet, soles. Blueness of finger nails. Heaviness of limbs, feet. Numbness of hands and fingers; legs, feet. Pain in limbs; rheumatic; joints. Gouty pains. Pain in upper limbs, rheumatic, shoulders, elbow, wrist, hands. Pain in lower limbs. Sciatica, worse at night. Pain in thighs; paralytic; knee, ankle, foot, heel. Aching in limbs. Drawing in upper limbs; thighs. Sore pain in limbs, upper limbs. Stitching in limbs; shoulders; hip, thigh. Tearing in shoulders, upper arms; thighs. Paralytic weakness of limbs. Restlessness of all the limbs, especially of the legs. Stiffness of joints of upper limbs, hands and fingers; of lower limbs, knees and feet. Swelling of upper limbs, hands; of knees, ankles and feet. Varicose veins of lower limbs. Weakness of limbs, joints; knees, legs, ankles.

Dreams anxious. Sleep restless. Sleepiness afternoon and evening. Sleeplessness before midnight. Sleepless with sleepiness. Waking early.

This remedy has chill, fever and sweat. Chill in morning, noon, evening, NIGHT. Chill even in bed. Quotidian; tertian. Chill with trembling. The fever is intense, and follows chill; aggravated in afternoon, evening, and highest at night. Fever after midnight. Fever without chill in afternoon, evening, night. Fever intermingled with chill. Dry Heat. Heat in flushes. The flushes rush upwards. Chronic intermittent fevers with enlarged spleen and liver. Internal heat and external coldness. Heat comes on after sleep. Perspiration day and night. Perspiration morning, night; during anxiety; in bed; CLAMMY, cold, on coughing, with great exhaustion, after eating, during slight exertion; long lasting; while lying; on motion; PROFUSE, morning. Perspiration during sleep, after sleep; offensive, sour, staining linen yellow; during stool. Symptoms aggravated while perspiring.

Burning of the skin. Coldness of the skin. Liver spots. Pale skin. Red spots. Yellow. Dryness of the skin. Sensitive skin. Sore feeling in skin. Swollen skin. Oedema. Ulcers, burning. Withered warts.

FERRUM IODATUM

Morning, afternoon, *evening*, NIGHT, after midnight. The patient feels better in the open air. Anæmia in a marked degree. General physical anxiety; *chlorosis*; choreic twitching of the muscles; constantly taking cold; congestion of organs and glands; external and internal dropsy. Symptoms are worse after eating. Emaciation. Markedly worse from exertion. Fainting in anæmic patients. Hemorrhage from many parts. Induration of glands. Lack of physical irritability. Lying down and lying in bed increases many symptoms. Sensation as of lying in a cramped position. Worse before, during and after menses. Motion increases many symptoms; desire to move. Catarrhal condition of all mucous membrances. Orgasm of blood even when quiet; pulsation in body and limbs; on waking from sleep; fast pulse. Many symptoms are worse from touch. The glands are swollen. Walking aggravates many symptoms. Worse from warmth and warm clothing. Weakness from slight exertion; during menses; from walking.

Very irritable and easily angered. Anxiety and aversion to company. Dullness of mind and concentration difficult, worse when reading; confusion of mind in the evening; over-conscientious about small matters; very excitable;

hysterical conduct and hilarity; changeable mood; indifference; irresolution; *sadness*. Restless at night; starting from sleep Stupefaction. Weeping. Vertigo while walking.

Heat and hyperæmia of the head; heaviness of the head; worse in a warm room; better in the open air; in the forehead. Itching of the scalp. Pain in the head in the morning; in the afternoon; better in the open air and worse in the house; worse coughing; with coryza; worse from the pressure of the hat; compelled to lie down; better lying; before menses; worse moving the head; better from pressure of the hand; *pulsating*; worse when reading; worse from smoking; worse from walking; worse from writing; worse in a warm room. Pain in the forehead; worse on the right side, in the evening; better in the open air; better when standing in a draft; worse from coughing, from pressure of the hat, when reading, when writing, from motion, in a warm room, from smoking, above the eyes; above the left eye extending to the top of head. Pain in the occiput; in the sides of head; worse on left side, in temples, in vertex. Cutting pain from bridge of the nose to the occiput. Pressing pain in forehead; worse in right side; worse in a warm room; in temples; in vertex. Sharp pain from below the eyes up through to vertex. Stitching pain in head; in temples. Tearing pain in head. Pulsation in head; forehead; temples.

Inflammation of the conjunctiva, with copious pus when forcibly opened; conjunctiva bluish-red; itching of eyes; lachrymation. Pain in eyes from light; aching, burning of lids; cutting, as from sand; stitching. Photophobia. Protrusion of eyes; exophthalmic goitre. Redness of eyes; bluish-red, of lids; *swollen lids*. Weak eyes. The eyes are jaundiced. A cloud of sparks before the eyes after breakfast.

Noises in the ears; humming, ringing, *roaring*. Cutting pain in ears. Hearing impaired.

Catarrh of the nose; morning; post-nasal discharge bloody, copious; *crusts*; EXCORIATING, *greenish, purulent, thick, watery,* yellow. Fluent coryza, worse in the morning, with copious mucus from larynx. Sensation of dryness in nose. Epistaxis on blowing nose; from coughing. Obstruction of nose; morning, night; better after blowing; cutting pain in root of nose extending to occiput. Sneezing at night. The nose is swollen; ulceration in nose.

The face is *pale, earthy,* even *chlorotic*; RED; circumscribed redness; sallow; sickly; YELLOW. Eczema and vesicles on the face; expression sickly. Countenance Hippocratic; swollen, puffed, bloated face; swollen submaxillary glands.

Bleeding gums. Coated thick, yellow tongue. Dryness in the mouth and throat; burning tongue; salivation; taste bad in the morning; bitter, insipid, metallic, offensive, putrid, like peppermint, sour, sweetish. Pain in the teeth.

Scraping of mucus from throat and nose; viscid mucus. Food seems to push up to throat as though it had not been swallowed; reversed action of æsophagus. Burning and pressing in the throat. Tickling and scraping throat and larynx. Swollen cervical glands. Exophthalmic goitre.

The appetite is variable; diminished, *increased, insatiable,* ravenous, wanting. without relish of food, easy satiety. Atonic condition of the stomach; aversion to food; to meat. Distension of stomach from gas. Eructations; bitter, after eating; empty, greasy, of food, rancid, sour, violent, waterbrash. Feels as though he had eaten too much, even after small meal. Flushes of heat in the stomach. Heartburn. Heaviness after eating. Loathing of food. Nausea after eating. Pain in stomach: after eating; burning; cramping, after eating; distress with nausea and headache; pressing after eating; soreness in pit of stomach with pinching in back behind stomach. *Pulsating* in stomach. Tension. Thirst in evening; strong thirst;

extreme thirst. *Vomiting*; on coughing; after drinking; after eating; of blood; of food. A feeling as of a cord drawn, connecting anus and navel, with a cutting pain every time he straightens up from a bent position. Distension of abdomen after food or drink· Enlarged liver and spleen without fever. Flatulence. Fullness or "stuffed" feeling. Heat in abdomen. Pain in abdomen; after eating; during menses; in hypochondria; in inguinal region extending across hypogastrium; in liver; spleen; in umbilicus; cramping before stool; pricking in side of abdomen, worse raising arms and worse walking. Stitching in hypochondria and in inguinal region when walking; soreness in inguinal region when walking. Rumbling in abdomen before stool. Abdomen feels like a rubber ball when pressed; swollen abdomen.

Constipation; no stool for a week, alternating with diarrhœa; difficult stool, ineffectual straining. Constriction of anus. DIARRHOEA; stool frequent; morning; after eating; bloody stool; mucus; watery. Flatus; external piles; itching of anus; sensation as though anus were compressed; as of worms in rectum; as though a screw were boring in anus; crawling in anus; pain in anus; burning after stool. Stitching during hard stool; tenesmus; urging after stool; stool bloody; brown, *hard* mucus, scanty, soft, watery.

Urination frequent, involuntary, with tenesmus. Pain in both kidneys but worse in left. Gonorrhœal discharge from urethra; with itching crawling. Burning on urination· Sensation as if drops of urine remained in fassa navicularis and could not be forced out. Urine albuminous and of low specific gravity. It has cured where sugar was found in the urine. Urine: dark, red, copious and pale, scanty, white. *Urine smells sweetish.*

Erections troublesome and painful at night; wanting. Relaxed scrotum. Seminal emissions. Sexual desire increased. In the female it has been used to prevent abortion.

Itching and soreness of the swollen vulva. It has cured dropsy of the ovaries. *Leucorrhoea*: acrid, hot, copious, *like starch*; before and after menses; thin and watery; menses absent, copious, too frequent or late, painful, SUPPRESSED. Metrorrhagia. *Bearing down feeling in the pelvis; while sitting she feels something pushing up.* It is a most useful remedy in prolapsus and displacements of all kinds.

Irritation and much mucus in the larynx and trachea. Pain in the larynx; burning. Tickling in the air passage. Hoarseness and aphonia.

Respiration asthmatic; difficult at night and on motion; rattling, short, suffocative, wheezing.

Cough in the morning, afternoon, evening, asthmatic, *dry*, during fever, from irritation in larynx and trachea, loose, from motion, short, spasmodic, from talking, from tickling in the air passages. Expectoration in the morning; bloody, *copious*, difficult, greenish, hawked, bloody mucus, offensive, purulent, tasting putrid, *viscid*, whitish, grayish-white, yellow.

Anxiety in chest and heart. Cancer of right breast was greatly benefited. Catarrh of chest. Congestion of chest and *heart*. Hemorrhage of lungs and air passages. Inflammation of bronchial tubes; of lungs. Cardiac murmurs. Oppression of chest. Pain in chest during cough; in sides of chest; in right side, from heart to axilla; stitching on coughing. *Palpitation* at NIGHT; *from least exertion; on motion*; on rising up; on turning in bed; during sleep.

Pain in the back during menses; in dorsal region; in lumbar region during menses; in sacrum; aching, as if broken, in lumbar region, at night; dull pain in dorsal region, each side of spine; extending through chest; stitching pain in back. Stiffness in back on rising from bed.

Cold hands and feet at night; cramps in feet. Heat of

hands; heaviness of limbs; lower limbs; of feet. Numbness of fingers, legs, feet. Pain in the limbs; in the joints; gouty, rheumatic; rheumatic in upper limbs; rheumatic in right upper arm; in elbow, in *hip*, in thigh, in right tibia; rheumatic pain extending upward from back of left foot, in evening. Aching in the shoulder. Drawing pain in lower limbs; in the thighs; in tendons of back of right hand and left foot. Sore-bruised lower limbs, thighs, legs, stitching upper limbs and shoulder; tearing upper limbs and hips. Paralysis of upper limbs; sensation of paralysis of shoulder; in right arm in evening when writing. Restless feet. Dropsical swelling in lower limbs; legs and feet. Weakness of limbs, of lower limbs. Trembling and weakness in limbs on using hands and on walking.

Dreams anxious; confused; of dead people; of fighting; of previous events; fantastic; of robbers; nightmare; unpleasant; *vivid*. Dreams that he is from thirty to sixty feet tall. Restless sleep. Sleepiness morning and evening. Sleeplessness; frequent waking.

Chill at *night*; coldness in and better rising from bed; chilliness in evening followed by heat and sweat; shaking chill; warm room does not ameliorate the chill. Fever in the afternoon and evening with chilliness. Dry heat. Flushes of heat; internal heat, with chill. Intermittent fever with desire to uncover.

Perspiration in the morning; in afternoon; at *night*; in bed; *clammy, cold, copious*, on least EXERTION, worse on motion.

The skin burns or is cold; jaundiced; liver spots. Dry skin. Urticaria. Swollen skin.

HAMAMELIS VIRGINICA

The striking features of this remedy are venous congestion and hemorrhages. Veins are distended in all parts, or only in single parts. Varicose veins of many parts, marked soreness in the varices. Bloody discharges from all mucous membranes. Purpura hemorrhagica has often been cured with this remedy. Dusky purplish appearance of the skin, with full veins. Inflammation of veins of any part, especially lower limbs and anus. Varicose veins about ulcers that bleed, a dark blood. Ulcers are dark, even black, and discharge black blood. Dark blood flows from any part. Bright red fluid blood is the exception, but has been recorded. Especially suitable in very nervous, sensitive, excitable patients. Sore, bruised feeling as in Arnica, all through the body, not only in single parts, Veins are especially sensitive to pressure. Extremely sensitive to a jar as in Belladonna, but: only in the muscles and veins that are inflamed and swollen. Much weakness with or without bleeding: out of proportion to the loss of blood. Vicarious hemorrhages are a strong indication. The patient is tired, mentally and physically; aversion to mental work; he forgets the word when talking; Irritable, depressed and stupid, with recurrent hemorrhages. Pulsating pain over the left eye. Feeling of a bolt from temple to temple. Bursting headache in the morning when waking, worse when stooping. Headaches are connected with venous congestion in other parts. The strange part of these cases and conditions is that the patient is often sensitive to cold and to cold air. Ecchymosis with extreme tenderness of head, eyes or face. Headache from straining eyes. Ecchymosis of eyeballs. Sore pain in the eyes. Congested veins of eyes with oozing blood. Inflammation and ulceration of eyeballs. Epistaxis of dark blood recurring frequently. With the menses, also when the menses fail. Epistaxis sometimes copious and clotted and very dark. Gums bleed easily and are very vascular. Throat is dark red, chronically congested and covered with varicose veins. Tonsils are covered with varices. Suffers much from soreness in the throat with oozing of dark blood. No thirst and aversion to drink. Nausea, vomiting blood, tenderness in the stomach. Pulsáting in the stomach. Vomiting black clots. Over the abdomen are found varicose veins that are tender to touch. Burning in stomach and abdomen. Dysentery when the stool is much blood rather than the scanty, bloody, mucous stool that belongs to dysentery. Copious dark blood from piles. Constipation a usual condition. Ulceration of intestine, rectum, and anus; with copious dark blood. Portal congestion and hemorrhoids, with much bleeding. Hemorrhoids that protrude, pulsate, and bleed much; also after confinement. The anus contracts spasmodically with intense burning pain. Itching of the anus. Urine; much blood every day, for weeks, was cured at once. Much urging to urinate. Much sexual excitement (male). With dreams and emissions; pain down spermatic cord to testes. Varices in spermatic cord. Tenderness in ovaries and uterus. Uterine hemorrhage with copious dark clots; sometimes with bright red blood. Active or passive uterine hemorrhage. Paroxysmal pain in left ovary. Vicarious menstruation from nose, stomach or lungs. Subinvolution with much uterine tenderness, and occasional bleeding. Menstrual flow copious, dark, clotted. Acute vaginitis with contraction and bleeding. Tenderness of vagina during coition. Spasms of the vagina. Recurrent hemorrhages in pregnant women. Hemorrhage occurring during parturition. Varicose veins during pregnancy. Has been useful in milk leg. Most useful in the cough accompanied by expectoration of much dark blood. Cough from varicose condition of throat. Scraping blood from larynx and trachea by the mouthful. Hæmoptysis in phthisis, especially recurrent. Tenderness of spine, cervical region. Breaking and tearing pain in lumbar region of spine. Bruised pain in all the limbs. Aching bruised feeling in thighs. Soreness in veins of thighs and legs. Varicose veins of legs; with or without ulcers; worse during pregnancy; can neither walk nor stand, limbs so painful during pregnancy. Pricking, stinging in the congested veins.

KALI ARSENICOSUM

This is a very deep, long acting remedy, and one greatly abused by traditional medicine in the form of Fowler's Solution. It was used extensively as an antiperiodic after quinine had failed, and as a tonic, for skin diseases of all sorts, for syphilis, for anaemia, etc. It is a most positive remedy in all of these complaints, when it suits the patient's symptoms. The toxicological symptoms following the traditional abuse have furnished a broad beginning for the homeopathist to build upon. How well it was known to the good old doctor that Fowler's Solution must be stopped if the patient became pale, waxy, puffed under the eyes and was weak. Who does not know the "fattening" powers of this drug! Horses become fat and shiny of coat after taking Fowler's Solution for a while. The jockey knew this too well. He traded off a broken-down horse as a fine animal, but the horse soon gave out; his wind was short; he would sweat easily, become weak and incapable of work. It was then said: "That horse must have been jockeyed up on arsenic." The old medical journals are full of effects of overdosing with this drug. A summary of old school drugging, a few pathogenetic symptoms, and extensive clinical observation with the use of this remedy in potentized form, have given the basis of this study. Not too much reliance should be placed upon the writer's clinical opinion; let the remedy be tested along the lines indicated until provings shall fix the finer action.

While it has morning and evening aggravation, the nights are full of suffering; midnight especially, and from 1 to 3 a. m., there are many sufferings. The chilliness is very marked. Extreme sensitiveness to cold, and complaints are aggravated from cold, from cold air and from becom-

ing cold, from entering a cold place. Aversion to open air.
Takes cold from a draft, and from being heated. Anaemia.
Chlorosis. Pale, waxy, and covered with sweat. Ascending brings on suffocation, cough, and manifests the weakness of body and limbs. Glands dwindle and the extremities become numb and prickly. Molecular death prevails
extensively. Cancerous ulceration has been restrained by
this remedy many times. It has cured lupus.

The weakness that it has produced is much like that
found in patients looking toward phthisis and Bright's
disease. Clonic spasms have been produced by it. Convulsive action of muscles with full consciousness is not
uncommon. It has cured epilepsy and hysterio-epilepsy.
It has caused abdominal dropsy and œdema of all the limbs,
face and eyelids. While taking it there is an increase of
flesh and weight, but after stopping it the prover emaciates. Most complaints are aggravated after eating and
after exertion. The muscles are flabby. Faintness and
fainting spells. Eating ice cream when overheated brings on
many complaints. Aggravated from cold foods, cold drinks,
milk and fat food. There is formication all over the body.
It sets up inflammation in many organs and glands, especially the stomach, liver and kidneys. Great dread of motion. All mucous membranes become catarrhal. It is a
most painful remedy; burning, stitching and tearing. The
most marked periodicity is every third day Pulsation
felt all over the body. It is a deep acting antipsoric, and
often useful in rheumatic and gouty affections. It has
cured syphilis in the hands of the traditional doctor, and
in the highest potencies it cures many specific complaints—
when the symptoms agree. Some symptoms come on first
falling asleep, but during and after sleep are also marked
times of aggravation. Rheumatic and gouty stiffness of
all the joints with œdema of legs and feet. Swelling from
inflammation of joints and glands. Trembling from noise, or
sudden unexpected motion. Tension of muscles. Twitch-

ing of muscles. Extremely sensitive to touch. Ulceration of skin, especially of legs and of mucous membranes, with burning and spreading. Uncovering brings on the pains, and increases many complaints. Symptoms aggravated on waking. Walking fast aggravates most symptoms, especially the breathing and weakness. Warmth ameliorates most complaints. He is so weak he cannot sit up in bed. The restlessness of arsenic is often present.

Arsenicum is stamped upon the mental symptoms. Anxiety even to great anguish, with great fear. Anxiety in the morning on waking, but most marked in the evening and during the night. He is anxious without cause, about his health; anxious before stool; wakens during the night with anxiety and fear. He fears to go to bed. He fears death, or a crowd of people, yet equally dreads being alone. Fear that something will happen. Fear of people. He is very easily frightened and startled. He has frightful delusions and sees images. He despairs of recovery. he sees dead people in his nightly delirium. His thoughts dwell upon death, and he is sure he is going to die. He is very fretful, and dislikes to answer questions. He behaves like a crazy man. Fickle-minded, with confusion. Constantly discontented. Very excitable. Mental exertion intensifies mental and head symptoms. Always in a hurry, and very excitable. Many hysterical symptoms, with cramps and fainting. Indifference to all pleasure. Cannot settle upon what he wants to do. Wakens up in the morning very fretful. He is irritable during chill, and during headache. He has impulses to do violence to his friends, to kill somebody. Lamenting and bewailing. His memory is weak. He grows morose and quarrelsome, fault-finding, and scolds those about him. He is restless of mind and body, evening and night; anxious tossing all night, during chill and heat; also during menses. Sadness in the evening when alone, and during the fever. Oversensitive to noises, and especially to voices. Becomes so beside herself that she shrieks. There are long spells of silence in which she refuses to answer questions; at these times she sits even with others near her and refuses to speak. Easily startled from noise, on falling asleep and during sleep. Thinks of death and of suicide. Suspicious of all her best friends. Persistent tormenting thoughts often keeping him awake at night, with feet and legs icy cold and head hot. He becomes increasingly timid. Weeping at night without cause. Weeping in sleep.

Vertigo in the evening, during headache, with nausea, and when walking in the open air.

The forehead perspires easily, and complaints and pains come on from uncovering the head. There are congestive, pulsating headaches, with electric shocks through the head. The head feels cold, and is sensitive to cold air and to drafts. The neck is stiff, and the head is drawn to one side. During the headache the head feels heavy and enlarged. Eruptions with crusts, dry or moist, form upon the scalp. It has cured many cases of eczema. From the suppression of eruptions on the scalp, many chronic periodical sick headaches have come, lasting a lifetime, or until cured with a similar remedy. These headaches begin in the afternoon and evening, very severe after midnight, worse from cold air and from a draft. Headaches caused by checking a chronic catarrh, or such as come with coryza, or with gastric disturbances. Rheumatic headaches. Congestive headaches during chill, during fever and during menses. All headaches of this remedy are aggravated after eating, while lying, during motion, from noise, after sleep, from standing, and walking in cold air; ameliorated from sitting, external heat and hot drinks, and wrapping up the head. The pains are paroxysmal, and the headaches are often periodical. The pains come in the forehead, over the eyes and in occiput, and in parietal bones. Sides of head become sore. Burning, stitching and tearing are most common pains. Pressing outward over the eyes, and

9

stitching on coughing. Tearing over eyes and in occiput. Many of these headaches come from suppressed malaria, and it will be stated that these headaches began after having been cured (?) of ague. This remedy is an excellent antidote to the abuse of quinine.

Catarrhal conditions of the eyes, excoriating mucous discharges, and the lids stick together in the morning. The veins are injected, the balls feel enlarged, and there is free lachrymation. The eyes look glassy, pale, fishy. Opening of the lids difficult because of dryness. Oedema under the eyes, and the lids are swollen. Ulceration of the cornea. The eyes are jaundiced, and tears acrid. Staring, fixed, startled look. Spots on the cornea. Redness of the eyes and lids. Pains at night, worse from motion and reading, and ameliorated from warmth. The pains are burning, tearing and pressing. Sensation of sand in the eyes. Smarting in eyes while reading. There are colors in the field of vision, green and yellow. Vision is dim and foggy. Sparks before the eyes. Asthenopia. Vision lost.

The ears tingle, and are hot. Ears swollen. Eruptions on ears. Ears cold. Otorrhœa, bloody, fetid and yellow. Itching deep in auditory canal. Ncises in the ears; buzzing, cracking, humming, ringing, roaring, rushing; after quinine. Earache evening and night, ameliorated by heat; aggravated in cold air. The pains are burning, stitching and tearing. The hearing is at first acute, later impaired, and finally lost.

This remedy cures chronic nasal catarrh that has lasted from childhood, when the discharge is excoriating, bloody, burning, greenish, thick, or yellow. It is purulent and offensive. Dryness in nose nights. The nose is obstructed. Epistaxis. Itching of nose, and inside of nose. Sneezing, frequent and violent.

Cachectic, anxious, frightened look. Pale, waxy and chlorotic. Lips pale. Lips bluish, or even black. Dark circles below the eyes. The face is sunken and pinched. Face covered with eruptions; eczema, herpes, scurfs, vesicles. Furfuraceous eruption in the beard. Eruptions on nose, and about the mouth. The face is sickly, haggard and suffering. Itching of the face. Inflammation of the paratoid and submaxillary glands. Much perspiration on face. Twitching of the muscles of the face. Ulcers on face and lips. Epithelioma of lips. Oedema of face. Swollen lips. Pain in face in cold air, ameliorated by heat. Rheumatic and neuralgic pains, coming periodically. The pains are burning, stitching and tearing.

Aphthæ and ulcers in mouth. Dryness of mouth and tongue. Tongue is red, and coated white. Inflammation of tongue. Bleeding gums. Offensive odors from mouth. Burning, raw mouth and tongue. Excoriation of tongue. Swollen gums and tongue. Taste bad, bitter, insipid, putrid, sour, sweetish. Vesicles in mouth and on tongue.

The teeth are sore, and there is pain on masticating. Pain in teeth from cold drinks, during menses, extending to ear, head and temples; ameliorated by warmth. Pulsating, tearing pains in teeth.

Sensation in throat and larynx as if forced asunder. Inflammation, with heat and dryness. Lump rising from stomach to throat, like globus hystericus, ameliorated by eructations. Choking, with copious flow of saliva. Roughness, and scraping the throat. Spasms of the œsophagus. Swallowing is very difficult and painful. There are burning, soreness and stitching in the throat. Ulcers in throat.

A multitude of sufferings is found in the stomach. Great anxiety. An anxiety from stomach to spine, with palpitation. Appetite ravenous, or wanting. Aversion to food and meat. Coldness in the stomach. Desires sour things, sweets, warm drinks. The digestion is poor and the stomach is easily disordered, with distension from flatulence. Empty, sinking sensation and faintness. Eructations after eating, bitter, empty, of food, of sour fluid; waterbrash. Fullness after eating. Heaviness after eating like a stone. Heartburn. The most obstinate form of gastritis, acute and chronic. Loathing of food. With most complaints there is intense nausea. It has nausea during chill, after cold drinks, during cough, after dinner, after eating, during headache, during menses, and during stool. It has cured nausea during pregnancy. The pains are burning, cramping, cutting, pressing, soreness, stitching; and they come on at night and are worse after food, and cold drinks; and ameliorated by heat. Retching on coughing. Pulsating in stomach. Tightness felt in stomach. Thirst extreme during heat, and for warm drinks during chill. In chronic complaints it is thirstless, like Arsenicum. Vomiting bile, food, mucus, sour, watery; aggravated morning and during night, on coughing, after drinking cold water, after eating, with headache.

Coldness felt in whole abdomen; must have much warmth. Distension of abdomen after eating. Tympanitic distension and dropsy. Flatulent distension. Inflammation of intestines with ulceration, and of peritoneum. The abdomen is very painful at night. Pain on coughing, during diarrhea, after eating, during menses, during stool. Pains all paroxysmal and violent, ameliorated by warmth. Pain in liver, hypogastrium. Gall-stone colic. The whole abdomen burns. Cramping before stool, and constant desire for stool. Cutting in abdomen and liver. Pressing pain in liver. Soreness in abdomen and liver. Stitching in abdomen, liver and groin. Pulsating in abdomen. Great uneasiness in abdomen. Rumbling before stool. Twitching of the muscles of abdomen.

There is some constipation, alternating with diarrhea. Constriction of the anus. Violent diarrhea at night, after midnight, after cold drinks, after eating, after milk. Much pain during and after stool. Involuntary stool. Itching and excoriation about the anus. Hemorrhoids, and bleeding from the anus. External and internal piles, aggravated walking. Burning as with a red hot iron, with piles, and diarrhœa, during and after stool. The pains are cutting, pressing, soreness, stitching. There is tenesmus during and after stool. Paralysis and ineffectual urging for stool. Catarrh of the colon.

Stool is acrid, black, bloody, brown, copious, frothy; or scanty, watery, white and frothy; or hard, dry, dark, knotty. Sometimes light colored, offensive, or purulent, yellow.

Inflammation of the bladder. Retention of urine. Urging to urinate at night, constant, frequent, ineffectual. Urination is dribbling, or difficult and painful. Urination frequent at night. Incontinence. He feels that he had not finished.

Inflammation of the kidneys. Pain, cutting and stitching. Cutting along the ureters. It has been of service in Addison's disease.

Hemorrhage from the urethra, and burning during urination.

Urine albuminous during pregnancy. Urine bloody, burning, cloudy. Color of urine is black, greenish or red. Urine copious. Urine scanty with pellicle on surface. Sediment copious, mucus, pus red. Specific gravity diminished. Urine watery and clear.

The testes are hard, painful and swollen. Seminal emissions. Erections feeble.

This remedy has greatly restrained the development of cancer of uterus. It is mentioned for cauliflower excresence with putrid discharge. Itching of vulva. Leucorrhea, excoriating, burning, offensive, putrid, yellow; aggravated after menses. Menses absent, acrid, bright red, copious, frequent, offensive, painful, pale, protracted, scanty, suppressed. Uterine hemorrhage. Burning in the genitalia. Pain in uterus. Stitching in ovaries. Prolapsus.

Catarrh of larynx and trachea. Sensation in throat and larynx as if forced asunder. Dryness in larynx. Rawness, soreness and scraping in larynx. Hoarseness, and voice lost.

Respiration is rapid, anxious and asthmatic at night, aggravated from 2 to 3 a. m. Difficult evening and night, and aggravated 2 to 3 a. m., on coughing, on exertion, on lying, on motion, when walking. Respiration rattling, short, suffocative, wheezing and whistling.

In the cold anæmic patient there is a morning cough with copious expectoration, and a night cough that is dry. The cough is aggravated after midnight, and at 2 a. m., and 3 a. m. The cough is a hacking cough during the afternoon and evening. The cough is aggravated in cold air, on becoming cold, after cold drinks; aggravated lying in the evening, and on motion. The cough comes during chill, and fever, and with coryza. It is a choking asthmatic cough sometimes. It is spasmodic and suffocative. Irritation to cough is felt in the larynx and trachea, and he coughs until exhausted.

Expectoration morning and evening, bloody, copious, difficult, greenish, purulent, viscid and yellow. It tastes bitter, sickening, putrid or sweetish.

In the chest there is great anxiety and oppression. It has cured obstinate cases of catarrh of the chest. It has constriction of chest and heart. Effusion of the pleural sac. Hemorrhage of the lungs . Inflammation of bronchial tubes, endocardium, pericardium, lungs and pleura. Cardiac and anæmic murmurs. Oppression of heart and chest. Anxious and violent palpitation. Weak feeling in chest. A most useful remedy in threatened phthisis, and especially when there are cavities in the lungs, and the patient can not get warm even with warm clothing and in a warm room. Cannot get warm in summer; and when cold drinks bring on many symptoms. The pain in the chest is aggravated from coughing, and from inspiration. It is felt most in the sides of chest, and in the heart. The pain is burning, cutting, soreness and stitching. The stitching pains are aggravated on coughing, and on the left side.

The back is cold, and sensitive to cold air and drafts. Pain in the back during heat, and during menses. Pain in the cervical region, scapulæ and between the shoulders. Pain in lumbar region and sacrum. Aching, bruised, burning, drawing in back. Tender spine. Stiffness in the back.

Cold hands and feet. Cold feet evening in bed. Cold extremities during fever. Knees bent up by muscular contractions so he could not move his feet. Corns on the palms, and soles. Cramps in the thigh and calf. Blueness of the nails during chill. Herpes on the shoulders. Pimples and vesicles on the extremities. Fissures on the elbows and wrists. Vesicles on the upper limbs. Pimples and vesicles on the hands. Eruption on thighs and legs. Vesicles on the soles. Excoriation between the thighs. Formication of the limbs. Burning heat of feet. Heaviness of lower limbs. Insensibility of the fingers. Itching of hands, lower limbs and feet. Numbness of the extremities, hands, fingers and feet. Rheumatic and neuralgic pains in the limbs during chill, in cold air, ameliorated by heat. Aching in the shoulder. Sciatica, extending downwards. Pain in hips, thighs, knees and legs. Pain in the knee as if bruised. Burning in hands and fingers, feet and soles. Drawing in lower limbs, knees, tibia, and feet. Stitching pains in the limbs when the legs are cold; especially knee, foot and heel. Tearing pains in shoulders, upper arms, elbows, wrist, hand and fingers; also in hip, thigh, leg and foot. Paralysis of limbs, upper and lower. Perspiration of feet. Restlessness of the lower limbs. Stiffness of knees. Dropsical swelling of hands and knees, legs and feet. Tension in the hollow of knee and hamstrings. Trembling limbs. Twitching in the thighs. Ulcers on the legs. Varicose veins on lower limbs. Weakness of all the limbs, but greatest in lower limbs.

The sleep is much disturbed by dreams, amorous, anxious, of the dead, of death, fantastic dreams, of fire, frightful, misfortune, nightmare, vivid. He is late falling asleep. The sleep is restless; he tosses and turns all night. Sleepiness afternoon and evening. Sleepless before midnight, but worse after midnight. Sleepiness, but cannot sleep. If he wakens cannot sleep again. Wakens early and cannot sleep again. Distressing yawning.

Constitutional coldness is a marked feature of this remedy. It has intermittent fever with chill, fever and sweat, The chill may come at any time, but most likely in the afternoon. Chilliness from drinking cold water, from walking in the open air, and from motion. The periodicity is not very regular. It has chill with perspiration. The paroxysm may be daily, tertian or quartian. It has a violent shaking chill. The time most common is 8 p. m., 4 p. m. and 1 a. m. Warm room ameliorates the chill This remedy has fever without chill. It has fever with chilliness. Dry external heat. Flushes of heat. It has been helpful in hectic fever. The heat is intense. It has internal heat with external chill. The perspiration is often absent. It is a very useful remedy in chronic intermittent fever. He sweats copiously at night from great weakness, as well as from fever. He sweats while eating, from slight exertion and from motion, and during sleep. The sweat is cold and offensive. When the sweat has been suppressed, from entering a cold damp room or cellar, complaints come on much like this remedy.

There are blotches on the skin. There are burning spots, and the skin burns after scratching. It is an excellent remedy to be used against the spread of malignant disease, as so often the symptoms are found in this remedy. The skin is cold. Desquamation, with or without eruptions. Pale waxy skin, or yellow skin. Liver spots, red spots and yellow spots. The skin is dry and burning. Inability to perspire. The complaints of this remedy are often associated wtih eruptions. It has moist, and dry eruptions. Blisters, and bloody eruptions. The eruptions burn. Eruptions that are furfuraceous and powdery, mealy. It has cured eczema many times. Itching, scaly herpes. The eruptions itch and burn violently. They are painful, and spread rapidly, often turn into phagadenic ulcers. Psoriasis, must scratch until moist. Pustules. Rash. Scabby, scaly eruptions. Stinging in the skin after scratching. Nodular urticaria. Vesicular eruptions. Vesicles come after scratching.

It cures erysipelas, when the symptoms agree. Intertrigo. Itching when undressing, and when warm in bed. Itching, burning, crawling, and stinging. Sensitive skin, sore to touch. Sticking after scratching. The dropsical swellings burn. Pain in the skin as if an ulcer were forming. Ulcers; bleeding, burning, indolent, phagadenic, suppurating, with ichorous bloody discharges, and turned up edges. Warts grow easily.

KALI BICHROMICUM

The following symptoms have recently been cured by Kali-bi. They are found under Kali-bi. in Allen's Encyclopœdia of Pure Materia Medica, page 237:

Weakness of digestion, so that the stomach was disordered by any but the mildest food (chrome washers). Incarceration of flatulence in stomach and whole lower portion of abdomen. (Zlatarovich).

Great feebleness of stomach in the morning. (Lackner).

Feeling of emptiness in the stomach, though want of appetite at dinner. (Marenzetler).

Feeling of sinking in the stomach before breakfast. (Dr. R. Dudgeon).

The patient wakes in the night with great uneasiness in the stomach, and soreness and tenderness in a small spot to the left of the xiphoid appendix, which is very similar to symptoms in Drysdale's proving.

Sudden violent pain in the stomach, in its anterior surface, a burning constrictive pain. (Zlatarovich).

The same patient complains of repletion after a mouthful of food, and he had taken Lycopodium without benefit.

There was also cutting as with knives, and he was unable to digest potatoes or any starchy food.

There were no catarrhal symptoms of nose or chest, and no thick, ropy, mucous discharges, therefore Kali-bi. was neglected. The stomach symptoms alone guided to its use, as he had no other symptoms of importance.

The relief is marked, and I think permanent.

It will be seen that I have made use of the language of the prover mostly, as it so perfectly describes the symptoms of the patients.

In looking over the proving, the patient underscored such symptoms as he had suffered from, and the remedy was furnished on these symptoms, which really lends value to the provings. Especially are these provings the more beautiful, as they are by several provers.

KALI-MURIATICUM

Symptoms appear in the morning; forenoon; afternoon; evening; *night*; before midnight; after midnight. Aversion to the open air and sensitive to drafts. The open air aggravates many symptoms. Asleep feeling in single parts. Dread of bathing and worse from bathing. Cold in general makes the symptoms worse; worse from cold air; worse from becoming cold; worse from cold, wet weather. It has been a useful remedy in many kinds of convulsions; clonic; *epileptic*; epileptiform; internal. Worse after eating and from exertion. Fainting spells. Worse from cold food, fat food, cold drinks. Formication in many parts. Sensation of fullness. Easy bleeding of any part; blood dark and clotted. Heaviness external and internal. *Induration of many tissues*; in glands; in muscles. Inflammation and the results of induration; infiltration following inflammation; hepatization after pneumonia (Calc. Sulph.). Marked lassitude. Desire to lie down. Complaints from lifting and straining of muscles and joints. Lying makes many symptoms worse; worse after lying; worse lying in bed; worse lying on the right side; worse lying on the painful side; better lying on the painless side. Worse before and *during* menses; worse from motion. Increased mucous discharges *viscid and milk white*. The pains are biting, bruised, burning, *cutting*, jerking, pinching, pressing, stitching. Stitching pains, outward, transversely in glands, *in muscles*. Tearing downward in muscles. Twinging and ulcerative pains.

Paralysis one-sided; of organs. Pulse full, hard, intermittent, irregular, slow; small, soft. General pulsation. Marked relaxation of muscles. Rising from sitting increases or brings on symptoms. Rubbing ameliorates symptoms. Sensitive to pain. Complaints one-sided; either side; mostly *left-side*. Complaints worse while sitting. Sluggish patients; feeble reaction; slow repair; slow convalescence. Swelling of parts; of glands. Feeling of tension in muscles. Aggravation from touch. Twitching of muscles. Warmth of bed makes some symptoms worse. Weakness of the whole body; in the morning; in the evening; after acute catarrhal diseases; from walking. Worse in wet weather.

Irritability and anger in the evening; anxiety: in the evening; about trifles. She has a delusion that she must not eat. Discontented and discouraged. Dullness of mind. Mental excitement. Fear that some evil will come to him. It has been used with benefit in imbecility. Indifference to all pleasure. Insanity and irresolution. Loathing of life. Moaning, MANIA. Obstinate. Restlessness. *Sadness*. Silent. Inclination to sit in complete silence. Talking in sleep. Unconsciousness in advanced states of brain and meningeal diseases. Vertigo; when rising or stooping; when walking.

Constriction of the scalp. Dandruff, copious, white. Eczema. Heaviness of the head; of the forehead; in the *occiput* with aching in trachea and hard cough; in the *occiput* as if full of lead; in occiput as if head would sink backwards; in *occiput* with hard cough. Sensation of looseness of the brain. Sensation of movements in the head. Pain in the head in the morning on walking; in the afternoon; *evening*; in cold air; in the open air; worse from binding up the hair; worse after eating; paroxysmal; worse from pressure; worse from stooping; worse from touch; worse walking; worse walking in the open air; worse from wine; better from wrapping up the head. Pain in the forehead. Pain in occiput, like a weight holds head fast to pillow (like Opium). Pain in the sides of head; temples; boring, bruised, burning in forehead; cutting; gnawing in occiput; jerking. Pressing pain in whole head; in forehead, outward; in *occiput*; in temples, outward. Shooting pain in head; in occiput. Stitching pain in head; worse stooping; in forehead; in *occiput*; in side of head; in temples. Stunning pains in head. Tearing pains in the head; in the forehead; in the occiput and sides of occiput; in *sides of head*; in the temples; in the *vertex*. PERSPIRATION ON THE HEAD. Pulsation in the head. Shocks in the head.

Catarrhal discharges with milk-white mucus or greenish or yellow purulent. Inflammation of the conjunctiva with thickening; PUSTULAS; of the *cornea*. Burning in the eyes; in the canthi. Pressing. Pain as if sand in the eyes. STITCHING pain in eyes. Photophobia. Protrusion of the eyes. Redness in the evening with pain. Staring. Swollen lids. Twitching inner canthi. Vesicles on the cornea. Vision dim. Double vision. Lights before the eyes when coughing or sneezing.

Closure of the eustachian tubes. Discharge from ears of milk-white mucus. Dry catarrh of the middle ear; the ears are hot. Stitching in the ears. Noises: buzzing; cracking on blowing nose and on swallowing; humming; reverberations; ringing; roaring; singing; snapping; tickling; whizzing. Pain in the ear; behind the ear; drawing; pressing; *stitching*; stitching behind the ear; tearing: tearing behind the ear. Pulsation behind the ear. Tingling in the ears. Twitching. Hearing acute; for noise; for voices; impaired.

Nasal catarrh; discharge copious; *excoriating*; purulent; thick; *white*; *milk-white*; viscid; yellow; posterior nares. *Coryza*; with cough; fluent, dry; *thick and milk-white discharge*. Dryness in the nose. Epistaxis in the afternoon; evening. Itching in the nose. The nose is obstructed with mucus. Frequent sneezing.

Epithelioma of the lips and lupus of the face. The face is bluish; pale; red. Dryness of the lips. Eruptions on the face; cheeks; lips; *around the mouth*; pimples. Suffering, sickly expression. Flashes of heat in the face. The face is hot. Pain in the face; worse in the right side; drawing; *stitching*; *tearing*. Paralysis of the face. Perspiration. *Sunken face*. Painful, swollen face; lips; glands of jaw. Tension. Twitching. Ulceration of face; lips.

Aphthae in the mouth of children and nursing mothers. Bleeding gums. Gum boils. The tongue is red or *white*. Dry mouth and tongue. Heat in the mouth. Inflammation of gums and tongue. *Mapped tongue*. *Milk-white mucus in the mouth*. Odor from the mouth offensive, even putrid.

Burning mouth and tongue. Sore gums and tongue. *Scorbutic gums.* Salivation. Speech wanting. Swollen gums and tongue. Taste: *bad; bitter*; metallic; *putrid*; *saltish*; *sour*; *sweetish.* Ulceration of *mouth* and tongue; *syphilitic.* Vesicles in the mouth. Teeth on edge and become loose. Pain in the teeth; stitching.

The throat is dry and red and there is choking. Heat in the throat and much mucus. Inflammation of throat; tonsils; *chronic.*   White exudate in the throat; gray patches. It has many times cured diphtheria. MUCUS: VISCID; thick; *milk-white*; covers pharynx; adherent. Pain in throat; on swallowing; burning; pressing; rawness; *sore.* Scraping in the throat. Swallowing very difficult. Swollen throat; *tonsils*; uvula, œdematous; parotid gland. Ulceration of the throat.

Anxiety of the stomach. The appetite is diminished or entirely lost or it is increased, even ravenous, after eating. Aversion to food; to meat. Constriction of the stomach. Emptiness not ameliorated by eating. Eructations: after eating; ineffectual; bitter; empty; of food; sour; waterbrash. Flashes of heat; heartburn, and sensation of fullness. Weight in stomach worse at night. Hiccough. Inflammation of the stomach. Loathing of food. Nausea after fats and rich food. Nausea and shivering. Pain in the stomach; aching; burning; cutting; pressing with emptiness; sore to touch; stitching. Tension. Thirst extreme; during chill. Vomiting: bile; blood; *food*; mucus, milk-white and dark green; morning diarrhœa with vomiting white mucus; sudden; incessant.

Distension in abdomen after eating. *Emptiness.* Ascites. Enlarged spleen. Flatulence: in day time; afternoon; night; prevents sleep. FULLNESS; AFTER EATING. Pain in abdomen; night; colic; griping with diarrhœa; during diarrhœa; after eating; as if menses would appear; before and *during* stool; in hypochondria, especially the right; burning in right hypochondrium. Cramping in abdomen; before stool; in hypogastrium with diarrhœa. Cutting in abdomen; in umbilical region. Pressing in hypochondria; in right better by passing flatus. Sore bruised abdomen; in right hypochondrium; in inguinal region. Rumbling before stool. Tension in abdomen.

Constipation; stool difficult; from inactivity of the rectum. The stool is dry, *hard,* large, light colored, clay colored. Diarrhœa; painful; morning; evening; after fats. The stool is excoriating; bloody mucus; copious; green; offensive; watery; white mucus. Dysentery with slimy stool or pure blood. Flatus during diarrhœa. *Formication of the anus.* Hemorrhage from rectum. Hemorrhoids: congested; *external*; large; SORE; worse walking. Involuntary stools; when passing flatus. Itching of the anus; *after stool.* Pain in rectum and anus; during and after stool. Burning during and *after stool.* Pressing in the anus. SORENESS; *after stool.* Tenesmus. Paralysis of the rectum. Urging with normal stool; constant.

Catarrh of the bladder with much mucus in the urine. Retention of urine. Urging to urinate; at night; constant; *frequent*; ineffectual. Urination *dribbling*; feeble stream; frequent, at night; involuntary at night; retarded. Must press long to start the urine. Inflammation of the kidneys. Pain in the kidneys. Suppression of urine. It has been used much in chronic gonorrhœa with gleety, milky discharge. It has cured violent chordee. Itching of the urethra. Burning and cutting during urination. Urine: albuminous; black; greenish black; *bloody*; burning; cloudy; dark; pale; red; copious at night; scanty; containing sugar; thick.

Inflammation of glans penis and testes. Indurated testes. Erections troublesome; violent. Stitching of the scrotum. Drawing pain in testes. Seminal emissions. Ulcers on the penis; chancres.

Leucorrhœa: excoriating; MILKY; white; VISCID.
Menses bright red; clotted; *frequent*; late; painful.
Metrorrhagia. Labor-like pain.

Irritation of larynx; inflammation; dryness; croup.
Mucus in the larynx; THICK MILKY. Larynx sensitive to
touch. Tickling in larynx. Hoarseness; voice finally lost.
Respiration rapid; *asthmatic*; deep; *difficult*; rattling;
snoring. Cough day and night; asthmatic; barking; from
deep breathing; croupy; dry; hacking; after eating; harsh;
from irritation in larynx and trachea; loose; paroxysmal;
racking; short; violent; whooping cough. Expectoration:
morning; bloody; mucus; white; gray; *milk-white*; yellow.

Catarrh of the chest and anxiety of the heart. Coldness in the region of the heart. Congestion and flashes of
heat in chest. Constriction of the chest; of the heart; as
from sulphur fumes. Hemorrhage of the lungs. Hepatization of lungs after pneumonia. Inflammation of *bronchial
tubes*; of *lungs*; *pleura*. *Oppression of the chest*. Pain in
the chest; on respiration; sides of chest, on respiration;
heart; *cutting*; pressing; *soreness*. Stitching on breathing; stitching in the heart. Violent palpitation.

Coldness in the back. Stitching of the back. Pain in
the back; on breathing; better lying; while sitting; while
standing; while walking. Pain between the scapulæ. Pain
in the lumbar region; better lying; while sitting and standing. Pain in the *sacrum* better lying. Pain in the coccyx.
Aching in the back; lumbar region; sacrum. Burning in
the back. Drawing pain in lumbar region; in sacrum.
Lightning-like pains in small of back to feet, must get out
of bed and sit up. Pressing pains in back; in lumbar
region. Stitching pains in scapulæ; in sacrum.

Cold extremities; HANDS; *feet.* Cracking in joints and
tendons of back of hand. *Cramps in limbs*; thighs; LEGS.
Eruptions in limbs; pimples; vesicles. Heat of hands and
feet: burning soles. Pains in the limbs; nightly; rheumatic

worse from the warmth of bed; rheumatic in joints; rheumatic left shoulder and elbow. Drawing pains in wrists; thighs; knees; legs. Pressing pains in shoulders. Stitching pains in knees, in legs. Tearing pains in shoulders; hands; fingers; in thighs, worse from heat of bed; in *knees*; *calf*. Paralysis of one side; perspiration of feet; *cold*. Stiffness of knees. Swelling of legs and ankles; œdematous. Tension in knees; calf. Twitching in limbs; in *thighs*. Ulcers on legs, warts on hands. Weakness of the limbs; of thighs.

Dreams: amorous; *anxious*; of death; of previous events; frightful; of misfortune; pleasant; vexatious; vivid. Restless sleep. Sleepiness afternoon; evening; after dinner; *after eating*. Sleeplessness all night. Waking early.

Chill morning; afternoon; evening; in *open air*; in bed; chilliness in evening; external coldness; shaking chill. Fever evening in bed. Perspiration morning; *night*; midnight.

Burning or coldness of skin. Dryness of skin. Eruptions: eczema; herpes; pimples; scabby; scaly; white thin bran-like scales; vesicles. Jaundice. Erysipelas. Excoriation; intertrigo. Formication. Itching in evening in bed; night; burning; crawling; better by *scratching*; stinging. *Ulcers* burning; suppurating, warts.

KALI-SiLICATUM

The silicate of potassium is a very deep acting remedy. Some of the symptoms are worse or come on in the morning, a few in the forenoon and afternoon, many in the evening, and very many in the *night,* and especially *after midnight*. Aversion to the open air and worse from the open air and from draughts. He dreads bathing and is worse from bathing. *He is sensitive to cold weather and worse from becoming cold*; after becoming cold complaints come on; worse in cold room and in dry, cold weather; cold, wet weather also makes him worse. He takes cold easily. After eating complaints are all worse; worse after slight exertion. Faintness, *emaciation*. He is worse after *cold drinks*, cold food, milk and fat food. Creeping feelings all over the body, but especially in the limbs. Induration in glands and muscles. His painful parts are very sensitive to a jar. Lassitude is very marked and quite constant. *Desire to lie down* all the time. After straining muscles the weakness lasts long. He dreads to move or walk and he is worse from motion.

Mucous secretions all increased. The blood surges from the body to the head. Stitching, tearing pains are numerous; he suffers if the perspiration is suppressed from a draft, or from insufficient clothing; he is worse from pressure and very sensitive to touch.

Pulsation in head and limbs; stiffness all over the body and in the limbs; he trembles all over, especially in abdomen; twitching of muscles. Symptoms all *worse from uncovering the body*; worse walking and from walking fast. Great weakness in the morning on waking, also in the evening; also after eating and after walking. *Weariness.* Worse in winter, in cold weather and better in summer.

Absent minded and becomes angered over trifles; anxiety in the evening, in bed and during the night; anxiety in the evening, in bed and during the night; anxiety with fear; anxiety after eating, about his health; during menses, about trifles, capriciousness. It is a very useful remedy for children in school when they can not learn their lessons. Difficult concentration of mind; he has lost confidence in his own ability. Confusion of mind in the morning on arising, in the evening, *after mental exertion*, while sitting. Consolation aggravates the mental symptoms; contrary and cowardly. His mind is full of imaginations; about dead people; illusions of fancy; sees images in the night; sees frightful images; sees ghosts and thieves. He is discontented and discouraged. Dullness of mind when reading and writing; in the morning on waking. Much excitement. Mental exertion aggravates many symptoms. Fear with anxiety; fear and dread of work; easily frightened; forgetful and heedless, which looks like approaching imbecility; many hysterical manifestations. He is very impatient, and indifferent to his friends and to pleasure; he takes pleasure in nothing. *Irresolution.* He seems not to care how things go, one way is as good as another. Has no opinions on prevailing questions. Extremely irritable; worse in morning and evening; *worse after coition;* worse from any attempt to console him. Memory very feeble; mistakes in speaking and writing; misplaces words. He is very obstinate and his moods are constantly changing. *Mental prostration.* Great restlessness during the night. Very sad in the morning. Seems at times to lose his senses. At times he is very sensitive to noises. It is a very useful remedy where these symptoms have been brought on by sexual excesses. Wants to sit still or sit around and do nothing; *very indolent.* Startled easily, from fright; from noise, on falling asleep, when touched. *Wonderful timidity.* Indisposed to conversation. Talking in sleep. Weeping much; weeping evening and night; weeping in sleep. Will power feeble; aversion to mental work.

Vertigo morning, afternoon, evening; inclination to fall backwards; vertigo during headache, as if intoxicated; must lie down; vertigo with nausea; objects seem to turn in a circle; vertigo almost constant; while rising, *while sitting, while stooping,* while walking, while walking in open air. Coldness of the head, of vertex; the head is sensitive to cold and must be covered. Boiling sensation in the brain; anæmia of the brain; congestion of head at night on coughing; constriction of the scalp, especially of the forehead. Eruptions in margin of the hair back of head, moist-like eczema; fullness of the head and the hair falls out; heat in the whole head; worse in forehead; heaviness in the fore-head in the morning; sensation of movements in the head. Pain in the head *morning*, afternoon, evening, *night*; *after midnight*; pain *worse in cold air* and from a draft; *after coition*; from head becoming cold; from coryza; after eat-ing; when hungry; from being overheated; *worse from a jar*; from light; from *mental exertion*; from motion; from motion of head or eyes; from noise; during menses. Com-pelled to lie down. *Applied heat relieves.* The pains are pulsating, periodical and paroxysmal. Headache came on from sexual excesses; worse after sleep; from stepping heavily; *from stooping* and from *straining the eyes*. The pain is violent, worse from touch and when walking; *wrap-ping up the head relieves.* Pain in forehead daytime, morn-ing, *afternoon*, evening, night, above the eyes; pain in occi-put; pain in sides of head, worse on right side; pain in temples. Boring pain in forehead; bruised pain in whole head; bursting pain in forehead; drawing pains in whole head and in *forehead*; pressing pains; pains pressing out-ward; pressing in forehead, *outward, over eyes*, occiput, temples and vertex; shooting pains in forehead and occiput; *stitching pains in head*, forehead, occiput, sides of head and temples; stunning pains in head; tearing pains in head, fore-head, occiput, sides of occiput, *sides of head, temples* and vertex. Perspiration of whole scalp; perspiration of fore-head. Pulsating in the head, in forehead. Shaking or trembling sensation in the brain; uncovering the head in cool air brings on many symptoms.

The eyelids are stuck together in the morning. Cata-ract has been cured by this remedy. Discharges yellow and thick; dryness in the eyes; eczema around the eyes and in the eyebrows; the eyes feel hot; inflammation of the eyes, of the conjunctiva, of the lids; psoric complaints of the eyes; infected blood vessels; lachrymation in cold air. It has cured opacity of the cornea. Pain in the eyes, right most affected, better by warmth; the pains are *burning*, *pressing*, *stitching*, tearing; pain as if sand in eyes. It has cured paralysis of the optic nerve. Photophobia marked in daylight; redness of the eyes; spots on the cornea; staring, swollen lids; ulceration of the cornea; weak eyes. In the field of vision there are many colors, *floating spots* and black flies; dark colors, yellow. Dim vision. *Dazzling*. Complaints from *exertion of vision*; flickering before the eyes; thinks he is going blind; sparks before the eyes and weak vision. Discharge from ear, bloody, offensive, purulent, *thick yellow*. Scurfy eruption behind the ear; flapping sensation in the ears; the ears are hot; inflammation in the middle ear; intense itching deep in the ears; noises in ears with dizziness; flapping sounds, ringing, *roaring*. Pain in ear, mostly right, better by warmth; pain behind the ear and deep in the ear; aching, boring, cramping pain; drawing, *stitching*, *tearing*; drawing and tearing behind the ear. Pulsating pain deep in the ear; the ear feels stopped; ulceration in the ear. Hearing is acute for noise, later impaired. It has cured deafness from catarrh of the eustachian tubes and the middle ear.

Catarrh of the nose and posterior nares in chilly people who are weak and want to keep still and rest; very offensive discharge, offensive breath in syphilitic subjects; the discharge is bloody, crusty, acrid, *greenish*, purulent, thick, yellow. He is subject to frequent coryzas as he is taking cold constantly. Dryness in the nose; bleeding of the nose on blowing it; itching deep in the nose where many crusts form; the nose is constantly obstructed; pain in the nose, and in the bones of the nose; great soreness in nose; burning pain in nose. Smell acute, later diminished, finally lost. Frequent violent sneezing; the nose is greatly swollen; much swelling inside of nose; ulceration in the nose.

Discoloration of the face; bluish, red, pale; circumscribed red cheeks; the face is jaundiced; the lips are cracked and dry; face looks sickly and drawn with *suffering* expression. The face, chin, lips, upper lip, around the mouth, nose, extending down on the neck, covered with moist eczema. She was a sight to look upon and her friends all shunned her; she was comfortable only when in a very hot room. Herpes and pimples on the face. Indurated parotid gland; inflammation of the parotid gland. Itching of the face; drawing, stitching, tearing pain in the face; much sweat on the face; swelling of the cheeks, lips, parotid and submaxillary glands; ulceration of the lips; hard crust continues to form on the under lip.

Dry mouth without thirst; bleeding gums and white tongue; apthæ in the mouth; copious mucus forms in the mouth; odor from mouth offensive. The tongue is very sore. copious saliva flows into the mouth; swollen gums and tongue; taste is bad, bitter in the morning, bloody, sour.

Sensation of dryness in the throat with copious mucus; sensation of a lump in the throat; pain in the throat on swallowing; stitching pain in throat on swallowing; burning, rawness and soreness in the throat; much swelling in the throat and tonsils and swallowing is difficult. Swelling of cervical gland.

Sensation of anxiety in the stomach with aversion to food and especially to meat; ravenous appetite; appetite entirely lost; sensation of coldness in stomach; most troublesome eructations, worse after eating; bitter, empty sour, water brash; eructations ameliorate the stomach symptoms; heart-burn and fullness of the stomach; hiccough and weight in the stomach. Loathing of food. Nausea after eating and during headache; nausea with dizziness. Pain in the stomach at night, after eating; the pains in stomach are cutting, burning, cramping, gnawing, *pressing* and stitching; sore, bruised feeling in stomach; pressing in stomach after eating; pulsating in stomach after eating; retching when coughing. Sensation of tightness in stomach from flatulence. Thirst during chilliness and during fever; extreme thirst. Vomiting night and morning; of bile, of food, mucus and watery fluid; vomiting on coughing, after drinking *cold water*, *after eating*, and during headache.

The abdomen is distended after eating with obstructed flatulence; fullness, hardness and heaviness in abdomen; great heat in abdomen; pain in abdomen at night, during cough, after eating, before and during menses, after stool; warmth ameliorates. Pain in right hypochondrium, in the hypogastrium, in the inguinal region and in the liver; the pains in the abdomen are burning, cramping, *cutting, pressing, stitching* and *tearing*; pressing and stitching pains in the liver. Rumbling and tightness in the abdomen. *Constipation with very difficult stool*; difficult soft stool; insufficient stool. Constipation during menses. Stool dry, *hard, knotty, large*, light colored. Diarrhœa in the morning and at night; painful diarrhœa during menses, with stool bloody, frequent, offensive, purulent, watery; dysentery with scanty mucus, purulent and bloody stool; constriction of the anus. It has cured fistula in ano. Passing flatus ameliorates; formication of the anus. Hemorrhoids that protrude, ulcerate and bleed; inactivity of the rectum; itching of the anus after stool; ineffectual urging of stool; pain in anus during stool; burning during and after stool; burning after a hard stool. *Cutting*, pressing, sticking, stitching, pains in the anus; tenesmus, *extreme soreness* in the anus.

Catarrh of the bladder. The urine is cloudy, red, copious or scanty, with much mucous sediment; pressing pain in the bladder; urging to urinate; night, constant, frequent, ineffectual; the urine dribbles; urination frequent during the night; feeble stream; he cannot quite empty the bladder; slow in starting; he feels that he has not finished; involuntary at night. Burning in the urethra during urination.

Erections in the morning and during the night, painful, even violent, without desire; induration of the testes; itching of the scrotum; *seminal emissions*. Sexual desire at first increased, then diminished, later lost; swelling of the testes.

Eruptions and itching of the vulva; leucorrhea, *excoriating* and *yellow*; worse after the menses. Menses bright red, copious, *frequent, intermittent, late, offensive*, painful, pale, scanty, short, *suppressed*; metrorrhagia between the menstrual periods; dragging down feeling in the pelvis; burning in the genitals; labor-like pains at the menstrual period; soreness in the genitals; prolapsus of the uterus.

Catarrh of the air passages; irritation of the larynx and trachea; much mucus in the air passages and especially in the larynx; scraping in the larynx, tickling in the larynx and trachea. The voice is hoarse and rough. It is a very useful remedy in asthma. Difficult breathing from exertion, while lying and when coughing; rattling in the chest; short, suffocative, whistling breathing; cough in daytime, morning, forenoon, evening and most severe and constant during the night; cough worse after eating, during fever, lying; the cough is asthmatic and suffocative, racking and spasmodic; dry cough during the night; hacking cough during the night; cough from irritation in larynx and trachea; cough from tickling in the larynx and trachea; the cough is violent, spasmodic and paroxysmal, like whooping cough. Expectoration in the morning, bloody, copious, greenish, mucus, *purulent*, putrid-looking, tough, *viscid, yellow*.

Catarrh of the chest; abscess of the lungs; abscess of the axilla. Tightness of the chest. Dropsy of the pleura. Hollow sensation in chest; hemorrhage of the lungs; chronic inflammation of bronchial tubes; weight on the chest; pain in chest during cough on deep inspiration; pain in the sides of chest on deep inspiration; burning, pressing, stitching pains. Rawness on coughing, soreness in chest, stitching on coughing and on inspiring, extending to back; stitching in sides of chest on breathing; stitching in mammæ; tearing pain in the walls of the chest. Palpitation on excitement and on slight exertion. It has been a most useful remedy in phthisis. Swelling in the axillary glands. Feeling of great weakness of the chest much like stannum.

The back feels cold. Itching of the back. Pain in the back *during menses*, while sitting and when stooping; pain in the back of the neck, between the scapulæ, in the *lumbar region* and in the sacrum; pain in coccyx; the whole spine is painful. Aching in lumbar region and sacrum; burning in the lumbar region; drawing pain in cervical region, lumbar region and sacrum; pressing pain in lumbar region. The whole spine is sore. stitching pains in scapulæ, *lumbar region* and sacrum; tearing in the cervical region; stiffness of the neck; tension in the back; weakness in the lumbar region.

The hands are chapped in cold weather; the hands and feet are cold; cramps in hands and calf. There are vesicular eruptions on the hands; pimples on the lower limbs; many eruptions on the thighs. Felons on the fingers. The hands are hot. Marked heaviness of the lower limbs, legs and feet. *Hip joint disease.* Itching of upper limbs, hands and palms; itching of lower limbs, thighs and legs. Jerking of the muscles of lower limbs; numbness upper limbs, hands and fingers; numbness of lower limbs, legs and feet. Pain in limbs during chill, better by warmth. Rheumatic pains in limbs; hard pain in the joints; gouty pains in joints; pains in shoulder and fingers, in hips, thighs and knees; pain in the sciatic nerve. Aching in the legs; burning soles; drawing pains in limbs; upper limbs, shoulder, elbow, forearm, wrist, hands, fingers, lower limbs, thighs, knee, leg, ankles, feet; pressing pains in thighs; sore, bruised pain in all the limbs; upper limbs, lower limbs, hip, leg; sprained feeling in all the joints; stitching pains in all the limbs and in the joints, stitching in shoulder, upper arm, wrist, hand, fingers; stitching in thighs, knees, legs ankle, *foot, heel*, toes, first toe; tearing pains in all the limbs and joints; tearing in shoulders, upper arm, elbow, forearm, wrist, hand, fingers, finger joints; tearing in hip, thigh, knee, leg, calf, ankles, foot, soles, toes, first toe; paralysis of upper and *lower limbs*. Sweat of palms; profuse, cold, *offensive* sweat of feet and between the toes. Stiffness of the joints, shoulders, knees; swelling of feet, legs and knees; tension in the knees and calves; trembling of all the limbs, of hands and legs; twitching of all the limbs, *thighs*. Ulcers on the legs; weakness of the joints, thigh, knee and ankles.

Dreams *anxious*; of dead people; of death; events of the previous day; horrible, fantastic, fire, *frightful*, ghosts, nightmare, visionary, vivid, of water. Sleep is restless, sleepiness in the afternoon, *evening*, after dinner. Sleepless before midnight, after midnight, after 2 a. m., with sleepiness. Sleeplessness from thinking, after waking. Waking frequently and too early; frequent yawning.

Chill morning, forenoon, noon, afternoon, evening, night, in open air, in cold air, in a draft of air; chilliness in evening in bed, after eating; chill external and internal, worse from motion; chilliness with pain; *one-sided chill*; shaking chill in the evening; better in a warm room; external heat ameliorates.

Fever afternoon, evening and during the night, alternating with sweat; dry heat, external heat; flushes of heat; perspiration absent; *night sweats*. Perspiration morning, daytime and *during night*. Perspiration during and after eating, from slight exertion, from motion; *profuse at night*; sweat during sleep; offensive while walking. If perspiration is checked in cool air, many complaints come on.

Burning after scratching; old scars become painful.

The skin is cold much of the time. The skin cracks; discoloration of the skin; blotches, liver spots, red spots, yellow skin; dry skin, dry, burning skin with inability to perspire. Blisters on the skin; burning eruptions; chafing skin; desquamating eruptions; eruptions moist and eruptions dry. It has cured most stubborn cases of eczema where sulphur and graphites seemed indicated and failed. Herpes that burn and are corrosive, scabby and itch and sting; eruptions that are painful, itching and spreading; itching pimples and pustules; scabby eruptions after scratching; scaly eruptions dry or moist; smarting after scratching; stinging after scratching; *nodular urticaria.* Vesicular eruptions; excoriation after scratching. Erysipelas. Indurations in the skin. *Intertrigo.* Itching, burning, crawling, smarting and stinging after scratching. It has cured lupus. Moisture of the skin after scratching, he scratches the skin until it is moist or bleeds; sore sensation of the skin. After scratching, the skin is swollen and burns, looks œdematous; sensation of tension in the skin; ulcerative pain in the skin. The ulcers that form upon the skin are characterized by *bleeding*, burning, spreading, pulsating, smarting and suppurating; ulcers are very indolent; the discharge from ulcers is bloody, copious, ichorous and thin. Tearing pain in the ulcers. Injuries and small wounds of the skin refuse to heal and suppurate. Warts that are painful, stinging, suppurating and withered.

NATRUM SILICATUM

The times of aggravation of the symptoms of this remedy are morning, *forenoon, evening, night,* and after midnight; he feels amelioration sometimes during the forenoon. Formation of recurrent abscesses; it relieves the pain and hastens the flow of pus in abscesses. AVERSION TO THE OPEN AIR; the symptoms are worse in the open air and he is extremely sensitive to a draft of air. The symptoms are worse from stimulants. He is sensitive to every change of weather from warm to cold and to cold damp weather. He feels all used up after coition. He is worse from cold in general, from cold air, from becoming cold, and after becoming cold; he is always taking cold. He feels worse and his symptoms are worse after eating. He is worse from slight exertion. He emaciates rapidly. Symptoms are worse after cold food, cold drinks, fat food, and milk. *There is a marked lack of vital heat.* Heaviness felt in body and limbs. Formication through the body. Induration of glands. Inflammation of external parts; of bone, excessive physical irritability and sensitiveness to jarring. Great *lassitude and desire to lie down*; lying ameliorates and motion aggravates. This remedy is full of pain; pain in the bones; the pains in the body are boring, burning, *cutting*, pressing, sore, *stitching and tearing*. Pressure ameliorates many symptoms. There is a marked pulsation felt all over the body and in the limbs. Pulse fast in the evening and until 2 a. m. There is marked sensitiveness in the remedy. The bones and glands become very sensitive. The symptoms are worse after sleep, worse from touch, when walking and after wine. Trembling and twitching. Great weakness in the morning, from walking; NERVOUS WEAKNESS. He is weary throughout the proving.

He becomes angry when contradicted. Anxiety in the evening and during the night but especially before midnight; anxiety at night in bed; after eating; on waking; during the night. Concentration of mind is difficult. He has lost all confidence in his own judgment. There is confusion of mind in the morning and in the evening; after eating; FROM MENTAL EXERTION; on waking. He is over-conscientious and there are moments of being discouraged and sometimes despair. Dullness of mind on waking. Worse from reading or any *mental exertion*;

all of the mental symptoms are worse from *mental exertion*. He is very excitable. He wakes up with anxiety and fear. His memory is very weak; he forgets almost everything. He is *easily frightened*. The female provers become quite hysterical. The first stage of imbecility is the general character of many mental symptoms. He is very indifferent to his friends and surroundings; irresolution is a strong feature and he cannot conclude to do one thing or the other. Irritability in the evening; after coition; after sleep. He no longer desires to live and seems to loathe life. A high degree of mental prostration prevails. Restless during the night driving him out of bed and with it there is great anxiety. Sadness during menses, with weeping. Extreme sensitiveness to noise. Starting from fright; *from noise*; from sleep. Indisposed to take a part in any conversation. Vertigo at night; with headache; from mental exertion; while walking; when turning in bed.

The following particulars will always yield to this remedy whenever the above generals strongly predominate.

There is tension of the scalp and especially of the forehead; *falling of the hair*; hyperaemia, fullness and heat of the head at night, felt especially in the forehead; heaviness of the head and forehead. It is wonderful headache remedy; the headaches are of many kinds and the circumstances numerous. Pain morning, afternoon, *evening* or night; pain worse after eating; from motion; *from exertion*; MENTAL EXERTION; before and during menses; binding up the hair in women; *from noise*; rising from sitting; sitting; after sleep; stooping; straining eyes; walking; wine. Pressure ameliorates; very hot applications are grateful. It is very useful in periodical headaches. With coryza there is severe pain in the forehead especially on the left side; comes on in the morning; pain in forehead above the eyes; pain in OCCIPUT; sides of head;

temples; pain bursting; drawing in forehead; dull, jerking. Pressing from mental exertion in forehead, as if brain would be forced out; pressing in occiput, temples, forehead; stitching in forehead; sides of head; temples; stunning pains in the head; forehead, sides of head, temples; perspiration of forehead; pulsation in head; forehead, vertex twitching of the head. Uncovering the head brings on headache.

The lids are stuck together in the morning. Fistula lachrymalis. Heaviness of the lids; inflammation with ulceration of the cornea; inflammation of the lids; itching of the eyes and lachrymation. Biting, burning, pressing, sore, stitching pains in eyes. Paralysis of the optic nerve. Photophobia, especially in daylight. Staring appearance; swollen lids; dark colors before the eyes; sparks in the field of vision. The vision is dim. Symptoms are worse from exertion of vision.

Itching in the ears; noises in the ear with vertigo; humming, ringing and roaring in ears; pain in ears and behind ears; stitching. Tearing in and behind ears; pulsation in ears. Stopped sensation. Hearing is acute for noise. Hearing is impaired.

Fluent coryza with cough. It cures catarrh of the nose with crusts and greenish, *offensive, purulent, thick* or *yellow* discharges. Epistaxis in the morning and on blowing the nose. The nose is obstructed during the night. Smell acute at first, later lost. Much sneezing. Ulcer high up in nose.

The lips are cracked; the face is pale, even earthly, or red with headaches; sometimes yellow. Eruptions on face worse on nose; herpes around lips; vesicles on lips; itching. Some pain in face. The glands of lower jaw swollen; *swelling of the submaxillary gland* and lips; ulcer on the lip.

Bleeding gums; *dryness of the mouth*; saliva flows

freely; speech is difficult. Taste is bitter, bloody. Metallic; sour. The teeth are painful during the night, and after eating; better from warmth. The pains are boring, digging, pulsating and stitching. The teeth are sensitive.

The throat is inflamed and red, *very dry*. He hawks much to clear the throat of thick, yellow mucus; sensation of lump in the throat; pain in the throat on swallowing; burning and stitching in the throat. Swallowing is difficult. It cures goitre and swollen cervical glands.

The appetite is increased and even ravenous; aversion to meat; a sensation of emptiness in the stomach. Eructations after eating: empty, tasting like food, sour; waterbrash. Many symptoms of stomach are better after eructations. Fullness after eating. Heartburn. Weight in the stomach and hiccough after eating; loathing of food; nausea morning and evening, and during diarrhœa; pains in stomach after eating; cramping, pressing, after eating; stitching pain; sore and tender to touch. Pulsation in the stomach. Retching. Sensation of a stone in the stomach. Extreme thirst, worse at night; during chill. Vomiting on coughing; after milk; bile, bitter; mucus.

Distension after eating; obstructed flatulence; fullness and gurgling; a commotion in the abdomen. Hard, heavy abdomen. Pain in morning, afternoon, night; after eating; in hypogastrium; in hypochondrium; burning, cramping, cutting, stitching in hypochondria, liver and spleen; rumbling in bowels. Sensation of tightness in abdomen.

Constipation with difficult even soft stool; fruitless urging to stool; inactivity of the rectum; unsatisfactory stool. Constricted anus. Diarrhœa morning and evening, from milk, painless; stool bloody, frequent slimy, thin, watery; constipation with stool hard, light colored, soft, scanty. Formication of the anus and much flatus. Itching. Pain after stool; burning during and after a hard stool; soreness of anus, with cutting, stitching and tenesmus.

Pressing in the bladder; tenesmus; constant or frequent urging to urinate; worse during the night; urination frequent during the night. Involuntary urination at night. Must wait long for urine to start in the morning. After urination he feels that he has not finished. Emission of prostatic fluid during a difficult stool; enlarged prostate. Burning during urination. The urine is hot, cloudy, *copious*.

Troublesome, painful, violent erections; the glans penis is inflamed; itching of the penis and scrotum; pain in the testes; seminal emissions. Sexual passion increased. Swelling of the testes. It greatly restrains the progress of cancer of the cervix uteri. The desire is much increased. Induration of the cervix. Leucorrhœa copious and yellow before menses: menses absent, copious, frequent or late; protracted, scanty. Bearing down in the pelvis as in prolapsus. Pain in left ovary during coition.

Irritation in the larynx; hoarseness; respiration is rapid; asthmatic, *deep, difficult, short.*

Cough in daytime, morning, afternoon, evening, *night*; dry, hacking cough in morning; loose cough in the morning; cough from irritation in the larynx; cough during chill, cough with expectoration morning and evening. Expectoration bloody, greenish; *offensive, purulent*; viscid, yellow, tasting putrid, salty.

Constriction and oppression of the chest; pain in chest on coughing. Pressing in the region of heart. Rawness in chest on coughing; chest feels sore and bruised on coughing; stitching in sides of chest, especially the right. Palpitation strong, worse at night, after eating. Swelling of the axillary glands.

Coldness of the back; itching of the skin of the back; pain in the back during menses; on motion; while sitting. Pain between the scapulæ; pain in lumbar region in stooping pain in sacrum; aching in back; lumbar region; burning in lumbar region; drawing in cervical region; soreness in spine; stitching between scapulæ; in lumbar region, in sacrum. Perspiration on the back; stiffness of the cervical region; during headache. Tension in the cervical region. Weak feeling in small of the back.

Awkwardness in using the hands and in walking. Coldness of hands, lower limbs, *legs*, FEET; evening in bed; corns that are sore and sting; cracked skin of hands and fingers. Cramp in calf, foot, toes. Vesicles on fingers and lower limbs. Heat of hands; of feet; of soles. Heaviness of upper limbs; *lower limbs*; feet. Itching of upper limbs; lower limbs; legs, *soles*, toes. Jerking of limbs during sleep. Jerking of lower limbs. Numbness of the right arm in the morning; of the arm lain on; of feet. Pain in joints, pain in shoulder. Bruised pain in limbs. Drawing pain in elbow; forearm; lower limbs; thighs; knee; leg. Stitching in hip, thighs, knees, legs, ankles, soles, heels. Tearing in limbs; joints; upper limbs; shoulders; upper arm; elbow; wrist; fingers. Tearing in *hip*, thigh, knee, leg, foot, toes. Paralytic weakness of side of body; right arm and right lower limb. Perspiration of hands and *feet*. Restless arms and feet. Stiffness of the limbs. Oedematous swelling of feet and legs. Tension of calf. Tingling of fingers. Trembling of hands and lower limbs. Twitching in limbs; upper limbs; forearm; thighs. Weakness of limbs; upper limbs; hands, lower limbs; thighs; *legs*, ANKLES; feet.

Dreams ANXIOUS; previous events; frightful; of ghosts; nightmare; murder; pleasant; VIVID. Falling asleep late. Restless sleep. Sleeplessness before midnight, *after midnight*; with sleepiness. Sleep unrefreshing; waking too early; too frequent. Sleepless during nightly fevers.

Chill morning; forenoon; evening in bed. Chill in cold air; after eating; one-sided, chilliness. Shaking chill. Internal chill. Flushes of heat. Fever without chill or

11

sweat from 9 p. m. until 2 a. m. with very red face and hot skin.

Perspiration nights; cold, on *least exertion*; profuse. Biting of the skin after scratching. Blotches here and there in the skin. Burning skin. Coldness of the skin. Desquamation. Dry burning skin. Eruptions; Boils; burning, moist; dry; herpetic; itching; painful; pimples; stinging; urticaria; vesicular. Formication. Itching, biting, burning, crawling worse after scratching. Itching stinging. Moisture after scratching. Sensitive sore skin. Unhealthy skin.

NATRUM SULPHURICUM
AND SYCOSIS

As its name indicates, it is the chemical combination of Natrum and Sulphur, Glauber's salts, Sulphate of soda. It partakes of the wonderful properties of both Sodium and Sulphur, and some day will become a very frequently indicated remedy. It is a remedy which typically corresponds to many of the complaints of a bilious climate. Natrum sulphuricum combines, in a measure, the wonderful effects of Natrum muriaticum and of Sulphur in the Western climate, as an active malarial agent. Malarial climates are all more or less bilious. Of course, I do not mean every man or every woman that comes to you and says: "Doctor, I am bilious." We never know what that means. It means more or less liver; it means more or less stomach; a general derangement of the system. Any kind of sickness may be called biliousness, but where the liver and stomach combine to effect disorders, we have true biliousness.

It is a most wonderful combination in its symptoms, because it not only pertains to muscular debility and disturbances of the general structures of the body, but also combines that which gives it consideration mentally. Its complaints are those that are brought on from living in damp houses, living in basements, and in cellars. They are generally worse in rainy, wet weather; hence it was called, primarily, by Grauvogl, one of his hydrogenoid remedies. It produces a profound impression upon the system in a general way like sycosis and a deep-seated or suppressed sycotic disease. Therefore, it is one of the grandest remedies underlying asthma, asthmatic and inherited complaints. In fact, Natrum Sulphuricum is one of the best, one of the clear-cut indicated remedies for those constitutional conditions in children that result in chest catarrhs and asthmatic complaints. This shows you only one of its hereditary features. Now, if we take into consideration the sycotic nature, the hydrogenoid condition of the constitution—always worse in wet weather— and this heredity, we have one of the grand features of this medicine.

Its next grand sphere is its action upon the liver and stomach, producing a bilious disturbance. We have, corresponding with this liver excitement a long list of mental symptoms marked with irritability, anxiety, desire to die, aversion to life and to things in life that would generally make people pleasant and comfortable. Now, if I begin on this mental state and go down through it, we will see more of it.

A good wife goes to her husband and says: "If you only knew what restraint I have to use to keep from shooting myself you would appreciate my condition!" It is attended with wildness and irritability. No remedy has that symptom like Natrum sulphuricum. You may examine the various remedies in our drug pathogenesy and you will find almost every kind of mental symptom, but here is one that stands by itself—this wonderful restraint to prevent doing herself bodily harm, is characteristic of Natrum sulphuricum. The satiety of life, aversion to life; the great sadness, the great despondency, coupled with the irritability and dread of music—music makes her weep,

makes her sad, makes her melancholy—this symptom runs
through the Natrums which it receives from the Natrum
side of its family; Natrum carbonate, Natrum muriaticum,
Natrum sulphuricum, all have it. Anything like melan-
cholic strains aggravate her complaints; mild music, gentle light, mellow light that pours through church windows,
these little glimmers of light that come through the colored glass, all these make her sad. Now, such are the mental characteristics of Natrum sulphuricum.

With the constitutional troubles there are important
head symptoms—mental symptoms from injuries of the
head. A young man in St. Louis was hurled from a truck
in the fire department. He struck on his head. Following
this for five or six months he had fits; I do not know what
kind of fits he had; some said epilepsy. Some said one
thing and some another, and some said he would have to
be trephined. He was an Allopathist, of course, as these
firemen all are, for it is hardly ever that you can get one
to go outside of Allopathy and try something else. He
was a good, well-bred Irishman; so he had to have some
good stout physic. Some of his friends prevailed upon
him to stay in the country for a while. He did so, but he
did not get better; he was irritable; he wanted to die. His
wife said she could hardly stand it with him; always
wanted to die; did not want to live. His fits drove him to
distraction. He did not know when he was going to have
one, they were epileptiform in character. Well, in the
country he ran across a homeopathic doctor, because he
had one of these attacks and the handiest doctor at the
time was a Homœopath. That Homœopath told him
that he had better come back to St. Louis and place himself under my care. He did so. At that time it had been
about six months that he had been having these fits.
When he walked into my office he staggered; his eyes were
nearly bloodshot; he could hardly see, and he wore a shade
over his eyes—so much was he distressed about the light

—such a photophobia. He had constant pain in his head.
He had injured himself by falling upon the back of his
head, and he had with this all the irritability that I have
described. There was nothing in his fits that was distinctive of a remedy, and the first thing that came into my
head was Arnica; that is what everybody would have
thought. Arnica, however, would not have been the best
remedy for him. Had I known no other or better remedy,
Arnica would have perhaps been the best. As soon as he
had finished his description, and I had given the case more
thought, I found that Natrum sulphuricum was the best
indicated remedy for injuries about the head, and I have
been in the habit of giving it. So I gave it in this case.
The first dose of Natrum sulphuricum cured this young
man. He has never had any pain about the head since.
He has never had any mental trouble since, never another
fit. That one prescription cleared up the entire case. If
you will just remember the chronic effects from injuries
upon the skull—not fractures, but simple concussions that
have resulted from a considerable shock and injuries without organic affections—then Natrum sulphuricum should
be your first remedy. Now, that may not be worth remembering, but when you have relieved as many heads as I
have with Natrum sulphuricum you will be glad to have
been informed of this circumstance. Ordinarily, Arnica
for injuries and the results of injuries, especially the neuralgic pains and the troubles from old scars; but in mental
troubles coming on from a jar or a knock on the head or a
fall or injury about the head, do not forget this medicine,
because if you do many patients may suffer where they
might have been cured had you made use of this remedy.

It has violent head pains, and especially so in the base
of the brain; violent pains in the back of the neck;
violent crushing pains as if the base of the brain
were crushed in a vice, or as if a dog were gnawing
at the base of the brain. These symptoms have led me to

prescribe this medicine. In the spinal meningitis of to-day, if all the remedies in the Materia Medica were taken away from me and I were to have but one with which to treat that disease, I would take Natrum sulphuricum, be-cause it will modify and save life in the majority of cases. It cuts short the disease surprisingly when it is the truly indicated remedy. In relation to the symptoms that you are likely to find in spinal meningitis, there is a drawing back of the neck and spasms of the back, together with all the mental irritability and delirium already described. The violent determination of blood to the head we find in this disease, clinically, is readily relieved.

The next most important feature is in relation to the eyes. That is characteristic, and is equaled only by one other remedy in chronic diseases where there is an aversion to life with photophobia, and that is Graphites. You take these cases of chronic conjunctivitis, with granular lids, green pus, terrible photophobia, so much so that he can hardly open his eyes; the light of the room brings on headache, distress and many pains. Here Natrum sulphur-icum should be compared with Graphites, because Graph-ites has also an extreme aggravation from light in eye ef-fections. Of course, this classes it entirely away from Belladonna and the other remedies that have acute photo-phobia, of acute determination of blood to the brain, be-cause it gives you a chronic state and condition that you must study.

Natrum sulphuricum produces a stuffing up of the nose, red tongue, irritable mucous membrane of the eyes, nose, and ears, with great dryness and burning in the nose. Pus becomes green upon exposure to the light.

The mouth always tastes bad. The patient says: "Doctor, my mouth is always full of slime." That is a common expression of the patient when he comes to you. And the provers, all of them, said that they were troubled with a slimy mouth. Thick, tenacious, white mucus in the mouth. Always hawking up mucus; it wells up from the stomach; mucus from the œsophagus; mucus by belching; mucus coughed up from the trachea, and it is always foul and slimy.

There is a distended feeling in the stomach; a sense of a weight in the stomach; almost constant nausea; vomiting of slime, bitter and sour. These are the characteristics: bitter and sour.

A sensation of weight in the right hypochondrium, in the region of the liver; aching pains; sometimes cutting pains, and a great amount of distress in the region of the liver. Engorgement in the region of the liver. He can only lie on his right side, his complaints are aggravated from lying on his left side. When lying on the left side, the congested liver seems to pull and draw; the great weight increases the pain and uneasiness and he is compelled to turn back on the right side. Now, it is from these symptoms, whenever a patient comes into my office and says, "Doctor, my mouth is so slimy and tastes so bad, and I think I am bilious," that he always gets Natrum sulphuricum.

Natrum sulphuricum produces great flatulence, distention of the abdomen, cutting pains in the abdomen, associated with congestion of the liver. In this tympanitic condition of the liver that sometimes comes on in the inflammatory conditions in bilious fever, you will find Natrum sulphuricum your remedy.

I began the use of this remedy with Schussler's remedies some years ago, and find the indications well carried out by the higher and highest potencies. Bell says that if the thirtieth potency of Arsenic is equal to a complete knowledge of the drug, crude Arsenic would be equal to complete ignorance.

There is a condition of the chest that is characteristic, and that is in relation to the cough. It has a cough with a sensation of "all-goneness" in the chest. In this it competes with Bryonia; both hold the chest when coughing. Bryonia holds the chest because he feels as if it would fly to pieces; there is such a soreness that he feels the necssity of steadying his chest. The complaints of Bryonia are relieved by pressure. Natrum sulphuricum has this same desire to hold the chest; but in Natrum sulphuricum the muco-pus that is expectorated is thick, ropy and yellowish green, looking like pus—purulent—and there is an "all-gone," empty feeling in the chest. He feels a sense of weakness there; that his lungs are all gone, that he must die in a few days with consumption or some other failing like that, and that it is coming on in a short time.

Bryonia corresponds more to the irritable states with the cough, where there is great rawness, great constriction, great sense of tearing in the chest; burning in the chest; while Natrum sulphuricum corresponds to a case that has been going on for perhaps a week; every cough brings up a mouthful of purulent sputa with a desire to press upon the chest to relieve the weakness; Natrum sulphuricum is then your remedy.

Another condition is that of humid asthma. If a child has asthma, give Natrum sulphuricum as the first remedy. Asthma, when hereditary, is one of the sycotic complaints of Hahnemann. You will not find that in your text-books, so do not look for it, but it may be an observation worth knowing. I have cured a very large number of such cases of asthma, although the text-books would discourage you if you should read them under asthma, because they will tell you that cases of asthma are incurable. For years I was puzzled with the management of asthma. When a person came to me and asked: "Doctor, can you cure asthma?" I would say, "No." But now I am beginning to get quite liberal on asthma, since I have learned that asthma is a sycotic disease, and since I have made judicious application of anti-sycotics I have been able to relieve or cure a great number of such cases. You will find in the history of medicine that wherever asthma was cured, it has been by anti-sycotic remedies. That is one of the first things I observed, that outside of sycotics you will seldom find a cure for asthma. There is that peculiarity that runs through sycosis which gives you a hereditary disease, and asthma corresponds to that disease. Hence it is that Silicea is one of the greatest cures for asthma; it does not cure every case, but when Silicea corresponds to the symptoms, you will be surprised to note how quickly it will eradicate it. While Ipecac, Spongia, and Arsenicum will correspond just as clearly to the supervening symptoms and to everything that you can find about the case, yet what do they do? They palliate; they repress the symptoms; but your asthma is no better off, your patient is not cured. Arsenic is one of the most frequently indicated remedies for the relief of asthma; so also are Bryonia, Ipecac, Spongia and Carbo veg., but they do not cure; though they relieve surprisingly at times. Where a patient is sitting up, covered with a cold sweat, wants to be fanned by somebody on either side of the bed, dyspnoea is so distressing that it seems almost impossible for the patient to live longer, to get another breath, then Carbo veg. comes in and gives immediate relief and the patient will lie down and get a very good night's rest. But what is the result? On comes the asthma again the very next cold. Natrum sulphuricum goes down to the bottom of this kind of a case. If it is hereditary, that is, not long-lived, if it is in a growing subject, Natrum sulphuricum goes down to the bottom of such a case and will cure when its symptoms are present; and the symptoms will so often be present. It is because of this deep seated anti-sycotic nature, we find in the combination of Natrum and Sulphur, that we have a new state and combination running into the life. When the chest is filling up with mucus, rattling of mucus, expectoration of large quantities of white mucus, with asthmatic breathing in young subjects, this remedy must be thought of.

In relation to the genito-urinary organs, we have some very valuable symptoms. In chronic gonorrhœa, with greenish or yellowish-green discharges. Instead of gonorrhœa running off into white, gleety discharge, it keeps up a yellowish, thick, greenish discharge. It competes here with Thuja and Mercurius, both of which are anti-sycotics. When Natrum sulphuricum is indicated there is generally very little pain, it is almost painless. There is chronic loss of sensibility in the part.

The urine is loaded with bile, is of a pinkish or yellowish color, with a "corn-meal" sediment, or it looks like stale beer and is extremely offensive. Offensive urine is not in the text.

Like sulphur, it has burning of the soles of the feet at night, and the burning extends to the knees; burning from the knees down. It has also, like sulphur, great burning in the top of the head; it has tearing, rending, cutting pains from the hips down to the knees; worse at night. The stomach symptoms are worse in the morning, and so also with the mental symptoms, they are generally worse in the morning.

Now, upon the skin we have some eruptions; we have those cases of so called itch, scabies or vesicular eruptions, vesicular eczema, with a thin, watery discharge exuding from the fingers, and the fingers are swollen stiff and stand out stiffened by the swelling; they are swollen so stiff they can hardly be gotten together. (Baker's itch and barber's itch come under this head). Natrum sulphuricum cures where the palms of the hands are raw and sore and exude a watery fluid. Also vesicular eruptions around the mouth and chin and various parts of the body; little, fine water blisters, very much like Natrum muriaticum and very much also like Natrum carb. So you see it runs into the Natrums. The other disease that I incidentally mentioned a moment ago—the barber's itch—is a sycotic disease, a sycosis menti, a disease of the hair follicles. It is sometimes even contagious. It is one of the highest types of sycosis; the next highest type of sycosis is the venereal wart known as the gonorrhœal warts. This medicine corresponds to this state and condition of the body.

Now, we have said considerable about sycosis. We know in sycosis, which is a constitutional miasm, that we have venereal warts or gonorrhœal warts; that we have another sycotic state that comes upon the female in cauliflower excresences. We have also hereditary asthma, a constitutional disease that depends upon sycosis, and this peculiar barber's itch is one of the highest types of sycosis; they are all due to one cause, and some day this cause will be demonstrated to be latent sycosis. Gonorrhœa will will some day be known to be the true offspring of this sycosis. It is the contagious part of the sycosis. It is the means by which the disease is handed from generation to generation. This thing you will not find in the books, and it is, perhaps, only a private opinion and, therefore, worthless. But some day you will remember that I told you this. I have seen things in my observation that astonished me. I believe I have solved what Hahnemann called sycosis, though he has never described it. To me it is very clear from the cases I have cured, with this theory in view or this doctrine in view. The cases I have cured lead me to believe that I am on the right track.

Now, I say that gonorrhoea and all of these latent conditions of the body are one and the same thing; that primarily they date back to one and the same source. Of course, the books will tell you that gonorrhœa is not a constitutional disease; but when gonorrhœa will produce warts, and gonorrhœal rheumatism, and will last throughout life, and children be brought into the world with the same disease, how are you going to get around it? There was a young man in the St. Louis City Hospital who had been there many months, and who was so sore in the bottoms of his feet that he could not get around; he had to leave his business, he was a baker. Finally his old employer came to me and wanted to know if I could do anything for that young man. I did not know anything about the nature of his disease. I told him to bring the young man to me. He was brought, and I learned from his history that years before he had had gonorrhœa; that it had been suppressed with injections. I put him under such constitutional treatment as these theories that I have just mentioned guided me to, and I cured him. In our city I have cured twenty-five or thirty cases of this peculiar kind of sycosis that dated back to a latent gonorrhœa. Symptoms of a latent gonorrhœa are unknown to the books. You will find nothing of it. It is known only to such observers as have been able to make two out of two times one—by putting things together. By and by I shall have a complete chain of evidence to show that gonorrhœa is a constitutional disease and can be handed down from father to son, as can syphilis. It is one of the chronic miasms, and one about which very little is known. If this be true, it is as dangerous to suppress a gonorrhœal discharge before its time, as it is to suppress a syphilitic chancre before its time. You will never know if you go on treating these constitutional miasms by suppressing the primary manifestations—you will never know the harm you are doing.

The most of these are calculated by the process of evolution to wear themselves out, to roll out, or to evolve themselves into symptoms that are so depleting to the disease that they leave of themselves, or leave the patient very nearly free from the disease. Such is the calculation of Nature in a gonorrhœal discharge, and such has been the intention of Nature in the chancres that appear upon the genitalia. But poor ignorant man, believing he must do something, has made it his first business to cauterize these chancres—to dry up these discharges—and he does

not know how much harm he is doing. But this is only a
private opinion. I have observed this, that there are two
kinds of gonorrhœa—one is a simple urethral discharge,
which when stopped by injection, will not produce a constitutional taint, because that is not sycosis; and the other
form is the sycotic gonorrhœa, which, if suppressed with
injections, will appear in constitutional symptoms. Now,
it is for you to live and think for yourselves. If you can
make anything out of what I have told you, and it ever
helps anybody, I shall be amply repaid. You will most
naturally see that all these thoughts are in furtherance of
Hahnemann's teaching, based upon the facts observed by
him and his faithful followers. Unless guided by the light
of the dynamic doctrine of disease and cure, these things
would scarcely be observed. For the study of this sycosis
I might have taken up Thuja, but knowing how well the
master has performed his work, I have taken a remedy
that is scarcely second in importance to bring out as well
the use of a remedy as a miasm in relation to it.

SULPHUR IODATUM

This is a very profound and long-acting remedy affecting all parts of the body with aggravations morning,
afternoon, *evening*, NIGHT, and after midnight. Desires
open air, *which ameliorates* the most of his symptoms.
There is an indescribable feeling throughout the body like
a *general physical anxiety*, which compels him to hurry in
all his work and when walking. Atrophy of glands,
chronic jerking of muscles and a sensation of a band
around parts. He takes cold on the slightest provocation,
while he desires to be in a cool place, and in the cold air
he takes cold from becoming cold. There is a convulsive
tendency in the remedy; hysterical and epileptiform. The
cavities become dropsical. Some symptoms are better after
eating, and others are worse. Emaciation is marked, and

it should be of great service in marasmus of children, with increased appetite. Slight exertion brings on all the symptoms: Weakness and palpitation; faint and fainting spells, with palpitation; feels unusually weak when hungry, warm food brings on much distress; formication all over; full feeling in body and limbs; body feels distended, as if there were great vascular engorgement; hemorrhage from internal parts; *great heat of the body*, which is only a sensation; heaviness of body and limbs; INDURATION OF GLANDS; hard, knotty lymphatic glands in the neck like ropes; induration of muscles. This feature points to its usefulness in carcinoma of glands. When used early it is often able to cure promptly. Inflammation of organs and glands. Injuries with extravasations. Lack of reaction and marked lassitude. The symptoms are worse while lying, but sometimes better after lying a long time. Worse lying on the back and worse in a warm bed. It is an antidote to the over use of mercury. Though he is restless and desires to move, the motion increases his symptoms. From all mucous membranes there is an increased flow. There is numbness in single parts and in suffering parts. There is a marked surging of blood in the body with general pulsation and hot sensations. Pain in bones and glands. These bruised, burning, cutting, jerking, *pressing*, stitching and tearing pains; when heated he sweats much and cannot cool off without taking cold. Its complaints are such as are found in plethoric, full blooded, vascular people. Any kind of hurry or running creates a flush and surging in the body with palpitation and weakness. Many symptoms are one-sided, especially the *right*. Sluggishness is a marked feature of the whole complex of symptoms; many symptoms are worse sitting and better standing. He is much worse in the heat of summer, and in the sun's heat. *Swelling of glands*.

Its symptoms are such as are often found in the

advanced stages of syphilis, and it is especially useful in such as have been heavily charged with mercury. The symptoms are worse from touch and pressure. Throughout the body there is a feeling of tension. Trembling, internal and external. The muscles twitch and the limbs jerk. The symptoms are worse from walking. The symptoms are worse *from warmth; warm air, warm bed. warm room, warm wraps.* Marked weariness in the morning; from ascending stairs; after diarrhœa; during menses; from walking. He is worse in wet weather, and better in winter.

Anxiety driving him to keep on the go. Apathy. Aversion to company. When reading and thinking cannot control the mind, Lost confidence in his own ability. Confusion of mind in the morning and evening, and when he exerts the mind. Over-conscientious about small matters. Says he is becoming timid, even cowardly. There are times in the night when he is almost delirious. Illusions of fancy. Sees dead people. Despair, cannot see any brightness in life. Discontented and discouraged. Dullness of mind. Very excitable. The whole mental state is worse from mental exertion. Dread of exertion. Fear that some unknown trouble is coming to him; of insanity; of misfortune; of people. He finds himself doing things in a great hurry. Walks fast and in a hurry. Strongly inclined to hysterical conduct. Very impatient, cannot wait, but must keep on the go. At times indifferent to all surroundings. She becomes indolent and neglects her housework. She cannot compel herself to attend to her duties. Her mood is very changeable; irritable or mirthful. Mental prostration. Very restless, and forced to keep on the move although moving causes weakness and increases her bodily symptoms. *Marked sadness*, and dullness of the senses. Would like to sit, but too restless.

Starting during sleep. Stupefaction of mind. Persistent thoughts torment her. Weeps much in the evening.

Vertigo in the morning on rising, while lying, during menses, rising from bed, rising from a seat, *stooping*, walking.

The following particulars will yield to this remedy whenever the general symptoms above mentioned strongly predominate.

The scalp feels cold to the patient. Congestion on coughing and during menses. Eruptions on the scalp; crusts, eczema. Itching eruptions and itching without eruptions. Heat in the head and the hair falls out. The hair stands on end. The head feels heavy. Pain in the head in the morning on rising; in the forenoon; in the afternoon. Headache is better in the open air, by cold applications, by motion. Headache worse by binding up the hair, from fasting, from becoming heated, before and during menses, from heat of sun, from talking, from *warm room* and from warm wraps on the body. Pain in forehead, over eyes, in the evening, worse from motion. Pain in occiput in the afternoon. Pain in both sides of the head and again on only one side. Pain in temples and vertex. Pressing pains in forehead, over eyes; in occiput; *sides of head*; temples; vertex. Shooting pains in head; in the temples when stooping. Sore, bruised feeling in head; stitching pains in occiput; sides of head; temples; *vertex*. Tearing pain in temples. Perspiration on scalp; on forehead. *Pulsation in head*; in the temples. Tension in the forehead. Wrapping up head brings on headache.

Dullness of eyes, inflammation of conjunctiva. Catarrhal inflammation in psoric patients. The lids feel heavy. Inflammation of the iris in syphilitic subjects. Copious lachrymation in cold air. Pressing, sore, stitching pains. Protrusion of the eyes. Pupils dilated. Redness of eyes and lids. Staring eyes. Sunken eyes with swollen lids. Twitching of the lids. Jaundiced eyes. *Dim*, foggy vision, and there is *flickering* and sparks. Diplopia.

Discharge of pus from ear. The ears are hot. Inflammation of eustachian tubes. Buzzing, humming, ringing, and roaring noises in ears. Itching in ears. Aching, pressing, shooting, stitching and tearing pains. Stopped sensation. Hearing acute for noise. Hearing impaired.

It cures our most obstinate catarrhal conditions, with discharges, as follows: Bloody, *copious, excoriating, greenish*, hard, dry masses; purulent, *thick*, YELLOW. Excoriation and itching in nose. Redness of the nose. Coryza fluent in the open air, coryza with cough, long continued. It is a very useful remedy in hay fever. Burning in the nose on blowing it. Pressing pain in roof of nose, loss of smell, sneezing in the *evening*. The nose is swollen. There are small ulcers up in the nose.

Cold face. Discoloration; red, circumscribed redness, *sallow, yellow*. Drawn face. Eruptions, acne, boils, pimples, crusty eruptions on the nose. Dry and hot. The expression is haggard and *sickly*. The face is Hippocratic. Induration of the parotid and submaxillary glands. The face is sunken with pain. Burning heat of the face. Swollen glands. Swollen parotid and submaxillary glands. Twitching of the face.

Copious aphthæ. Bleeding gums. Tongue coated at base, red at points. Cracked tongue. The gums are detached from the teeth. The *tongue is dry*. It overcomes the bad effect of the mercury. Much mucus forms in the mouth. Offensive, even putrid, odor from the mouth. Burning tongue. Salivation. Stammering speech. *Swollen gums*. The taste is bad, *bitter*, putrid, sour. Ulcers in the mouth and on the gums. Toothache after eating. Tearing pain in teeth.

Choking, constriction of œsophagus. Dryness of throat. Gray exudation in the throat. Tough, viscid, yel-

12

low or white mucus in throat. Pain in throat on coughing; when swallowing. Burning in throat and œsophagus. Pressing pain in throat. Sore throat in the morning. Scraping in throat. Swallowing of liquids difficult. Swelling of throat and uvula. Ulcers in throat. It has cured goitre. It has cured indurated lymphatic glands in the neck where they were like knotted ropes. Sore lymphatic glands of neck. Swelling of the lymphatic glands of the neck.

Appetite INCREASED; RAVENOUS; *with diarrhoea*; with emaciation; with marasmus in children; without relish of food; appetite wanting. Aversion to food. Desires stimulants, acids, pickles and lemonade. The stomach is easily disordered. Marked distension from gas and sensation of emptiness. Eructations empty, sour, waterbrash. Eructations ameliorate. There is fullness, heartburn, heaviness after eating and hiccough. Chronic indigestion, nausea, at night after eating. Pain in stomach after eating relieved by eructions. Burning, cramping, cutting, gnawing, pressing, stitching pain in stomach. Tenderness of stomach. Pulsation in stomach. Retching from the cough. Sensation of tightness. Thirst in the evening; burning, extreme, unquenchable. Vomiting on coughing; with diarrhœa, after drinking; after eating; after milk. Vomiting bloody bile; food sour, watery.

Atrophy of the liver. Suppurating bubos. Tympanitic, distension of abdomen. Enlarged abdomen. Enlarged liver, mesenteric glands, spleen, lymphatic glands of groin. Much flatulence, HARDNESS OF LIVER, *spleen* and glands of groin. Inflammation of spleen. It cures many complaints of the liver. Pain in abdomen after eating, before and during menses. Pain in *liver*, in hypogastrium, in inguinal region; in *spleen*, in region of umbilicus. Burning and cramping in umbilical region. Cutting during stool. Pressing in liver, in hypogastrium, in groin. Soreness and stitching pains in liver. Rumbling and pulsation in abdomen. Suppuration of inguinal glands. Swelling of *mesenteric glands and glands of groin.*

Constipation with no desire to go to stool for a long time, and great straining to pass a stool. The stool is incomplete and unsatisfactory. Constipation alternating with diarrhœa. The stool is hard, knotty and light colored. There is diarrhœa in the *morning* and evening, worse after eating. Diarrhœa in emaciated people and in aged people. The diarrhœa stools are variable; black, brown, frequent, frothy, offensive, purulent, watery, white, yellow. There is also dysenteric stools of bloody mucus, frequent, purulent, scanty, with tenesmus. Hemorrhoids, heat and *itching of the anus* and much flatus passes. Burning in anus after stool.

Retention of urine. Frequent urging to urinate, worse during the night. The urine passes by dribbling, and there is involuntary dribbling. Frequent urination at night. Also in the morning. Prostate gland is enlarged. The urine is albuminous, cloudy, dark, red, copious, milky, offensive, with red sediment. The urine smells like raspberries. There is a cuticle on the urine, and it sometimes becomes scanty.

Erections incomplete, without sexual desire or wanting. Erections troublesome at night. It has cured hydrocele of small boys. Induration of the testes. Itching of the penis; in the urethra. Perspiration of the scrotum. Relaxed genitals. Seminal emissions. Swelling of the testes. It has cured tuberculosis of testes and spermatic cords.

It has cured predisposition to abort. In cancer of the uterus it greatly restrains the progress of the disease and palliates the sufferings where the patient is very vascular, is losing flesh, has a strong appetite and very sensitive to heat. Increased sexual desire. Inflammation of the uterus. COPIOUS LEUCORRHŒA, acrid, bloody, *burning*, *thick* and sometimes thin, *yellow*, before and after menses. Menses absent, *copious*, frequent, *irregular*, painful, of short duration, suppressed. Metrorrhagia. Hard pain in ovaries. Great tenderness of vulva and *ovaries*. Prolapsus of uterus.

Catarrh of larynx and trachea. Dryness, crawling and constriction in the larynx. Much hawking. Inflammation of the larynx. Irritation of larynx and trachea. Laryngismus. Much mucus in the larynx and trachea; dark purulent. Pain, soreness and stitching in the larynx. For laryngeal phthisis, is a most useful remedy; where the general symptoms are present. Roughness in the larynx. Tickling in the larynx and trachea in a warm room. *Hoarseness* in the morning. Voice rough, weak and lost.

Respiration is fast; *asthmatic, irregular, rattling,* short, *suffocative,* and wheezing; difficult at night, on ascending and from least exertion. Desire for deep breath.

It is a highly important cough remedy. Cough *morning* and evening, asthmatic, choking and very exhausting. It is *paroxysmal, spasmodic,* rattling and suffocative. Cough during fever. Dry cough in the morning. Hard cough during the early part of the night. It also has a less cough. Cough from talking and smoking. The cough is relieved in the open air, from becoming cold and from expectoration; worse lying down and better from sitting up. Short hacking cough. Irritation to cough in the larynx and trachea. Expectoration morning and evening; *bloody, copious,* difficult, *greenish,* mucous, *offensive, purulent,* sweetish, tough, *viscid, yellow.*

Feeling of anxiety in the chest. It is of great service in cancer of the mammæ. It is a most valuable remedy in catarrh of the bronchial tubes, *constriction of chest* and heart, dropsy of the pleura, eruptions of the chest. Great heat of chest. Induration of the mammary glands. Inflammation of lungs and bronchial tubes. Inflammation of the pleura, especially where neglected. Itching of the skin. Where the milk becomes suppressed in the nursing woman. Oppression of the chest. Pain in chest on coughing; pain in side of chest, worse on the right side. Pain in the region of the heart. Aching burning and cutting. Cutting in the region of the heart. Pressing in sides of chest on coughing. Stitching in chest on coughing. *Palpitation at night, on exertion,* during menses, on motion. It is a very useful remedy in phthisical conditions of the lungs; in ulcerative conditions and cavities. Swelling of the axillary glands. Feeling of weakness in chest.

Itching of the lumbar region. Pain and soreness under scapulæ. Pain in lumbar region during menses. Pain in sacrum and coccyx. Stitching in the back; in the lumbar region. Weakness of spine.

Painful gouty nodosities of the fingers. Coldness in upper limbs; hands; legs; *feet at night.* Convulsive action of muscles in upper limbs. Old corns become painful. Cramps in thighs, *legs*; feet. Vesicles on the limbs. Heat of hands. Heaviness of the limbs; feet. Itching of upper limbs; lower limbs. Numbness of limbs; fingers; legs. Gouty and rheumatic pains in the joints and bones. The soles ache and burn when standing. Pain in upper limbs, worse on motion. Rheumatic pain in limbs. Pain in elbow. Pain in hip; thigh; *knee*; calf; foot. Drawing pains in lower limbs; thighs; knee. Pressing pains in upper limbs. Sore bruised pains in shoulder, upper arms and thighs. *Stitching in knees.* Tearing in upper limbs; elbows; knee; leg. Paralysis of lower limbs. Perspiration of hands, cold palms; *feet.* Pulsation in limbs. Stiffness of limbs; fingers. Dropsical swelling of limbs; hands; lower limbs; knees; legs; feet. Trembling of all the limbs. Twitching in thighs, weakness of limbs; knees.

Dreams amorous; anxious; of dead people; distressing;

nightmare; vivid; sleep is restless. Sleepiness in the evening. Sleepiness during daytime and sleepless at night. Sleeplessness after midnight; waking too early.

Chill at night in bed, better after rising. Internal chill. Warm room does not relieve. Warm bed does not relieve. Shaking chill worse from motion. Quartan or tertian. Fever in the afternoon alternating with chill. External heat. FLASHES OF HEAT. It is a very useful remedy in hectic fever. Internal heat with external chill. Fever without sweat. Chill followed by heat. Wants to be uncovered during heat. Perspiration morning and night in bed. Clammy, cold, exhausting sweat. *Sweat from slight exertion*; from motion. Profuse sweat during the night. The sweat smells sour.

Anæsthesia. The skin sometimes burns; again it is cold. The skin desquamates. Discoloration; liver spots, red spots; yellow skin; yellow spots. The skin is dry. Eruptions; boils; blood boils; herpes; pimples; psoriasis; pustules; rash; scaly; urticaria. Where eruptions have been suppressed by ointments. Erysipelatous inflammation of the skin. The skin becomes excoriated easily. Excrescenses form upon the skin. Formication. Freckles. Inactivity of the skin. Itching, burning and stinging. Burning in swollen skin. Burning in erysipelas. Pale, spongy, dropsical swelling of skin. Tension of skin. Ulcers: Bleeding; cancerous, *indolent*; indurated; sensitive *spongy*; suppurating. The discharges from ulcers are bloody, copious, corrosive, thin, watery, yellow.

VESPA VULGARIS

A young man in perfect health was stung by a large number of wasps. Frequent convulsions followed, involving all the muscles of the body, with loss of consciousness; the convulsions disappeared after three years, leaving him subject to attacks of unconsciousness when walking about.

He often starts to go somewhere and finds himself several blocks beyond the place he started for.

The period of unconsciousness lasts several minutes. He does not fall nor does he drop things which he happens to hold in his hands.

If spoken to he does not answer nor seem to hear or notice anything; he looks into space. When he comes to himself, he has no memory of the moments that have passed; he is as bright as ever. He has no warning of the coming spell: A friend remarked that his eyes were glassy and bloodshot, and he looked as though he had no sense.

When standing upon the platform of a street car, he was noticed to grasp the iron railing and look wild; two men standing near him undertook to loosen his hands and put him in a seat, but they could not force him to let loose until he came to himself, and then he needed no aid. It was thought that he continued to grasp the railing about ten minutes, but time flies under excitement, and no one has timed this period.

He becomes sick and faint near a warm stove or in a close room; often gets up and leaves a close warm room to prevent vomiting; craves cold washing of hands and face which makes him feel better. Anger or excitement will bring on a spell.

The usual antidotes have helped for a while, and then the symptoms have returned with about the same general features.

Mentally he is not strong, and the tendency is to grow weaker.

WYETHIA

When in the autumn our hay-fever patients report to us with violent symptoms of coryza, great depression of spirits, symptoms worse in the afternoon, easy sweat and langour, extreme dryness of the mucous membranes of nose, mouth and throat, with burning acrid copious flow of mucus, constant swallowing, itching of the soft palate, and compelled to scratch it with the tongue, Wyethia will cure for the season, and it has cured permanently in some cases.

ZINCUM PHOSPHORICUM

The times of aggravation of this remedy are *morning*, forenoon, AFTERNOON, EVENING, NIGHT.

He has a strong craving for warm, fresh air and is markedly sensitive to drafts; the open air ameliorates in general; marked general physical anxiety; many symptoms are worse from ascending. Hands and feet and other single parts go to sleep and become numb. Many symptoms come on from bathing. Some symptoms are worse after breakfast. It has been a very useful remedy in the treatment of chorea; lack of vital heat; sensitiveness to cold air. Symptoms come on from becoming cold and in cold, wet weather There is constriction like a band around the body. There are convulsions: clonic; epileptiform; hysterical; internal; tonic. Some complaints are worse and some are better from eating. Complaints are worse after the least physical exertion. Frequent fainting spells. Several kinds of food seem to disagree: bread; milk; sweets; warm drinks; cold drinks ameliorate. Marked formication all over the body. There is marked *heaviness* in the body and limbs. Great sluggishness and *lack of reaction*. Violent JERKING in the body. Extreme LASSITUDE with desire to lie down yet lying in bed aggravates many symptoms. Worse before, DURING and *after* menstruation. Some symptoms are worse and some are better from motion. Most symptoms are worse on beginning to move: there is aversion to motion: NUMBNESS in many parts. Pains are very numerous; BITING; *boring*; bruised; burning external and INTERNAL; CUTTING; pressing external and INTERNAL; STITCHING; TEARING in MUSCLES and NERVES. Paralysis one sided; of organs; painless. External and internal pulsation. Pulse: FAST; *intermittent*; *irregular*; *small*; weak. He desires to be rubbed and most symptoms are ameliorated by rubbing. Sensitiveness prevails throughout the whole proving especially to pain. Electric shocks are quite common. From looking at the proving as a whole it may well be said that the symptoms resemble the results of sexual excesses. The symptoms are quite often one sided. The symptoms come on while SITTING, *standing* and during sleep. Throughout all the muscles a feeling of tension. Throughout the body and limbs extreme *trembling* and *twitching*. Uncovering aggravates. Walking ameliorates the restlessness and aggravates the weakness; ameliorates the pain in the back. There is marked weakness in the *morning* and evening; during menses; marked NERVOUS weakness; worse walking. A sensation of extreme weariness. The patient is very sensitive to wet weather to *wind* and to *wine*.

Becomes angry from trifles and even violent and his symptoms become worse from anger. Anxiety in morning; afternoon; night; with fever during menses; on waking. Wants things which he does not need. Aversion to being alone. Concentration of mind is quite difficult; confusion of mind in morning; on waking; evening; after eating. Much annoyed by presentiment of death. Delirium: frightful; raving; rasping with fingers; picking at the bed clothes; violent. Delusions of fancy and even sees dead people; fire; images at night. DULLNESS OF MIND. EXCITEMENT. Attempts to escape. Mental exertion aggravates his symptoms. Exaltation of fancy. Constantly APPREHENSIVE; evening; night; of death; ghosts; of robbers; on waking VERY FORGETFUL. His symptoms are worse from fright. He is heedless, impatient, impetuous, indifferent, extremely INDOLENT, and appears like one going into imbecility. It should become one of our most useful remedies in insanity. Marked irresolution. Irritability in the morning; EVENING; with headache; during menses. Silly spasmodic laughter followed by loquacity. *Loathing of life.* Malicious ideas come frequently. *Memory very weak.* Hilarity in the evening. Moods are very changeable. Morose, obstinate and easily offended. MENTAL PROSTRATION and aversion to work. Restlessness in the morning; evening; night; anxious. SADNESS in the morning; afternoon; evening. Marked dullness of the senses. Sensitive to music and to NOISE. Sexual excess aggravates the mental symptoms, shrieking out in sleep. Inclination to sit in perfect silence; indisposed to speak. Speech at times is incoherent. Starting easily during sleep. Marked stupefaction with much vertigo. Thinks much about suicide. His thoughts wander and vanish. He talks in sleep. Unusual timidity. Unconsciousness from fainting. Much weeping; during menses. Vertigo in the morning in bed; forenoon; noon; night; during headache; after dinner; tendency to fall; with nausea; before menses; while sitting; while standing; while walking.

The forehead is cold. There is constriction of the forehead and even of the whole head. Heat in the head especially in the evening; forehead. Hyperæmia of the brain. Eruptions on the scalp. The hair falls out. The head feels heavy in the morning and in the evening; forehead; occiput. The scalp itches. Pain in the head: in the morning in bed; *afternoon*; *evening*; at night; BETTER IN THE OPEN AIR; worse on ascending steps; binding up the hair; better from cold applications; worse after eating; from becoming heated; with desire to lie down; lying sometimes aggravates and sometimes ameliorates; before and during menses; *from mental exertion*; NERVOUS AND SPINAL HEAD-ACHES; worse from noises; paroxysmal; periodical every day; better from pressure; worse from the heat of the sun; from talking; while walking; warm room; WINE. Pain in the forehead in the morning; *above the eyes.* Pain in the *occiput*; *sides of the head*; *temples*; *vertex*. Burning pain in forehead. Sore bruised pain in the head. Bursting pain in the forehead. Drawing pain in the forehead; occiput; temples. Pressing outward in the *forehead*; over the eyes; occiput; sides of head; temples; occiput; vertex. Stitching pains in the head on coughing; forehead; sides; temple; vertex. Stunning pains in the head. Tearing pains in the head; forehead; occiput; SIDES; *temples*; vertex. Perspiration of the whole head; *forehead*. Pulsation in the whole head; forehead. The brain is very sensitive especially during menses. Electric shocks in head.

Agglutination of the lids in the morning. It has cured cataract. Thick muco-purulent discharge from the canthi. The eyes are very dry and lustreless. Heat and burning in the eyes. Inflammation of the lids. Itching of the lids and lachrymation in the open air. He lies with half open eyes Pain in the eyes; biting; burning in the evening; *pressing*; shooting; *stitching*; tearing. Paralysis of the lids; *optic nerve*. Photophobia in sunlight. Pupils contracted and then dilated. Redness of the margin of the lids. Staring and sunken look. Oedematous lids. Before the eyes there are floating spots; green colors; a halo of colors around the light. The vision is dim. Exertion of vision brings on many symptoms. There is flickering before the eyes. *Vision becomes foggy.* Bloody or purulent discharge from the ear. Itching in the ears. Noises: evening; night; with vertigo; buzzing; fluttering; ringing; *roaring*; whizzing. Pain IN THE EAR; behind the ear; burning; *stitching*; TEARING. Pulsation in the ear. There is swelling of the external ear and inside of the ears. Twitching of the ears. Hearing is impaired.

Catarrhal irritation of the nose with redness of the skin of the nose. Coryza worse in the evening; fluent alternating with dry. Discharge from the nose; bloody; *copi-*

ous; excoriating; purulent; thick; from posterior nares. A sensation of dryness in the nose. He blows blood from the nose. The nose feels obstructed. Itching inside the nose. Soreness inside the nose. Smell at first acute, later diminished. Frequent sneezing. The nose is red and swollen.

The lips are dry and cracked. Much discoloration of the face; bluish circles around the eyes; earthly or pale; sickly face. Eruptions on the nose; pimples on the face and forehead; vesicles. The expression is sickly and haggard. Much itching of the skin of the face. It has cured right-sided paralysis of the face. The face looks sunken and distressed. The lips are swollen. There is a twitching of the muscles of the face. Small ulcers of the lips and corners of the mouth.

The gums bleed and the tongue is cracked. The mouth is dry and the tongue is coated white. The gums are painful and sore and the tongue burns. The papillæ on the tongue are erect. Salivation with bloody saliva, scorbutic gums. The gums are much swollen. Taste, bad; bitter; insipid; metallic; saltish; sweetish. Small ulcers upon the gums. Vesicles upon the tongue. The teeth become loose. Pain in the teeth; masticating; from pressure; on going to sleep; burning; drawing; jerking; pulsating; sore; stitching; tearing.

Constriction and *dryness* in the throat; constriction of the œsophagus. Frequent hawking. Throat is much inflamed. Sensation of a lump in the throat. Constant formation of tenacious mucus in the throat. Constantly scraping the throat. Pain in the throat on swallowing; burning; pressing; rawness; soreness. Spasms of the œsophagus on swallowing. Difficult swallowing of solids or liquids. Swelling of the throat, tonsils, and uvula. Drawing and pressing in the sides of the throat externally.

Appetite is variable; capricious; diminished; increased,

even ravenous; ravenous after eating; wanting at noon; wanting with thirst. Aversion to food; to cooked food; to meat; to sweets; to warm drinks; to wine.

Constrictive sensations in the stomach. Desires beer and cold drinks. A SENSATION OF EMPTINESS IN THE STOMACH. Eructations; in the evening; ameliorated by; after eating; ineffectual; acrid; bitter; empty; tasting of the food eaten; sour after eating and after milk; water brash. Fullness after eating with heaviness. Hiccough after eating. Heaviness in the stomach. NAUSEA; in the morning; noon; after eating; during headache. Pain in the stomach: morning; evening; after eating; during menses; burning; cramping; cutting; gnawing; fuming; soreness; stitching. Sinking in the stomach with retching. Extreme thirst in the afternoon and evening. VOMITING: morning; after drinking; *after eating*; with headache; during pregnancy; *bile*; bitter; black; blood; brownish; food; green; mucus; sour; *watery*; yellow.

Sensation of coldness in the abdomen. Distension of the abdomen after eating. Enlarged liver. Obstructed flatulence. Fullness after eating. Heaviness in the abdomen; sensation of a weight in hypochondria. Sensation of movements in the abdomen with gurgling. Pain in the abdomen; in the morning; in the evening; as if diarrhœa would come on; after eating; before menses; during menses; paroxysmal; after stool; while walking; in hypochondria; in hypogastrium before menses; in the inguinal region; in the region of the umbilicus.

Cramping pain in the morning; in the sides of the abdomen; in the umbilical region. Cutting pain in the region of the umbilicus. Dragging pain in the abdomen. Pressing in the hypogastrium and in the liver. Soreness in the hypochondria. Stitching pains in the abdomen; in the right hypochondrium; in the liver; in the side of the abdomen. Tearing pains in the abdomen. A nervous feeling in the abdomen; tension in the abdomen with *rumbling*.

CONSTIPATION: alternating with diarrhœa; stool very *difficult*; rectum inactive; no desire for stool; unsatisfactory stool; ineffectual straining; the stool is dry, hard, large, light-colored. *Diarrhoea*; afternoon, evening; painless; involuntary; with brain affections. The stool is bloody; brown; copious; frequent; green; offensive; watery. Copious flatus which ameliorates symptoms; offensive. Formication and itching in the anus in the evening. Hæmorrhoids external; bleeding. Much moisture about the anus. Pain in the anus and rectum; during stool; burning, during and after stool; cutting; pressing; soreness; stitching; tearing; tenesmus after stool. Prolapsus of the anus. Inefficient urging to stool.

Pressing pain in the bladder. Paralytic weakness of the bladder. Retention of urine. Spasmodic contractions in the bladder. *Urging to urinate*; night; ineffectual; sudden; must hasten or will lose the urine; sudden urging after urination. Urination dribbling; dysuria; feeble stream; frequent but worse at night; with interrupted stream. Urination involuntary but worse at night; during sleep; on coughing; after stool; weak bladder.

Pain in the kidneys; cutting in the ureters; stitching in the kidneys; suppression of urine. Emissions of prostatic fluid during difficult stool. Hæmmorhage from the urethra. Burning in the urethra during urination. Cutting and stitching in the urethra. Urine: albuminous; bloody; burning; CLOUDY ON STANDING; dark; *copious*; SEDIMENT; cloudy; flocculent and sandy and red, sandy and white. It has cured where sugar was found in the urine. It has cured so-called nervous colorless watery urine.

Troublesome, painful, strong, even violent erections at night. Pain in the testes; drawing pain in the testes; stitching pains in the penis and glans. *Seminal emissions*:

without dreams. Sexual passions increased and even violent. Swollen testes. In the female the sexual desire is also *increased*. Inflammation of the ovaries. *Leucorrhea*: acrid; bloody; *after the menses*; *yellow*; white. Menses: absent; bright red; clotted; copious; frequent; late; scanty; protracted; suppressed. Pain in the vulva; in the ovaries; worse in the left; bearing down before the menses; soreness in the vulva. Prolapsus of the uterus.

Constriction of the larynx. A sensation of dryness in the larynx. Accumulations of mucus in the larynx. Burning, rawness and soreness in the larynx and trachea. Tickling and scraping in the larynx. Hoarseness with coryza. Rough, weak voice. Respiration is accelerated, anxious and asthmatic, worse at night; spasmodic asthma; *difficult*; evening, night and after eating; *irregular*; *rattling*; short; suffocative. Cough: daytime; day and night; morning; afternoon; evening; night; asthmatic; from deep breathing; constant; after dinner; dry evening and night; exhausting; hacking; from irritation in the larynx and trachea; *a nervous cough*; paroxysmal; racking; during rest; short; worse sitting; better rising and moving about; spasmodic; *spinal cough*; tickling cough; violent. It has been a very useful remedy in whooping cough. Expectoration: daytime only; morning; bright, red blood; blood streaked; difficult; frothy; *greenish*; *mucus*; purulent; tasting putrid and sweetish; viscid; yellow.

An anxious feeling in the chest. Constriction as of a band; of the heart; in spinal affections. Pimples on the chest. *Oppression of the chest*. Pain in the chest; evening; during cough; on deep breathing; in the heart; aching in the chest; burning in the chest with rawness on coughing; cutting; *pressing*; soreness on coughing; soreness in mammæ. Stitching pains in the chest; on coughing; deep breathing; sides of chest; worse in the left side; in the heart. *Palpitation*: she feels every beat of the heart; *anxious*; heart pounds like a hammer; on waking. When spinal affections change into phthisis. Spasms of the chest.

Sensation of great heat, even burning in the back. Itching and formication of the back. Convulsive motions of the muscles of the back even to opisthotonos. *Pain in the back*: during chill; before menses; *on motion*; *rising from a seat*; WHILE SITTING; while standing; some pains are ameliorated walking; cervical region. Pain in the dorsal region; between the scapulæ; in the spine. Pain in the lumbar region; during menses; on motion; rising from a seat; while sitting; better walking. Pain in the sacrum. Pain in the coccyx, during menses. Violent pain in the spine while sitting, better walking. Aching in the lumbar region. Bruised pain in the back; cervical region. Burning pain in the back and spine; lumbar region. Drawing pain in thè back; between the scapulæ; in the lumbar region. Pressing pain in the back; lumbar region. The spine is very sore to touch; dorsal region; coccyx. It is a most useful remedy in spinal irritation. Stitching pains in the back; in scapulæ. Tearing pains in the back; in the cervical region; in the scapulæ. Stiffness in the back; in the cervical region. Great *weakness* in the lumbar region.

Chilblains of the feet. A most useful remedy in chorea. Cold extremities; upper limbs; HANDS; finger tips; thighs in the morning; feet icy cold at night. Cramps in the lower limbs, calves and feet. Blueness of the hands. Dryness of the hands and fingers. Pimples and vesicles on the extremities. Formication, especially of the feet. Heat of the palms and feet; burning soles. Heaviness of all the limbs. Itching of the skin of all the limbs. Jerking of the lower limbs; worse during sleep.

Numbness of all the limbs. Pain of all kinds in the limbs; rheumatic; upper limbs; shoulders; lower limbs;

thighs and legs; in the heel. Pain down the sciatic nerve. Burning in the upper limbs; forearm; hands; lower limbs; thighs; feet; soles. Drawing in the limbs; upper limbs; upper arm; forearm; thighs, thighs in the evening ameliorated by motion, worse sitting, better walking; *knees*; legs. Sore bruised pain in the limbs; thighs; legs. Stitching pain in the limbs; upper limbs; shoulder; hands; lower limbs; hips; thighs. *Tearing pains in the limbs*; JOINTS; *upper limbs*; shoulder; *upper arms*; forearm; wrist; hand; fingers; *lower limbs*; hip; *thigh*; knee; leg; toes. Painless paralysis of the lower limbs. Perspiration of the hands; cold; lower limbs; FEET; offensive foot-sweat; suppressed foot-sweat. Restlessness of all the limbs, especially feet and legs. Stiffness of the lower limbs. Dropsical swelling of the feet. Tension in the hollow of the knee; in the legs; in the calf. Tension in the thigh; in the evening; worse sitting; better walking; better drawing up the limbs. Twitching of the upper limbs and thighs. Weakness of all the limbs but more especially of the lower limbs and legs.

Comatose sleep: Dreams, anxious, of falling; frightful, horrible; of misfortune; of great mental exertion; vivid. Late falling asleep. Sleepiness in the afternoon and after eating. Sleeplessness before midnight and after three (3) a. m.; sleepless after waking. He is unrefreshed in the morning after sleep. Wakes up too early; three (3) a. m.; frequent.

Chill: afternoon; evening; cold air; in bed; after eating; *external chill*; *shaking chill*; after sleep. Fever: evening; night; *alternating with chill* flushes of heat. Perspiration: at night; cold; profuse; during sleep.

Diminished sensation in the skin. Sensation of biting after scratching. Burning sensation in the skin after scratching. Objective coldness of the skin. The skin cracks easily. Red spots. Dryness with burning. Erup- .

13

tions: boils; burning; herpetic; itching; moist; rash; scabby; worse after scratching; *smarting*; SUPPRESSED; suppurating; urticaria, worse after scratching; vesicular. FORMICATION all over the body. Itching: itching, biting; itching burning; itching crawling; itching stinging; worse in a warm bed. Hyperæsthesia. Sticking pains in the skin. Ulcers; bleeding; burning; discharge bloody; *indolent*; itching; painless; smarting.

CHARACTERISTIC SYMPTOMS

Phosphorus—Patients in low fever want to be mesmerized, they are starving for vital energy. Sometimes Calcarea.

Lycopodium—deep furrows in forehead and face with flapping nostrils in pneumonia or bronchitis.

Camphor—Vomiting and purging with cold, blue, dry skin.

Camphor—When the fever is present or when there are pains in the abdomen he covers up, but after these (both fever and pains) pass the skin becomes cold and he uncovers. Camphor only.

Stramonium—Eyes fixed upon dark side of the room away from the light; violent speech with wrinkled face.

Cuprum—Sudden blindness followed by convulsions.

Arnica—He goes into a rage when he sees the doctor, saying: "Go home, I am not sick, I did not send for you." (Apis).

Selenium—Shining face, impotency, prostatic dribbling.

Lycopodium—Old misers with wrinkled faces, when they get sick need Lycopodium.

Arsenicum—She cannot go to sleep because things in her room are out of place, and the room is not tidy.

Sulphur—Always theorizing—Apis, *Cannabis Ind.*,

Kali Ars.—Copious, thin, brown, horribly offensive, acrid leucorrhœa.

Calcarea Ars.—Headache goes to the side not lain on.

Staphisagria—Headache with ball in forehead and hollowness in occiput.

(Copy these into your Materia Medica so as to have them when you can find them when needed.)

PART II.

LESSER WRITINGS

A CRITICISM OF DR. HOLMES

On page 602, this year, my friend Holmes relates a perfectly simple Veratrum case and cure; a case that a recent graduate would not fail to recognize at a glance. He further reflects upon experience when he states that he did not have his "library" with him, and he had loaned his wheelbarrow. If Dr. Holmes had told us what he would have given or done had he found a case of sickness that presented symptoms entirely unknown to him, I would refrain from asking him to please come out again frankly and state just what he would have done. I believe that Dr. Holmes is honest, and therefore believe that he would have been sorry he had loaned his wheelbarrow, and sorry he had not brought his repertory. Dr. Holmes would have us believe that he thinks that doctors carry their repertory simply to make a show, simply to look for such simple cases as he reports. I do not know a member of the International Hahnemannian Association that would need a repertory for so simple a case as the Veratrum case. Perhaps Dr. Holmes offers this as a stumper— a case that would puzzle the honorable members of the International Hahnemannian Association. If Dr. Holmes offers this case to show his own erudition, and the full extent of it, he has succeeded, but if he has offered it to show that the repertory is not a valuable life-saving plan, he has failed.

He intimates that his "rule of practice" is to give a medicine high, but if his "rule of practice" is based upon the same reasoning as his rule of leaving his library at home (because a low potency would be so heavy to carry in a hurry), we presume his potency, therefore, was very high.

He gives six powders, but does not say how much better six doses would be than one; therefore we infer that six powders, one every half-hour, must be also a "rule of practice."

He says: "I consider this a desperate case, as several such had died under old-school treatment."

"As several such had died under old-school treatment" was his reason for thinking it a desperate case, and the only reason for thinking it a desperate case, we have no evidence that the prescription cured. He may have lived simply because he did not get old-school treatment.

"In cases calling for immediate action, it seems to me a risky piece of work to either take out a library at the bedside or to go back to one's office to study it up."

We therefore infer Dr. Holmes thinks it not risky to stay at the bedside of a violent sickness, even if one knows not the remedy for this sickness. What will Dr. Holmes do in the absence of knowing what to do that is right? Will he look on and let the patient die? Will he guess at one or several remedies? Will he break the law and give allopathic drugs, or what will he do? Does Dr. Holmes mean to have us infer that he, a young man, has so much wisdom and materia medica in his head that he is never puzzled? He attempted to convince us of that at Niagara, but made a signal failure.

"I have not, as a rule, been able to find just what I wanted when I was in a hurry." He means that he is not accustomed to the repertory so that he can find what he wants in a hurry. This is a criminal confession for a professed follower of Hahnemann. The confession means negligence or laziness when human life is at stake.

"Let those use their books who want or need them." By this Dr. Holmes says, in substance, that he does not want books and does not need them. This is an astonishing statement. I would like to study materia medica under Dr. Holmes.

A STUDY IN MATERIA MEDICA

There is a physician in this city, or at least he has a sign on his door, going about day and night seemingly not in his right mind, or if he be perfectly sane, what he does and says might be attributed to buffoonery (Stram.) with desire to calumniate (Ipec.), but if a very generous view be taken of the matter, he is not responsible for his words and conduct. He bellows on the street (Bell., Canth.), and assumes an air of importance (Hyos., Stram.). Some of his friends have observed great anxiety with sweat (Ars., Graph.). There is a great awkwardness about his movements and he drops things (Apis). He is advanced in years prematurely (Bar-c., Ant-c.) ; he is said to be astute in his madness (Anac.), and is much worse in his mental aberrations when alone (Elaps., Phos., or Stram.) with no one to talk to. He is given to alternations of humor (Ignatia), *i. e.*, irritability with cowardice (Ran.-bulb.). He is very jealous (Hyos.) and seems to have an aversion to his own business (Sep. or Kali-c.) because he attends so diligently to that of others. He has not manifested any desire to destroy his own clothing, but often rips his neighbor's coat up the back (Verat.). In all his ravings he is fearless, yet he is anxious from a slight noise (Caust., Silic., or Aurum), and he seems to dread a storm (Nat-c., Phos.). He has at times shown great apprehensiveness (Hyos.) with an active cerebral hyperæmia (Glon.). He sees faces from every corner (Phos.), and was known to make rapid movements in the street at the sight of a hand organ (Phos-ac.), so great is his aversion to music. Sometimes he thinks he sees cats (Puls., Stram.) and is said to be childish in his behavior (Crocus). Again he imagines he sees far into the future (Acon., Phos-ac.), and his comprehension is decidedly difficult (Lyc.) especially of what he hears. (Cham., Nat-c.). He frequently manifests a lack of self-confidence. (Bar-c., Kali-c.), because he knows that there are people living who know the real cause of his insanity (Phos.). Occasionally his conscience troubles him (Ars., Cocc.), and a small boy frightened him the other day by saying "rats!" (Calc.). He often looks back as if pursued by enemies (Dros., Lach.). He went home and looked in the looking-glass and thought he saw a goose (Hyos.). At times he is of a slanderous turn of mind (Nux) and lacking in moral feeling (Anac.). His pride is wonderful (Plat.). He often walks in his sleep (Phos.) and starts at a slight noise (Borax) and has a dread of thieves (Ars., Lach.). Perhaps a nosode would cure him if the product of his disease could be run through a potentizer. The remedy that causes the totality of symptoms does not appear, even after long study. Even "Christian Science" has failed to make a man of him. It has recently been reported that he has resorted to stimulants, and still he fails. Is there no saving a man who will not save himself? Echo answers, "no saving!"

LECTURE

A physician advanced in years looks back upon many failures. The faithful homœopathist recalls a man, a woman, a child, and realizes that these, among his past failures, would now be simple cases. Prescribing the homœopathic remedy is such a process of growth and progress that it may be said that "the best of the wine is saved for the last of the feast." In the beginning of one's practice many acute diseases run their course, in advanced years they are nearly all aborted.

The young man looks upon the successful years of long experience, and wonders if he will cure as he sees cures made—as Hahnemann made them. It is well to hope—for all to hope—that, with experience, each may attain the high degree of perfection in healing that Hahnemann attained. Much can be done now that Hahnemann could not do, because we have a greater number of remedies, and a greater number of potencies, and higher potencies. It is doubtful if the technique of prescribing has made much progress. It is in this direction that all need most to meditate. None of Hahnemann's pupils lived since Hahnemann who could do what he did. Few have lived since Hahnemannn that could do what he did. It was what he was able to do in his ripe old age that appears so wonderful.

If we would make progress, we must dwell upon the teaching of THE ORGANON.

1. We must dwell long upon what it is in the human being that must be changed, in order to restore man from sickness to health.

2. We must meditate long upon what it is in remedies or drugs that constitutes a healing power or principle. (§3.)

To some it will seem to be an old story even to refer to this question, which has been heretofore so fully considered; but it may also surprise some to learn that many of our so-called faithful friends are thinking and acting as if the patient is sick because his liver, or heart, or stomach, or some organ, is improperly functioning.

So long as one thinks that man is sick because his organs are not doing proper work, just so long he cannot construct a treatment that accords with THE ORGANON. So long as one regards the results as causes, so long the true idea is obscured. So long as one thinks in this way, he will take symptoms accordingly and work the repertory in such manner, and, although his results may satisfy himself, yet they will not compare with results obtained from thinking that sick organs are but the results of a disordered state of the man himself, who is composed of mind and physical being and, last, of organs and extremities. (ORG. §§ 10-11, 15.)

Traditional nosology may be useful so long as we have a public sphere to maintain, but it is useless in the homœopathic art of healing. It must be clearly settled what it is in man that is first, and what is last; what is highest, and what is lowest; what is innermost, and what is outermost; before we can perceive what are causes and what are ultimates. So long as one thinks of pathological conditions as causes, so long will he act in directions that are the opposite of healing, and toward destruction.

All nutritive processes are commanded and conducted from center to circumference, therefore all healing processes must go on from centralized efforts. Pupils have often heard these statements, and wondered at their meaning. I have kept a watchful eye over such pupils for many years, and all of them who have failed have wondered at the meaning of such statements. They who can perceive the meaning are the ones who are able to perform the works directed in THE ORGANON of Samuel Hahnemann, and heal the sick as he taught, viz: to cure the patient, and then the organs will also return to normal function. Men who give Bryonia for pneumonia, Nux Vomica for the stomach, Kali-iod for syphilis, and Belladonna for cerebral congestion, seldom learn to individualize from the patient to his parts and organs. The best they can do is to individualize from organs and parts, hoping to get somewhere. "Lucky hits" are their sole joy and success. Their successes would be failures in the minds of men who can follow Hahnemann in all he means in emphasizing the mind symptoms above all others in any given totality of symptoms of a sick man. (ORG. §213.)

1. DIAGNOSIS OF WHAT IS CURABLE

The true physician must know that whatever it is in man that is morbid can represent itself by signs and symptoms only. These he must meditate upon earnestly, patiently and wisely, that he may find in the Materia Medica symptoms most similar. If he is heedless of the best interest of sick people, or careless in discovering and writing down their symptoms, or too indolent to search for corresponding symptoms in the Materia Medica; or if he is given to making light of the symptoms he hears the patient speak of, or of the symptoms he reads in the

Materia Medica, he will never prosper or grow wise with age, but will go the way of all such men into indolence and levity, depending upon hired laboratory findings for the basis of a prescription. The last state of that man will be worse than the first. The man who believes that he is directing his remedies against germs, or against worms, or against a tumor the patient may have, is in extreme darkness, if he cannot perceive that a healthy man will have healthy tissue, healthy blood, and therefore there can be no soil for germs and worms or morbid growths. (§§7, 11, 12, 14, 70, 84, 89, 98, 107-9.)

On one side we have the laboratory to furnish a basis for prescribing; on the other hand is the ORGANON. One class of prescribers is demanding enormous expenditures for laboratory fixtures in our colleges, while giving no credit for our Materia Medica opportunities, though the latter are ten times greater than any found in the colleges of the former class. This clearly indicates the trend of traditional medicine and of the ignorant homœopath following in this line. They should be permitted to have their enormous and surplus laboratories in peace; but we must demand that we have our full privileges in Materia Medica and therapeutic philosophy. This demand has never been made upon State Boards that stand over our colleges with uplifted hands. The requirement of our Hering College should be entirely different from that of Rush or the P. & S. The basis of our knowledge in practice is Philosophy and Materia Medica, while theirs is laboratory. Both must have clinical advantages the same in quantity, but differing in character and quality.

The reverse of all these whims and imaginations are Hahnemann's substantial doctrines, based upon facts, and now confirmed by a century of experience, viz: *It is impossible to conceive of anything but symptoms that are to be removed or cured in order to establish health.* Look back upon our century of experience, and what have we cured. Nothing but symptoms. The results of disease disappear themselves when the symptoms are cured. When the symptoms are removed by a homœopathic remedy, the patient is cured.

The physician must perceive when the symptoms represent a complete image of a sickness. When only a few symptoms are observed, Hahnemann calls it a one-sided case, and says that no great things should be expected of a remedy chosen on a few symptoms. ORG. §§ 172-6, 185.) The homœopathic physician *clearly perceives* when he has a *clearly defined image,* and then he knows how certain the remedy is to act curatively. (§§3, 104.) Defective education is often revealed by professed homœopathic physicians bringing cases for advice with only a few clinical symptoms, or a few particulars, or the results cf disease, all mental symptoms and generals being omitted. The physician who administers a remedy on such a one-sided case will have a high percentage of failures; but he often struts like a peacock over his lucky hits.

All curable sicknesses make themselves known to the intelligent physician in signs and symptoms. (ORG. §§ 14.) Diseases are, therefore, incurable when they do not make themselves known in signs and symptoms. Whether the physician fails to find the symptoms, or whether there are no symptoms, as in malignant growths, or whether the patient conceals the symptoms, they are unknown to the prescriber.

2. MATERIA MEDICA.

Every effort is being put forth to re-establish the science of medicine upon a positive basis, yet these efforts are based upon pure theory. What can be more positive or matter-of-fact than the written declaration of the interested patient, or the prover? These are assertions of fact, and they are daily confirmed by thousands of experiences. How can a more substantial basis be expected?

The records of confirmed and verified provings stand as so many recorded facts.

The symptoms of the sick man are recorded as so many facts.

The similarity between these two is the only variable quality, and this is a matter of art; and art is always a variable quality.

Then all that remains is to find an artist—a physician —and all the questions are solved. Is this grade of intelligence too high for which to work? Can it be true that educated men and women wish to compete for a prize much lower in the scale of human accomplishments?

Whatever it is in medicine that heals the sick, nothing that represents the healing principle in each individual drug can ever be known but the symptoms obtained in healthy provers. The laboratory and microscope must ever fail, because these can discover only the ultimates, while the curative power is only a tendency, or *conatus*, of an invisible substance evolved into activities by circumstances. So long as men search in the laboratory for causes of disease, so long they will search in the laboratory for curative powers, which must always end in failure. (ORG. §§ 24-2, 108.)

The study of the homœopathic pathogenesis, which is so extensive, requires so much time and perseverance that men who are given to carelessness, indolence and levity, can do very little to make a showing for professional glory; hence the stupid, the flippant and the "smart" must always seek the material method and make it the basis of his efforts, thereby associating with, or placing himself on the same level as, the mechanic. Of course, all liquid substances seek their own level.

3. USE OF POTENCIES. APPLICATION OF REMEDIES TO SICKNESS.

And lastly, the physician must know how to adjust the one to the other, in order to gain the ends of healing. (ORG. §§ 146 *et seq.*) Our pathogeneses have expanded into enormous proportions, so vast that no mind can encompass them, yet this once may be expanded very many times by a full knowledge of the uses of the various potencies. The physician who knows how to use the various potencies has ten times the advantage of the one that always uses one potency, no matter what that potency is.

After thirty years of careful observation and comparison with the use of the various potencies, it is possible to lay down the following rules:

Every physician should have at command the 30th, 200th, 1m, 10m, 50m, cm, dm and mm potencies, made carefully on the centesimal scale.

From the 30th to the 10m will be found those curative powers most useful in very sensitive women and children.

From the 10m to the mm all are useful for ordinary chronic diseases in persons not so sensitive.

In acute diseases the 1m and 10m are most useful.

In the sensitive women and children, it is well to give the 30th or 200th at first, permitting the patient to improve in a general way, after which the 1m may be used in similar manner. After improvement with that ceases, the 10m may be required.

In persons suffering from chronic sickness and not so sensitive, the 10m may first be used, and continued without change so long as improvement lasts; then the 50m will act precisely in the same manner, and should be used so long as the patient makes progress toward health; then the cm may be used in the same manner, and the dm and mm in succession.

By this use of the series of potencies in a given case,

the patient can be held under the influence of the simili-mum, or a given remedy, until cured. *When the simili-mum is found, the remedy will act curatively in a series of potencies.* If the remedy is only partially similar, it will act in only one or two potencies; then the symptoms will change and a new remedy will be demanded.

Many chronic cases will require a series of care-fully selected remedies to effect a cure, if the remedy is only partially similar; but the ideal in prescribing is to find that remedy similar enough to hold the case through a full series to the highest. Each time the patient will say that the new potency acted as did the first one re-ceived. The patient can feel the medicine when it is act-ing properly. Some have intimated that suggestion is a help to the action of the remedy; but it is wise to know that suggestion fails when the wrong remedy has been given.

ADDRESS

Fellow Members of the International Hahnemannian Association: It is with pleasure that I welcome you to your eighth annual meeting; to one which promises to exceed in interest and profit even our last session.

In the past, this Association has accomplished some very useful work for the cause it espouses. Let us hope it will do even more in the future. And what *is* the cause we espouse; or in other terms, why this Association.

It was certainly for no idle purpose, nor for any sense-less caprice, that our oldest and most respected members left the American Institute and formed this separate Asso-ciation; it is equally true that we of the junior profession did not join this Association for any selfish or useless purpose. Was not this Association formed solely for the purpose, as expressed, of perpetuating and developing true Homœopathy? Was it not felt at the time of its organization that the hour had come for true men to arouse themselves, and work for the science they loved?

Had they not heard all the principles which Hahnemann had taught, and which the experience of many had proven to be true, villified and abused; had not, in short, all true Homœopathy been driven from the Institute? The Homœopathic school, then as now, was divided into two parties—the one representing Eclectic methods and practice, the other the principles and practice of Hahnemann, of Gross, of Boenninghausen, of Hering. The time had come when all practitioners had to decide which of the parties they should assist. And let it be to the eternal glory of these men that they chose rather to be right than to be with the majority!

In the history of the American Institute, we may read a warning for us. In its first years the Institute was composed of able and true men, and its purpose was for truth and usefulness. But little by little Eclectics were allowed to creep into its membership, and soon, behold! the whole body is Eclectic. Let us then beware whom we elect members, let our censors be even over-scrupulous lest a wolf creep in in sheep's clothing. Let no member sign any application for membership unless he knows the physician personally and is *very* sure he is qualified to serve with us. Too great caution cannot be observed in this matter. It is not great numbers that we want, but men of truth and purpose.

While much caution may be judiciously exercised in this matter of electing new members, let us not repel those who though not yet with us, are in sympathy with our purpose, and whose presence would be welcome. Let us not therefore erect any Chinese Wall of exclusion, but merely exercise all proper precaution to prevent evil. Let no good man be excluded by personal malice; nor any useless man elected to serve personal ambition. As well stated in the preface of our last volume of transactions:

"Personal interests or ambitions have no place here, but only *what* is truth."

14

Without doubt all will assent to this assertion, but many will inquire, and most rightly too, *What is truth?* This question has been asked many, many times, and of all subjects. In this case, limiting our statement to what is true in therapeutics, we unhesitatingly assert the law of similars to be true; to be a proven *fact*. Has it not been found operative in all diseases and in all countries? Can fuller demonstration be needed?

"*It is true; let it stand*," we all exclaim.

It may be well to remark that while our law is a fixed fact, we must never forget that our school is not to be stationary. The law is complete and perfect; our knowledge of the extent of its usefulness is very incomplete and imperfect. The law is fixed, the school is progressive.

Eclectics, building upon the uncertain sands of *theory*, need to be continually rebuilding, as each new theory causes a shifting of their foundation. Homœopathists, building upon the unchangeable rock of *law*, need never rebuild.

Our foundation then being firm, we need only develop and improve the superstructure. Our knowledge of the extent and usefulness of the law of similars has increased since Hahnemann's day; let us see to it that we continue to improve, and always in the right way.

The law, being of divine origin, is complete, perfect, and fixed; the school, being composed of erring humanity, is incomplete, imperfect, and changeable.

While many willingly concede this much to the Homœopathic law, yet they desire something more; they would like to have *liberty*, license, "to use their best judgment;" to be free to treat anomalous cases by non-homœopathic measures if, in their judgment, such may at any time be needed.

There is growing up such a tendency to the so-called

scientific that our young men stand in danger of being drawn into this vortex of confusion. This scientific vortex looks wonderful; it is so strong! What can there be in the science of medicine but a knowledge of how to cure the sick? The scientific physician, when asked what he knows, must say: *l know how to cure the sick*. If he really knows this he has the knowledge and is scientific. If he has not this knowledge, which he pretends to possess, he is a pretender and a fraud.

What is there of value in this word "scientific," when all the pretenders in medicine make use of it? These, most of all, cry "We are the scientific." "We teach science." The amount of science depends entirely on how much the instructor possesses, for "a stream cannot rise higher than its source."

The "Eclectics" claim to teach the most scientific (?) of all, because they select the good from all schools of medicine. Who has guided them to this great wisdom? Do they pretend to have a law or a philosophy to enable them to select the wheat and leave the chaff? No. Such a thing does not belong to their pretensions. They even claim the greatest empiricism to be the highest order of science. The greater the chaos and confusion the greater the science.

The cry of the unbelieving does not strengthen their scientific position when their only appeal is to the miscroscope and to common sense. *Common sense is opposed at all times to cultivated intelligence*. The man of lowest intelligence can prove that he must have a dose that can be seen and handled to cure him of his aches, by appealing to common sense. The mongrel makes use of the same reason and argument to condemn us that the Allopathist resorts to, to convict the mongrel—appeal to common sense and belief.

Ten men may stand and affirm each, "I did not see."

and one man states "I did see," and who of the eleven would the meanest court in the land accept as competent to give evidence? The one knows what the ten did not know.

The ten declared they have tried the high potencies and have failed to secure curative results. What have they demonstrated? *Nothing but their own ignorance* of the manner of using these potencies. But they say they cure with the low. I do not believe they cure with the low, because of the best reasoning. It is logical to suppose or presume that a physician who can cure with the high, can cure with the low, but the demonstration is entirely wanting to show that the physician can cure *with the low* and cannot cure with the high. Men who know how to select a remedy have confidence in that remedy and go on gaining yearly in this knowledge; men who are ignorant of the powers of the selected remedy of course have not gained the confidence necessary to cure with it, and they mix other means and other medicines.

It has been recently stated in a medical journal that there are logical reasons for deserting Homœopathy for Allopathy; that is, for abandoning law for empiricism. The idea is fallacious, and no sensible reason has ever been adduced in its support. There can only be one excuse for this change—and that is *failure*! And this failure has never yet been shown to be due to any insufficiency of the homœopathic law, but is always easily traced to the incapacity of him who uses it. All men are liable to err. Let him who thinks he cannot sin cast the first stone at our law.

Concerning the oft-made plea for liberty of medical opinion and action, we would remark that no one is free from the obligations of law; the greater your work, the higher you advance, just by so much do you rivet the chains of responsibility. Only the beggar in the gutter

is free to do as he will. No one can grant a physician
success in practice whose practice does not of itself secure
success.

If one practice Homœopathy he will secure Homœopathic success; if he practice Allopathy, he will gain only
the meager results of Allopathy. No results of learned
bodies can change this rule. We are freemen; free to do
and practice as we please; but our success will be
measured by our practice, and our title as Homœopaths
or Eclectics be given accordingly as we practice the one
or the other, and we all know the greatest measure of
success is attained by a strict adherence to the law of
similars, the minimum dose, and the single remedy. The
Homœopathy of Hahnemann gives the greatest success,
the greatest freedom, and the greatest honor. No man
can practice empiricism and honestly claim to be a Homœopath; such are "living a lie," as an Allopath has asserted.
The Eclectic is a slave, bound by error; the Homœopath
is free, emancipated by truth. A great poet declares, "He
is a freeman whom truth makes free, and all are slaves
beside."

Let not this Association harbor or indorse in any way,
even by absence of rebuke, any form of false teaching. Let
it be distinctly understood that we do fully and honestly
believe, collectively and individually, the resolutions of this
Association, as adopted. We have declared that these
resolutions "completely and fully represent the therapeutic
opinion and practice" of this Association. Let it be shown
to the outside world that we mean what we have said.
We do most assuredly believe Hahnemann's *Organon of
the Healing Art* to be the only true guide in therapeutics.
Let us not, then, tolerate any teaching which seeks to
pervert or abridge this master-work in any way. We
have asserted, as our belief, that the only true guide for
a prescription is the totality of the symptoms and the

proven drug. Let us not, then, prescribe upon any other basis; it cannot be Homœopathic nor wise to do so. We cannot allow to be true any teaching which seeks to controvert this fundamental principle of Homœopathic practice. He who recommends the building of therapeutics upon any new theory or upon any other basis than that prescribed by this law, is no Homœopath and has no fellowship in this Association. Successful practice cannot be based upon pathological theories. Whether these theories teach one to prescribe for a pathological condition or for a presumed dyscrasia, it matters not; both are un-homœopathic and both are unsuccessful.

The adoption of drug proving by Hahnemann, first introduced two great features into medicine, and these are *certainty* and *prevision*. We are sure a drug will cure in the sick such symptoms as it has produced upon the healthy; we are enabled by this certainty to *predict*, before the trial of a drug, what it will cure. For these grand features of its art, medicine is indebted to Samuel Hahnemann—see to it that no fault of ours destroys his noble work. In short, it is to be remembered that the basis of a homœopathic prescription is the symptoms of the patient, the question of the dose is secondary. The size of the dose can never make the remedy homœopathic in this case.

In this matter of dose, some err upon one side and some upon the other. So we see that while some believe an imperfectly selected drug may be made to do the work of the perfect similimum if it be "pushed" or exhibited in crude doses; on the other hand, we find some who are disposed to assent to almost any prescription so it be given "high" enough. Both these parties are in error. While we cannot dogmatize upon this question of dose, all here will agree that the better selection, *i. e.*, the nearer we come to the perfect similimum, the less medicine we need give. This proposition may be stated again in other words. It is the experience of our best prescribers that the similimum will cure most cases best if given high and in one dose, or at most a few doses. Indeed, experience tells us that the high potencies are always best; this is experience, however, and not law. But the converse of this proposition is *not true*, that a badly selected drug may be made to do good work by giving much of it. This idea is the cause of most of the mongrelism of the day.

In published reports of clinical cases, we find evidence of the necessity for careful examination of the patient. Hahnemann laid the greatest stress upon this examination, telling us how to do it, and saying, in effect, that a patient well examined was half cured. Unless this careful exam ination be made, one cannot get all those peculiar characteristic symptoms which Hahnemann has declared must be the deciding symptoms. All cases have many symptoms, which are to be found under many drugs, and are hence of little value in deciding our choice of a remedy. Each case should have, and probably does have, some peculiar symptoms; these we are to get. These we *must get*; and our examination of a patient is incomplete so long as we possess only a list of common and general symptoms. It should be our task to question and examine the patient until such peculiar symptoms are found. We hear much complaint of the insufficiency of our *Materia Medica*, of the uselessness of our repertories, but most generally the failure to prescribe correctly and even easily is not due to the want of good books, but to this lack of careful and thoughtful examination of the patient. Forget not this, that the greatest cures the world has ever witnessed have been made by the earlier Homœopaths with a much less complete library than we now possess. After selecting the proper remedy, we must not forget that it is of prime importance to give it in proper dose, and not to change too soon nor to repeat too frequently. Never change a remedy unless the changed symptoms call for another; never repeat the dose (or change remedy) when the patient is improving. For a fuller and a better understanding of the true healing art, you are to study and to restudy the *Organon*. Our purpose in these few remarks has not been to teach this art, but merely to call attention to a few salient points; to give admonition upon a few prominent features which cannot be too steadily kept in view.

This Association, it has been said, was organized for an especial purpose, and that purpose was to promulgate and develop Homœopathy. In pursuance of this work, the purifying and completing of the *Materia Medica* must be our chief concern. It is the foundation of our art. Our *Materia Medica* once corrupted and perverted, clinical success becomes impossible. We may again take warning by the fate of the American Institute, for it, too, started forty odd years ago, to do this same work, and for some years the Institute did good service in this study. But as it grew Eclectic, the Institute became enamored of the false siren named *progressive science*, and all truth was abandoned. Let us beware lest a like fate overtake this Association.

The *Materia Medica* is to be developed by careful and thorough provings of new drugs; we repeat, careful and thorough provings, for most of the modern provings are worthless, having been carelessly and improperly made. One is afraid to prescribe upon them; afraid to trust valuable lives to such careless work. How differently do we feel when we prescribe one of the old, reliable remedies. Then security begets quiet reliance and success crowns our efforts.

At our last meeting, a good beginning was made in this study of the *Materia Medica*, and your bureau gives promise of great usefulness and interest for this meeting. In all of our work we must strive to emulate the energy and zeal of Hahnemann and of his early disciples; they were indeed masters. Nowhere does one's knowledge of therapeutics and medical ability show forth to better advantage than in this proving of drugs and revising the *Materia Medica*. To do it well the best talent and the greatest zeal are required, but this need not deter us from the work, for ability and zeal are easily to be found in our ranks.

The *Materia Medica* is to be enriched by clinical observations, and here also we may again take pattern by Hahnemann's careful work. The admission of clinical symptoms into our *Materia Medica* must be done with the greatest caution. They can only be incorporated after the most searching inquiry, and then should always be so marked that we can tell the clinical from the pathogenetic. The hasty and inconsiderate adoption of clinical symptoms is certainly an evil; and if pursued to any great extent will render the *Materia Medica* unreliable. Every practitioner is not a reliable judge of the value of a clinical confirmation. Even reliable clinical confirmations need only be noted when peculiar or characteristic; of common, general symptoms we have an abundance.

The clinical symptom is only admissible to fill up the gaps left by imperfect provings, or in cases where provings cannot be obtained. Though some of the best symptoms now in use are of clinical origin, as a general rule they cannot be considered as certain and reliable as the pathogenetic.

Besides the provings of drugs and the careful, conscientious noting of clinical symptoms, we can also do a useful work in marking clinical verifications of pathogenetic symptoms. A symptom produced upon a healthy person and cured in a sick person becomes doubly reliable,

There can be no doubt about the value of such symptoms.

The most dangerous manner of perpetuating Homœopathic truth is to mix it with uncertainty or mystery. There are some things about the art of healing that pertain to the scientific, of which not one is more important than the *proven drug*. A member may state that he has cured somebody with an unproved drug, and he may fail to demonstrate the homœopathicity of the so-called cure, because of the lack of evidence that can only be obtained from the provings. There are many good things involved in mystery that the time is not ripe to discuss them. The relations of Homœopathy to them must be first demonstrated or this organization cannot recognize them. The Allopathist reports cures on unsupported opinion, and we reject these because he has no demonstration. If this same Allopathist reports a cure of vomiting by *Ipecac*, the Homœopathist can accept it as a real cure, because it is what can be expected. Experiment as you may on the healthy with new medicines, the sick man demands a remedy for his sickness the likeness of which has been found in a pathogenesis.

In no way can we perpetuate pure philosophy but by adhering to the proven drug in all our discussions. Better rule out all the fragmentary guesswork and make every report show its relation between drug and disease in the manner designated in our philosophy. The Publication Committee should reject, without fear or favor, all papers with reports of cures where we have not had access to the record of provings. Of what value is the cure without the proving? Save the cures until you have given us the proving.

By thorough and careful work we will some day complete a *Materia Medica* whose every symptom will have been repeatedly verified. Then, indeed, will our art become the exact science predicted for it. Such is the end for

which we labor. A great stride toward such an end will be
made when we have in completed form the *Guiding Symptoms*, by the late Dr. Hering. These are now promised,
and if given us as that master mind left them (not as
some lesser mind may think they should be given), our
school will secure a treasure. The very opposite of this
great work of Hering's is the so-called *Encyclopoedia of
Drug Pathogenesy*, which seems to be a confused mass of
mangled provings. We have more than once attempted to
gather assistance from its garbled and condensed pages,
but have always been baffled. That it has any value we
are unable to see. It is to be hoped it has a purpose, as
much labor seems to have been spent upon it, and much
expected of it.

There is another point to which your attention may
be profitably directed, and that is to secure greater care
in selecting our medicines and more care in manufacturing
our potencies. It seems as though carelessness were also
creeping into our pharmaceutics.   The greatest discretion
must be exercised in selecting proper material for our
pharmacopœia and in their preparation. The same preparation, especially in the use of our vegetable remedies,
should be used in the prescribing as was used in the
proving. We do not mean the same potency, but the same
pharmaceutical preparation. Impure or uncertain drugs
will, of course, not correspond in their effects upon the
sick to the action of a purer drug used in the proving.
The physician and the prover should use the same preparation. Without doubt, many of our failures may be justly
laid to some imperfection in our drug preparations.

During the past year little worthy of note has occurred in the medical world. In the old school new theories
have arisen and old ones have died. This is the old, old
story with these scientists. Among ourselves the work
seems to be steadily progressing for the better. The suc-

cessful meeting held a year ago at Saratoga has been productive of much good, has shown the outside world that this is a *working* association of genuine Homœopathists. Such successful meetings cannot fail to have a beneficial effect upon the Homœopathic school.

And now we meet for the eighth time to greet each other, and to work for the perpetuation of the art of healing known as Homœopathy. We have come together from the remote quarters of the land to sharpen a common faith by another year of busy experience. This organization has been separated from the masses of all grades in medicine, a mere handful, that has been called a respectable minority, and it can even now see the gulf that yawns behind it. With independence we are able to go on climbing the mountain of Homœopathic *truth*. Some say we are at the top. Be not so sure; we have but climbed a foothill; soon will we see a mountain beyond, with but the faintest trace of human footprints. We follow on, though the mountain side be steep and thorny, led by the light of truth. Soon the toilers grow weary and their number becomes smaller. In the distant past there is a multitude, while the valleys below still throng with conflicting millions. The few toil on up the steep and rocky mountain side, steeper, more rocky as they press onward. The distance brings to view the heavens, dotted with nebulous sky and space beyond. There is to be seen another mountain far away, and much higher, which is yet to be climbed, upon which, through the clear sky, above the clouds, behold the immortal Hahnemann.

ADDRESS—THE RELATION OF GOUT TO THE VOLUNTARY SYSTEM

When four to six years old she hated her sisters and her mother.

When fourteen, she began menstruating and fainted

with the violent cramping uterine pains at each period. When thirty, she had gouty finger joints.

When she was a child we could not call the mental state gout, nor at puberty could we think of gout, but was she not then afflicted with the beginning of what was later a gouty condition? When she was a child Fluoric acid would most likely have cured her. When she suffered at puberty she needed Lapus albus. When she became gouty she was cured of her lifelong sufferings with Silica fluorica calc. In many similar cases I have noticed that gouty conditions begin and continue along the course above described. Must we stretch our imagination, then, to say that the same remedy would have cured her if she had had it in infancy?

Why not let such cases lead us to things first, instead of things last:—the diagnostic symptoms or ultimates? Is it not possible to perceive that we have not fully taken the symptoms of any adult case, if we have neglected the symptoms from childhood to the present? Drugs may have obscured the recent symptoms, but if the mother can describe the mental state of the child we have a good beginning, and can sometimes see what remedy was needed before the drug doctor or the near-homœopath obscured the case.

To cure the results of disease—the ultimates—we must be guided by the symptoms that represent causes and first periods of developing sick constitutions. The man who waits for pathology to guide him to a remedy for a constitutional sickness is most unwise. We sometimes see the remedy shining through the pathology, but generally only the smallest hints are visible. These hints may strengthen the indications, but it is better to strengthen the indications with the early symptoms. If we are to arrest gouty formations we must look for early mental symptoms, as the gouty concretions give small clew to the remedy.

WHY IS CANCER INCURABLE?

In other words: What must be discovered, to lead to the cure of cancer? When a case has been cured, why was it possible when other cases, and most cases, have resulted in failure?

It is true that in some cases there are hold-over symptome enough to lead to the remedy, *but in most cases there is nothing discoverable but the malignant growth and its associated features of hardness, stinging pains, ulceration, enlarged glands and the tendency to involve the surrounding parts in its own development.* A neophyte could say that such a growth is malignant, without the aid of a microscope. Then, in most cases, the paucity of symptoms is the present state of the situation. If the child's mental symptoms could be fully ascertained, and the symptoms from the childhood to adult age, something might be done. Cancer generally comes on in after life, when childhood actions have been forgotten. The patient does not know her own childhood mental state, the parents may be dead, sisters and brothers may describe the antics of the child.

Many of our patients come to us with a history of old-school drugging from childhood; every childhood morbid condition has been suppressed; eruptions have been suppressed; symptoms have been changed by crude drugs; no clear-cut representation of the constitution has been permitted to evolve. We do not know whether the child was obstinate, hateful, ungovernable, hysterical, violent, slow in school work, or the opposite; we can learn only the commonest features of puberty, which is a most important time to investigate in all women. If the symptoms that have appeared from birth to the present date are undiscovered, it is no wonder that cancer is incurable.

To cure any condition *we must base the prescription on the totality of the signs and symptoms and not on the pathology.* The cancer is the ultimate. The symptoms from the first are the outward image of the patient. If they have been suppressed or changed by drugs that are not homœopathic, there is nothing left for the homœopath to do, and the surgeon can do no better. Palliation and prolonging life are not curing.

"*All curable diseases make themselves known to the intelligent physician in signs and symptoms.*" (Hahnemann.) Pathological conditions, as also the patient, are incurable when there are no signs and symptoms, and so long as there are no signs and symptoms these remain incurable. *In proportion as the pathology progresses the signs and symptoms decrease.* This is marked in cancer, in tuberculosis, in diabetes, in Bright's disease, and in all of the organic conditions of the body. In some instances, the remedy that was once indicated by mental and physical symptoms will cure even in moderately advanced pathological conditions; again, such a remedy will soon reveal that the patient has been sick too long and the pathology has progressed too far, and the reaction is so feeble that he sinks rapidly and the remedy must be antidoted.

I remember a patient who had long suffered from tuberculosis of the lungs; cavities were present; several hemorrhages had occurred; the mental and physical symptoms had called for Phosphorus from the early history, and even at the time he came this remedy fitted the symptoms. PHOSPHORUS was given in high potency, as I had not then learned better, and there followed a high fever, involuntary diarrhœa, and sinking. It was apparent that this patient would soon die, but ARSENICUM antidoted the over-action of Phosphorus and the patient lived several months. The patient must have the reactive ability when the similar remedy is administered, or become worse after such a remedy than before.

Therefore, *it is a homoeopathic remedy when the patient can react from it, otherwise it is only a similar agent and not a remedy.* When a similar remedy is not a homœopathic remedy is quite a new problem to many good thinkers. It is never such when the patient lacks that reaction which is always depended on and so promptly noticed in all curable cases. Some patients have lost this reaction when there is no visible or discoverable organic disease. This is what comes to the aged who die of senile debility and it may be said, as a fact, that the deceased had no disease.

We often see, in the last days of the aged, a quick response after the remedy, but it holds only a few hours and he sinks to his final rest. Quite similar is this lack of reaction in some feeble, young, and middle-aged people. Whether it comes from constitutional debility or pathological conditions, the lack of vital reaction is the same.

When we think of the curability of cancer or tuberculosis, this is the question to be considered. We can judge the measure of his reaction by watching the symptoms after the administration of the remedy. No two patients react the same. It is generally safe to conclude that so long as signs and symptoms are present good vital reaction continues, but after the signs and sypmtoms have departed, and pathology has taken their place, it is impossible to predict what the quality of his reaction may be, until the patient has been tested by the similar agent. When this is known, it will be easy to understand why old symptoms return, in chronic cases, after the administration of the similar remedy. Patients having only feeble reaction are only palliated, while those of strong reaction go through all their past symptoms in the reverse order of their appearance.

In patients with cancer or tuberculosis, we may be

quite certain of their ultimate recovery, if old symptoms return after administration of the remedy. These patients seldom have the vital reaction strong enough to develop former symptoms, hence they are incurable.

To be able to perceive the remedy from the signs and symptoms in the present or history is one item of cure, but another and quite different item is the vital reaction of the patient. To find a remedy that will restore his lost vital reaction is thus far impossible. Even the surgeon's knife has been a failure.

TUBERCULOSIS

A three-year old boy was brought to my office to be treated for adenoids. There was a history of several deaths from tuberculosis on the father's side. After long and earnest questioning, the mother continued to conceal the boy's mental state. She seemed ashamed to reveal his mental symptoms. It came to my mind to test his condition with Tuberculinum bovinum, as he had such a history of disorder, and I had many times seen this remedy cure adenoids that followed such a history. I then forcibly put a powder of the remedy on the child's tongue, after a struggle. He refused to put out the tongue or open the mouth. The mother attempted to persuade him to open his mouth; then the time came for the boy to exhibit himself.

He was voilently angry, eyes became glassy, appeared as if he would have a convulsion, attempted to spill the pellets out, turned upon his mother and said, "I will kill you, when I get home I will kill you." He frothed at the mouth. Then the mother was persuaded to relate the child's disposition and mental symptoms. She said that they were unable to govern him or persuade him to do anything he did not want to do. He would fly into a fit of rage and threaten to kill his father or mother, and would

froth at the mouth whenever they attempted to force him
to obey a command.

While the child was in my office the mother forced
him to open his mouth, and the dose of Tuberc, 10m was
put on the tongue. Four weeks later another dose of the
10m was given and later the 50m was given. Within a
month the child began to change and became a perfectly
gentle and orderly child. The adenoids had entirely gone
in three months. The child is a most promising boy, now
ten years old. No other remedy was required.

After observing a large number of consumptives from
the beginning to the ending, I am unable to say that the
corresponding mental relation is fixed and positive.

The mind is always out of balance in children who are
constitutionally affected from inheritance. Sometimes the
will is most disturbed and sometimes the understanding.

When the lungs, kidneys and intestines are the seat
of the localized disease, the understanding is predominantly disturbed. When the liver is the seat of the localized
disease, the will symptoms are most prominent in early
history.

All cases present early mental symptoms, and there is
always a trail of symptoms, mental and nervous, until
the development of tuberculosis is well established; then
the mental symptoms disappear, and in most cases there
has been an absence of mental symptoms for a period
before the beginning of the deposits. This leads to the
opinion that there is in nearly all cases a predisposition
to tuberculosis, and it is this predisposition that is inherited. If this is absent, protection is quite positive.

The predisposition is marked in many cases from
birth to the onset of the localized disease or ultimates.
We should not wait for the onset of the pathology, but all
cases should be prevented by study and tests. If parents
were aware of the possibility of testing and absolute pre-

vention, they would aid toward the final closing out of the "white plague."

NOSODE:

The nosode tendency is becoming altogether too extravagant. I have known Medorrhinum to be given and fail where Thuja would have cured promptly, because the symptoms were predominantly Thuja and not Medorrhinum. I have known Psorinum to be given because the case was supposed to be due to psora, where Sulphur was well indicated. It is a great error to prescribe for the miasm instead of the totality of the symptoms.

If the symptoms are very scanty and the remedy is doubtful and the patient has a history of gonorrhœa, his symptoms having come on since, it is a hopeful experiment to give Medorrhinum. In similar manner, if there is a history of syphilis with a paucity of symptoms, it is a good experiment to give Syphilinum. Most certainly we must rise above miasmatic prescribing, yet the miasm should be held in view and the remedies should be held in view, and the remedies that fit the symptoms should also be deep enough to cure the corresponding miasm.

THE MODERN TENDENCY TO RE-PROVE OUR MATERIA MEDICA

There is a general call for our old remedies to be re-proved; but nothing has been done as yet to improve any of the old provings made in the early days. We need not expect our Materia Medica to grow except in the hands of good observers.

When we have noted *all that can be observed by the physician himself, and felt and observed by the prover, and observed by companions*, we have gathered about all that is worth knowing for the purpose of prescribing.

Provers do not push a drug until tissue changes are

found, hence the expert examinations have been useless
and these laboratory examinations do not add to the information that is desired either in the patient or the
prover. The simple-minded patients and provers give us
the best symptoms for use. The so-called pathological
prescribing is all done on clinical symptoms or on the toxic
effect of drugs, yet most of the pathological prescribers
are so ignorant of the sources of symptoms that they oppose prescribing on clinical symptoms as a basis of the
prescription. Such ignorance is characteristic of mongrelism throughout.

In the wonderful re-proving of Belladonna, absolutely
nothing was added to the grand old Belladonna. Many
have urged that re-proving be made under the eye of
specialists with all laboratory tests, blood tests, blood
pressure, etc., thinking that this highly scientific procedure and display would cause Homœopathy to be accepted by the representatives of traditional medicine. In
my opinion we would only subject ourselves to ridicule.
If we would think more of the grand old method of proving
followed by Hahnemann, our minds would be clearer as
to what would be best to record—what would be needed.
These so-called modern provers are ignorant of the philosophy, and therefore do not know what is required for
a successful study of a drug, nor study of a sick man for
a successful prescription. The modern demands for proving reveal complete ignorance of the requirements for
prescribing. They aim at bringing forth the common symptoms and neglecting the symptoms that characterize the
patient. This defect is stamped upon all modern provings.
Materia Medica students should master the ORGANON first
and make provings later. The methods of Hahnemann
have never been improved. Let all compare the modern
provings with Hahnemann's provings and note the difference.

Our well-proved remedies do not need re-proving. Many of our scantily-proved drugs should have further provings, but in the same method followed by Hahnemann. Remedies should be proved in low, medium and high potencies. As soon as the prover begins to experience the symptoms, administration of the drug should be stopped until there is no manifestation of drug action, else confusion follows. The confusion has spoiled many otherwise good provings.

THE DEFINITION OF A HOMŒOPATHIC PHYSICIAN

"A homœopathic physician in one who adds to his knowledge of medicine a special knowledge of homœopathic therapeutics and observes the law of similars."—A. I. H.

"The homœopathic physician is one who prescribes the single remedy in the minimum dose in potentized form, selected according to the law of similars."

The superficial observer would not criticize either form of definition. The astonishing part of the first formula is expressed in the first part: "who adds to his knowledge of medicine."

Of what does the knowledge consist? Is it what all tradition count as up-to-date use of drugs, such as cathartics, ointments, depressants, compound tablets, coal-tar products, crude drugs in general, etc? Does it mean that the homœopathic physician must know these so that he can have something to which to add the special knowledge of homœopathic therapeutics in order to be a homœopathic physician?

It would be supposed that the homœopathic physician had abandoned the first to become a physician of an advanced and scientific order. It must be acknowledged that all of this knowledge of medicine, to which he is to add his homœopathics, is traditional ignorance and absurdities. Now to this ignorance he is to add a knowledge of homœopathic therapeutics. Would it not be better and wiser to say that a homœopathic physician is one who has abandoned traditional absurdities and adopted the science and philosophy of healing according to the Law of Similars? Men who depend upon the diagnosis, the laboratory findings, the pathology, the bacteriology, for selection of their remedies are expected to add to such knowledge (?) a special knowledge of homœopathic therapeutics!

It has been our experience to meet a large number of these so-called homœopathic physicians, but we have never met one who had added any knowledge of materia medica or the art of prescribing to his so-called general knowledge of medicine.

The astonishing part of the formula is that it frames into the definition just the part that prevents every man from becoming a homœopathic physician. So long as he holds on to the traditional absurdities, even when called modern scientific medicine, so long as he is incapable of learning the true art of healing according to the Law of Similars. So long as he believes that these absurdities are valuable knowledge, so long he feels no need of going into real knowledge of homœopathic therapeutics. It is not sin to know these absurdities so long as he realizes that they are such, but the formula calls them "knowledge of medicine." It cannot refer to anatomy, physiology, chemistry, ets., because to these he does not add, as they are part of doctors' rights and possessions.

If we look over the country and take note of the men who sail under this flag, and we ascertain their methods, it will be found that many of them scarcely differ from the allopath in the use of drugs and methods. The most of them believe in the Law of Similars, but are too ignorant of materia medica, of the use of repertory and of the philosophy, to practice Homœopathy.

In their ignorance they use drugs in the same crude

form as they were used for proving, whereas the sick man who has the corresponding symptoms is a thousand times more sensitive than was the prover. It is well to know that if these ignorant pretenders really administered a true homœopathic remedy, they would intensify the illness in hand. I have known them to do this many times, and in their ignorance they would change for another remedy, instead of stopping the drug to permit the patient to make a quick recovery. I have met many of these crude physicians, and they have generally blamed the college which turned them out with only a crude knowledge of materia medica, no knowledge of how to use the repertory, and without any homœopathic philosophy, although they had plenty of pathology, plenty of diagnosis. They saw ointments applied to the skin, in a very large skin clinic, by one of these physicians who professes to add to his stupid ignorance a knowledge of the law of cure.

Was not the adoption of this definition for the sole purpose of giving standing to men whose requirements were a knowledge of fads and traditional absurdities, and ignorance of Hahnemann's ORGANON and the PURE MATERIA MEDICA? It is a question that must come to the mind of every thinking homœopathic physician.

It is equally evident that the second definition, mentioned above as the description of a genuine homœopathic physician, could find only a small minority in the American Institute to favor it, as we all know. It has often been asked why Homœopathy grows so slowly. Is it not apparent that the reason is to be found in the sentiment that caused the adoption of this first definition of the homœopathic physician, which so misrepresents the true followers of Homœopathy? When such men are in the majority what is there to be seen in their prescribing that would attract the attention of any suffering man? No wonder that the world is slow to accept Homœopathy when the people see so little convincing proof of its usefulness. What better is it than the traditional medicine? How often do we hear our own faithful patients say: "If we could not find a genuine homœopathic physician I would call an allopath?" These are the patrons that know the difference. The patron knows better than to trust a man who alternates remedies, gives compound tablets and tinctures. Yet the A. I. H. definition permits the fraudulent misrepresentation to pose as a genuine homœopathic physician.

HIGHER USE OF PRIMARY BRANCHES IN MEDICAL EDUCATION

Learn well the anatomy, pathology, chemistry, diagnosis, and the symptoms and course of every disease and all disease ultimates, that common symptoms may be quickly and certainly known.

By this means it will be easier to say what symptoms are not common to the case in hand, and thereby to perceive that all symptoms present in a given case which are not common must be *uncommon* and *predicated* (in general or particular) *of the patient*. These must be foremost in guiding to the remedy and the common symptoms may fall in, taking their place naturally where they belong in each individual case of sickness. When this method is mastered, prescribing becomes easy, with experience.

If we are homœopathicians, how shall we discover it and prove it to ourselves and others?

We may give the single dose or repeat our remedies;

We may give potentized remedies in high or higher potencies;

We may wait ever so long on the action of our given remedies and yet fail to cure sick folks, and if we fail to cure sick people we are not homœopathicians.

The curing of sick people permanently, gently and quickly is the first and best test of a homœopathician.

This is easier said than done. It is often only a pretension. It is one thing to cure chronically sick people and another to cure acutely sick people, or sicknesses, or diseases as some would have us say.

If the remedy is properly chosen and properly administered in typhoid fever, how soon should the patient recover? This is a question that every homœopathician should ask himself, and by it should be willing to have himself measured.

Looking back over thirty years I can answer the question better than a young man. My cases of continued fever with prostration, tympanitic abdomen and sordes on the teeth recovered inside of two weeks in the first ten years of my homœopathic practice. In the last twenty years they have all been aborted in seven to ten days. Not one has continued to progress according to the usual course of the disease, therefore not one could be proved to be typhoid by the Weidal test.

The homœopathician will never have a case that will stand the eighth day test, therefore, according to modern science, he will never have a typhoid;

Hahnemann says that all acute diseases should be aborted. Why should we not expect to do this if Hahnemann did so a hundred years ago? Why call ourselves Homœopathicians if we cannot do as well as Hahnemann did?

Why not offer this as the test of our ability and skill, and consciously admit that we must abort all acute diseases or cease to call ourselves homœopathicians?

There can be no better test for our work and for our position than to announce to the world that we do this, if we do it, and let all others compare their work and stand or fall by the test of clinical experience.

Let the near-homœopath, the highly scientific laboratory doctor, the christian scientist, the eclectic, the osteopath, or whatever he may be, come in and show what he can do to abort acute diseases. We must stand by the test. All our homœopathicians know how to do this work and make good. Hahnemann says in his ORGANON OF HEALING, paragraph 149:

If we profess to follow Hahnemann, let us display to man what we do to entitle ourselves to the name and to disfranchise pretenders. Pretenders will at once come to the front and reveal themselves by denouncing us and affirming that it cannot be done. They thereby only declare that they cannot do it, and hereby convict themselves of being only fraudulent or pretended followers of Hahnemann. Even if they affirm that they are only modern homœopaths, they must disclaim on the work they do, pretensions. "The proof of the pudding is in the eating and not on the plausibility of their scientific methods or of it."

Homœopathicians abort all acute diseases—what do others accomplish? It only remains for us to educate the people so they will know what to expect, and what can be done, and who can do it. But first the education must begin with the physician, so that he can meet the requirements. Some will say "We do not believe it," which simply means that they have not seen such results, and this only signifies that they do not know how to apply the remedies homœopathically. Then let the education begin at home. That there are many professed Hahnemannians who are not doing this work in this way is no reason for our silence. It is enough to know that Hahnemann did it, that many others are doing it, that we should all do it. If we cannot do so, let us give up our pretensions.

ADOPTION OF HOMŒOPATHY

Homœopathy will not be universally adopted for many centuries. There are many people in the world who cannot

believe a great truth however much evidence is presented
in its favor. We are all encumbered with tradition. Unbelief in new things is our strongest tendency. The tendency to ridicule what we do not understand is born in us.
A few refined and educated minds that have been opened
by circumstances are prepared to examine our principles;
others have accepted the truth by force of circumstances.
All who really love Homœopathy have an unlimited desire
to teach it to associates and to their patients. They are
often astonished that the door is closed to their willing
efforts.

Our literature has been defective, to a large extent
as a teaching medium—that which has been prepared for
the laity as much as that which has been prepared to
teach the medical student and practitioner. Looking over
our literature of the past we observe its incongruities.
Here and there we find hints. Hahnemann's ORGANON is a
strong, rich source of knowledge, but it is in long sen-
tences, and very condensed, and difficult for many to understand. When one has fully comprehended the principles,
he then reads Hahnemann's ORGANON with the deepest
satisfaction. The subject is so deep, so difficult to comprehend. A most scholarly, deep-thinking man said to me,
"I have read your PHILOSOPHY five times and am still
reading it, and now I begin to understand Hahnemann's
ORGANON. When this is known it may not be a surprise
that so many fail to comprehend our principles. This has
been said to indicate how important it is to have our principles clearly taught in all our colleges. Yet nearly all our
colleges fail to teach these principles; the Chair of Philosophy may be filled by a man who knows nothing of the
subject. Such a state of affairs delays the spread of
Homœopathy. Homœopathy would develop faster if the
physicians were all true to its principles. So many use

the compound tablets, and prescribe tinctures in physiological doses, telling people they practice Homœopathy.

BOOKS

Homœopathy is slow to win its way because of the defective use of books, as well as because of defective books, thus producing results that are not striking but merely ordinary. There are books in existence that seem to foster the idea of pure Homœopathy which have done much harm along with much good. The Therapeutic Pocket Book has rendered all our old men a grand service, but it is most defective and yet has caused many good men to shun repertories. It has in most instances furnished only a moderate exhibition of results.

Its generalizing of all particulars has destroyed its worth in so many instances. When we see the circumstance of *lying*, shall we conclude that lying shall apply to headache, to vertigo, to dyspnœa, to palpitation, to backache, in the same degree? Shall we take the Mag-m. *aggravation of liver symptoms when lying on the left side* applicable to headache, to vertigo, to dyspnœa, etc., and all in the same degree? Must we have all our circumstances in the same degree in generals as in particulars?

All who have learned the better way look back with surprise at the faith reposed in the Pocket Book. One who is familiar with the materia medica can make very good use of this small book, but it will misguide the young man and lead him to drop the use of repertories, and thereby hinder the spread of Homœopathy.

When all our books are arranged so that the whole being comes into view, from generals to particulars, when taking the case; when working out the case; when reading the materia medica and when studying the philosophy; then may we hope that our cause will march on by healing

the sick and by teaching all who have the desire to learn it
and the ability to understand it.

THE POSITION OF THE SPECIALIST IN
THERAPEUTICS

The specialist assumes, and no doubt believes, that
the chronic complaints and symptoms of human being are
due to the disordered condition of the particular organ
which he has selected as his particular speciality. The
gynecologist tells the woman that all her suffering in the
various organs and parts of the body are due to the disordered pelvic organs. The cardiac specialist tells her that
all her complaints are due to her heart. The oculist tells
her that all her troubles are due to the eyes. The neurolo-
gist tells her that all her troubles are due to the spine.
Each one promises that the patient will be well when the
organ which he treats has been properly treated.

It would appear that this perverted idea of the specialist prevents him from ever learning to be a successful
homœopathic physician. It appears never to have dawned
upon one of them that the organs are sick and out of
order because the patient is sick. Each specialist gives
local treatment to the part that is his specialty, if he
can get to it to treat it locally. If he cannot reach it with
local treatment, he feeds the patient with drugs, supposed
to act upon such organ, in physiological doses.

THE LOCAL TREATMENT OF NOSE AND THROAT, VAGINA,
EYE AND EAR, IS NO DOUBT THE MOST DANGEROUS
OF ALL THE WORK DONE BY SPECIALISTS.

The specialists appear to think that all there is to
be learned about the human body is the anatomy, pathology, and local treatment of the part selected. With the
exception of a few specialists who do not work in this
way, it is evident that more harm comes thus to human
beings than the homœopath can counteract.

Any homœopathist who does careful and honest prescribing will have constantly on hand a lot of patients who have had discharges from ear, vagina, or eyes, suppressed by local use of strong drugs. If the specialist would only consider first *the patient as a whole,* while he is advising about the part that he has pre-empted as his own, and cease using the strong lotions, he would be a useful man, but he then would only be a physician and seldom a specialist.

The smallest part of the body should never be treated except by *a remedy that fits the symptoms of the entire constitution, organs and parts.* It is a complete loss, if not a damage, to a patient to take a remedy for the eye, unless it fits all the symptoms of the mind, body and parts, yet we cannot object to a physician choosing to be a specialist if first of all he is an all-round physician.

Let us picture to ourselves a weakling in medical college, who thinks he can cut down his work by confining his study to the treatment of a single part. Even if he goes to Germany and amuses himself for a year, watching the local treatment in the clinic of some celebrated specialist, he finds the same lotions used in the same manner and with the same results as in the medical clinic of his own home. Is it a wonder that so often in our hearing it is said the specialists are all humbugs?

The same lotion is used for every patient with a slight variation only in appearance. The great specialist and the small specialist are all the same in treatment and they all use the lotions that may be the latest fad. If they have found a more successful lotion it is only one that will do the patient a little more harm. In proportion as it relieves (?) the organ, in that proportion it injures the patient.

Homœopathic patients should be instructed so that they will know, when going to a specialist, whether he is treating them constitutionally or locally. When the patient is consulting a specialist for spine, heart, or brain trouble, he should know whether it is one who will give crude drugs for physiological action, or who is a genuine homœopathic prescriber and will take all the symptoms of mind, body, organs and parts and select that remedy which corresponds to the *totality of the symptoms*.

beware specialists

We have been too long silent on this subject.

The consequences of vicious suppressive treatment should be made known to all our patrons in no uncertain language. If the homœopathician is outspoken in all the matters that are for the people's good, it will be seen that we are not approaching the old school sufficiently to lead any person to predict a near conjunction of the two schools.

Why should a specialist who relies on local treatment expect to associate with homœopathic physicians? Can local treatment in the hands of a professed homœopath be any different from local treatment in the hands of a traditional doctor?

When this treatment is the same as that used by the old school doctor why should he call himself a homœopath?

ADDRESS

An address delivered before the Boenninghausen Society, Philadelphia. Pa.

Prostration coming on slowly.	Agar., Arn., Ars., Arum-t.,
Continued fever.	Bapt., Bry., *Carb-v.*, Chin.,
Zymosis.	Cocc., *Colch.*, Crot-h., *Gels.*,
Sordes in the mouth.	Hell., Hyos., Kali-bi., *Kali-ph.*,
Tympanitic abdomen.	Lach., Laur., Lyc., Mur-ac.,
Diarrhoea.	*Nit-ac.*, *Op.*, Petr., Phos-ac.,
Delirium.	Phos., *Psor.*, Rhus-t., *Secale*,
Petechiae.	Stram., Sulph., *Sulph-ac.*, Ver-
	at., Zinc.

Epidemic

Typhoid

TYPHOID FEVER.

Mr. President, Ladies and Gentlemen:—When I was asked to present the subject of the therapeutics relating to typhoid fever it occurred to me to present the subject in a general way, but as I thought about it and considered the epidemic now in the city, progressing and increasing to intensity, it seemed to me that it would be more profitable to study especially such remedies as relate to the present epidemic. Of course, this consideration cannot be taken up without a general extensive survey of typhoid; but to make the subject comprehensive would require a dozen evenings rather than one, so I will consider tonight only those remedies that belong to our present epidemic in Philadelphia. I shall not have time to go over the subject of diet, hygiene or prophylaxis, nor the numerous things that every well disposed and intelligent physician should know for himself, but will confine myself to the therapeutics, the homœopathic remedies that relate to the present form of typhoid.

On the black-board we have a general summary of the pathognomonic sypmtoms of typhoid fever, those that run through all cases, those that are present more or less all through the fever. You could scarcely have a group of cases of typhoid that did not exhibit these conditions. Then if we go into our Materia Medica we readily group the remedies that correspond. These on the black-board, if considered in a general way, you will find look like the symptoms we have placed opposite them. You see that in this group individualizing and differing symptoms are left out, only those that are common to them all are included. They all have prostration, they all have in degree a continued nature of the febrile condition; they all have, some higher than others, the zymotic tendency; they all have the sordes and the distension known as tympanitic abdomen; they all have more or less a diarrhoea, and most of them have petechiae. In a general way the group on the left equals the group on the right and vice versa, but this is the general and common consideration. But now as that entire group of remedies in complex is equal to that group on the left in complex, so is each one a likeness of the group on the left. Each one has in its nature a species of typhoid or continued fever and yet none of them produces true idiopathic typhoid fever. Only a likeness is found, but we deal only with similars, and while we recognize that the typhoid, the Agaricus and the Zincum are all individuals, yet we recognize that they are all similar. Not all, however, have the symptoms in the same form and hence the necessity of individualization comes up before us. Some have the diarrhoea at one time of the day, some have it at another time of the day; some have continued fever in very high degree and some have continued fever in low degree. Arn., Bry., Lach., Stram., sul-ac., have continued fever in very high degree, but China's most characteristic feature is intermittent fever, and it has continued fever in low degree. China has in a very high degree many of the symptoms and much of the nature of typhoid fever, the prostration, the tympanites, the zymosis, the sordes, the diarrhoea, the delirium, but as to a continued fever it is in a low degree, and hence China comes in in intermittents and remittents which are going towards and becoming continued. Primarily Gelsemium is a remittent remedy, but in a moderate degree it takes on continuance as it progresses, and hence has been found especially suitable for those fevers that are remittent in character in the earlier stages, but, as the disease advances, progresses towards a continued fever, and hence it is suitable for bilious and remittent fevers that take on the continued type, or, strictly speaking symptomatic typhoids.

Some remedies have delirium in the fore part of the night and some in the after part of the night. These questions have to be considered, and the only way to consider them is by a carefully prepared repertory. Even the fever has its time of aggravtion. It is important to find the time at which the fever is highest; in some rem-

16

edies it will be in the afternoon, some from 3 o'clock to midnight; in some the sharpest time is from 9 o'clock to midnight, etc.

Those remedies having highest fever at certain times are as follows:

Afternoon: Agar., Apis, Ars., Bry., Canth., Chin., Colch., Dig., Gels., Hyos., Ip., Lach., Lyc., Nit-ac., Nux-v., Ph-ac., Phos., Puls., Rhus-t., Stram., Sulph., Sul-ac.

Evening: Ars., Bry., Carb-v., Cham., Chin., Hell., Ign., Ip., Lach., Lyc., Mur-ac., Nit-ac., Nux-v., Phos., Phos-ac., Puls., Rhus-t., Sul-ac., Sulph.

4 to 8 p. m.: Lyc.

4 p. m. till midnight: Stram.

5 p. m.: Kali-n., Rhus-t., Sulph.

7 p. m.: Lyc., Rhus-t.

8 p. m.: Hep., Mur-ac., Phos., Sulph.

9 to 12 p. m.: Bry.

10 p. m.: Lach.

Night: Am-c., Apis, Ars., Arum-t., Bapt., Bry., Calad., Carb-v., Cham., Chin., Chin-a., Cocc., Colch., Kali-bi., Lach., Lyc., Merc., Mur-ac., Nux-v., Op., Ph-ac., Phos., Puls., Rhus-t., Stram., Sul-ac. Sulph.

Temperature running very high: Bry., Hyos., Rhus-t., Stram.

Midnight: Ars., Lyc., Rhus-t., Stram., Sulph., Verat.

Midnight, before: Ars., Bapt., Bry., Calad., Carbo-v., Lach., Lyc., Nux-v., Stram.

After: Ars., Bry., Chin., Chin-a., Lyc., Nux-v Phos., Rhus-t., Sulph.

These points as to the highest temperature are important. Remedies select a particular time. You may ask, "Why?" I am not here to answer that, but we observe the fact, and by observing we act accordingly. Find out from the nurse, or by your thermometer, at what particular

ime the temperature is the highest, and then examine
uch medicines as have this increase of temperature.

But these are only most common and general consid-
rations. The most important symptoms to consider for
he selection of a remedy are such as are not necessarily
ound in most cases of typhoid, such as belong to the
atient himself, such things as stamp upon the sickness
he nature and state of the patient. According to Hahne-
nann the sole duty of the physician is to pay attention to
he patient, not to treat his disease, but the sick man.
Iveryone suffering from this fever has only what might
e called a species of typhoid.

When the physician enters the room he should begin
o observe and gaze at everything for symptoms; for the
ymptoms are to the intelligent physician the index of the
isease.

What this patient is doing is certainly an important
hing for the physician to observe. Does he desire to move
r remain quiet? If he is worse during rest he will move,
nd if he moves continuously we at once examine a certain
lass of remedies, that may be called the moving remedies,
r restless remedies, such as Arn., Ars., Bapt., Hyos., Lach.,
yc., Rhus-t., Stram. It is important to examine into the
ause of his restlessness, and by observing him a little, or,
he be able to talk, by questioning him we will find that
ne (the Arnica) patient moves because he is sore and
ruised and wants to get off the sore spots; he often says
lat the bed is hard, but if he describes his sufferings
oncretely he will say he is sore and bruised and moves to
nd relief, only to become sore and bruised again, and so
e keeps on moving. Arsenicum is continuously moving.
is said in the text he moves from the bed to the chair,
ad from the chair to the bed, but you see by his face
lat it is an anxious restlessness that possesses him. His
ental state is one of anxiety, and is depicted upon his

countenance; and you will see that this mental state drives him to move and he cannot keep still. We sometimes see the Baptisia patient restless and moving, although many times curled up in a bunch and doing nothing, but when he moves it is like Arnica, to get off the sore place. Hyoscyamus moves from restlessness. Rhus tox. moves because he aches; he is sore and bruised and the longer he keeps still the more violent is that aching, and so he moves and tosses and lies but a moment; after moving he thinks now he is going to be comfortable, but the soreness soon returns and causes him to move. How does that differ from Arsenicum? Arsenicum has the mental anxiety and it is depicted upon the face. Rhus tox has that also in a less degree, but the anxious restlessness in Rhus. is not so severe as are his pains. Arsenicum is mental, Rhus tox is physical Stramonium moves and moves with the delirium and wildness of his mental state; his anxiety and awful state of frenzy keep him in continuous motion. This then expresses a difference, no two are alike.

But if after long watching the physician sees that the patient lies in one position and desires to be quiet, does not want to move, is not restless, he must study Bry., Cocc. Colch., Hell., Phos. These all lie perfectly still as if dead Bryonia in a high degree wants to be let alone, does not want to talk, is worse from motion, has a scowl if asked to move, lies there as if tired and dreads to move. Cocculus does the same lying on the back, eyes partly open knows a good deal that is going on, but does not want to be spoken to, with a great state of paralytic prostration. There is a strong key to it, viz., if you talk in his presence about his food, and how we will go about it to feed him. he is nauseated at once; Colchium has the same state, and it is only by further consideration that we will be able to distinguish between these two remedies

Cocculus has more of the paralytic weakness. Colchicum has a characteristic diarrhœa. In Cocculus it is the brain that is troubled; we will look in the abdomen for the symptoms of Colchicum. Hellebore also lies still with the head thrown back, the limbs drawn up upon the abdomen, rolling the head in delirium, but otherwise wants to keep perfectly still, and the physician has only to observe a few days to see that there are wrinkles coming in the face and brow showing cerebral disturbance of the gravest character. Or the mental weakness and increasing prostration, with thirst for ice cold water which gurgles through the bowels, will enable you to distinguish that he is needing Phosphorus.

Many patients have carphologia, as it is called, picking at the bed clothes or his lips or at flocks. The remedies having these symptoms are Arn., Ars., Cocc., Colch., Hell., Hyos., Lyc., Phos-ac., Phos., Psor., Rhus-t., Stram., Sulph., Zinc. They all make such motions, but if it is observed that he picks his bleeding lips, regardless of the fact that they are raw and sore and bleeding, and he tears off the crusts and still they bleed, and yet he picks them, Arum triphyllum is of great importance and must be added to the list, for it has this symptom along with two remedies already included, Phos-ac., and Zincum. If the physician continues to gaze, he observes the stupor. This state of stupor, profound or otherwise, is covered by quite an extensive list of remedies, such as: Arn., Ars., Bapt., Bry., Carb-v., Cocc., Colch., Crot-h., Gels., Hell., Hyos., Lach., Laur., Lyc., Mur-ac., Op., Petr., Ph-ac., Phos., Rhus-t., Sec., Stram., Sulph., Sul-ac., Verat., Zinc. They have varying degrees of prostration and if we had time it would be delightful to go through them all, but I will mention only a few. The peculiar prostration of Baptisia is noticed very early: the patient will be lying upon the right side quite stupid, quite prostrated, hardly able to answer, but usually he can be aroused. Sometimes he will finish what he is saying, but oftener he will not finish the sentence he has begun but will drop back into sleep or stupor, in the midst of it. The stupor of Muriatic acid is especially worthy of consideration, as it comes on gradually and is attended with a great degree of prostration. It comes on late in the progress of the disease, because it succeeds the muscular prostration which we will speak of later. In contra-distinction to this Phos-ac. becomes stupid early in the progress of the disease, and from the stupor of mind he progresses toward weakness of body, and hence we observe in Phos-ac., that which is peculiar, viz., copious diarrhœa of a watery character that is often cerebral, and yet there is no evidence of prostration. The physician wonders how such a copious watery ejection of fluid can be present without prostration, it is a nervous diarrhœa.

If the physician gazes sufficiently long he notices, also, the muscles and of parts trembling all over, quivering, jerkings, twitchings, called subsultus tendinum. The trembling early expressed is a strong indication of a severe nervous state quite analogous to Zincum, but if it is primarily of the tongue that the trembling is noticed, and not especially of other parts, it is found under Ars., Gels., Lach., Lyc., Phos., Rhus-t., Secale, Stram., Zinc. In Lachesis the tongue trembles on putting it out, and the sensation of trembling of the tongue in the mouth is also Lachesis. If, when he attempts to talk the lips quiver, that is, the effort at motion makes the lips quiver, we must study Lach., Phos., Stram., and Zinc.

A great degree of weakness is present when the jaw falls down, so that the mouth is wide open, and the tongue shows its bleeding and sordes. This patient will soon show a tendency to slide down in the bed with a great degree of paralytic weakness. For the symptom, jaw hangs down, we find the following: Arn., Arsen., Bapt., Carb-v., Colch., Hell., Hyos., Lach., Lyc., Mur-ac., Op., Phos., Secale, Stram., Sulph., Zinc.

The patient's expression will also be observed by the physician. When he sees an expression of anxiety depicted upon his countenance then these remedies come into his mind: Ars., Bapt., Crot-h., Lyc., Nit-ac., Stram., Sul-ac.; but if the patient puts on an appearance as if he had been intoxicated, looking as if he had been on a debauch, he must consult Bapt., Cocc., Gels., Lach., Mur-ac., Op., Stram. If he tries to rouse the patient and get him into conversation he may rouse up perfectly bewildered, and then the physician thinks of Nux-m., Phos-ac., Stram., Zinc. Or he sees that the patient gazes off in one corner in a vacant, fixed look, says nothing, answers no questions. This is like Arn., Cocc., Op., Phos., Stram., Sul-ac. For the idiotic expression seen in some patients he must study Lach., Laur., Lyc., Secale, Stram. The look of a typhoid patient is said to be sometimes very similar to a vacant stare, then it is that Cocc., Phos-ac., and Stram. are to be examined to see if all the rest of the symptoms agree.

As the physician looks into the mouth he sees the gums and the teeth and the tongue, and he finds that brown exuded blood has dried upon the various parts and upon the lips. Sordes are built upon the teeth, containing decomposing blood, and here we find in a high degree the following remedies indicated: Ars., Bapt., Bry., Chin., Gels., Hyos., Mur-ac., Phos-ac., Phos., Rhus-t., Secale, Stram., Sul-ac. If the tongue is more particularly examined, and it is found to be black, and the blood that exudes is particularly black, such remedies as Ars., Carb-v., Chin., Hyos., Lach., Lyc., Op., Phos., Secale, Sul-ac., are to be thought of. When the tongue is more brown than black Ars., Bapt., Bry., Carb-v., Chin., Colch., Hyos., Kali-ph., Lach., Lyc., Phos., Rhus-t., Secale, Sulph., Sul-ac., must be examined. The tongue is sometimes very red later on in the stages of typhoid. After it has cleaned off its thick heavy exudations it becomes very red, sometimes glistening with red sides, sometimes with red tip, but if generally red Ars., Bapt., Colch., Crot-h., Gels., Hyos., Kali-bi., Lach., Lyc., Nit-ac., Phos., Rhus-t., can be thought of; they all have red tongue. Later in the disease after the fever has to great extent subsided, or even though there still be fever, the tongue becomes denuded, is glossy, shiny, looking as if varnished, a glistening tongue, then we must examine Kali-bi., Lach., Phos. When there is a very red stripe down the center of the tongue Kali-bi., Phos., Phos-ac., Verat-v., become useful. When the tongue becomes very red and dry at the tip, Ars., Lach., Lyc., Nit-ac., Rhus-t., Sul-ac., become very important. Perhaps you may have noticed in these zymotic states that the tongue is generally dark brown or red, very seldom white or yellow; the yellow tongue belongs more to bilious or remittent fever. The tongue is generally dark, and in the more violent forms of the disease, blackish or brown. With the very heavily coated dark tongue, where these exudations pile up the following remedies will be found useful: Arn., Ars., Bapt., Bry., Carb-v., Cocc., Kali-bi., Lach., Mur-ac., Nit-ac., Phos., Phos-ac., Rhus-t., Secale. In very low forms of advanced typhoid with a great degree of prostration after the fever has somewhat subsided leaving a state of tremulous prostration, the tongue becomes cold and it is said often by the patient that the tongue feels cold; it is then that such remedies as the following must be examined: Carb-v., Laur., Verat., Zinc. When it feels cold to the touch of the physician, Ars., Carb-v., Colch., Laur., Phos-ac., Verat., Zinc., are the remedies. Then again the tongue becomes cracked, bleeds and is raw; oozing of blood appears about the mouth, about the tongue and upon the lips; for this bleeding, cracked appearance of the tongue, the following remedies must be examined: Ars., Arum-t., Bapt., Carb-v., Chin., Crot-h., Hyos., Kali-bi., Lach., Lyc., Mur-ac., Nit-ac., Phos., Rhus-t.

In some cases of typhoid either early or later in the disease, the tongue is as dry as chips, as dry as leather, dark brown or very black and it is tough like leather or wood. The patient has almost no use of it. This is found in the following remedies: Ars., Arum-t., Bapt., Bry., Carb-v., Chin., Cocc., Hell., Hyos., Kali-bi., Lach., Lyc., Mur-ac., Nit-ac., Nux-m., Phos., Phos-ac., Rhus-t., Secale, Sul-ac., Verat. If particularly the centre is dry as a board and withered, and upon the sides it is moist, looking more like a tongue, we think of Bapt., Crot-h., Lach., Phos., Stram., Sul-ac.

The physician then brings in his nose for the further consideration of his patient. The putrid odors from the mouth that the physician observes, call especially for Arn., Ars., Arum-t., Bapt., Bry., Carb-v., Crot-h., Kali-bi., Lach., Lyc., Mur-ac., Nit-ac., Phos., Rhus-t., Secale, Stram.

In this way we consider what has been observed by the physician himself throughout the entire body and appearance of the patient, and next we proceed to examine what the nurse has to say concerning this patient. The physician cannot examine all of the passages from the bowels and bladder, and he must rely upon what the nurse can relate concerning the things that take place during his absence; these, of course, are very numerous, but a few general things can be talked about. The diarrhœa, when it is of a nondescript character or a mere typhoid diarrhœa, coming as a pathognomonic part of the disease, is not a very important feature, but at times it becomes very severe, very exhaustive, and then the time of the aggravation must be considered. Some have the diarrhœa only at night, like China; some have it in the day time only, like Petroleum; some have it day and night, and of these exhaustive diarrhœas, the feature which is of most importance is the involuntary nature. Involuntary diarrhœa is found under Arn., Ars., Bapt., Bry., Carb-v., Colch., Crot-h., Gels., Hell., Hyos., Lach., Laur., Mur-ac., Op., Phos., Phos-ac., Rhus-t., Secale, Sul-ac., Verat. Quite a list to be examined, but the physician must examine well all of these. Sometimes we have a still greater degree of prostration in which there is involuntary discharge of both stool and urine, taking place simultaneously, and then Arn., Ars., Carb-v., Colch., Hyos., Laur., Mur-ac., Phos-ac., Phos., Rhus-t., Secale, Stram., must all be looked into. Copious flow of blood with the stool, hemorrhage from the bowels, will require an examination of the following remedies: Arn., Ars., Carb-v., Chin., Colch., Crot-h., Kali-bi., Lach., Lyc., Mur-ac., Nit-ac., Phos., Rhus-t., Secale, Sul-ac.

The nurse further relates in her description of the stool that it is very putrid, that it is cadaveric, like dead things, like stinking meat, horribly offensive. It is an unnecessary individualization in this typhoid state to go into the fine differences of the odor, because it is often only a difference in the nose to measure an odor. Putrid stools would call to mind Ars., Bapt., Carb-v., Crot-h., Lach., etc.

The very copious thin exhaustive stools often require such remedies as Phos-ac., Phos., Secale, Verat.

Then we notice another state, which is commonly worse in the night and may be observed also at times when the fever is at its highest, or when the patient is unconscious, viz., twitchings. He twitches and jerks; sometimes it is so marked that it is like a chorea, when it becomes like Agaricus, but when only in the finer muscles, Ars., Carb-v., Cocc., Colch., Crot-h., Hyos., Lach., Mur-ac., Phos., Psor., Rhus-t., Stram., Sul-ac., Zinc. become the remedies.

When the prostration becomes so marked that the patient slides down in bed until his head is perfectly level with the body, right off from the pillow, it is then that the following remedies must be examined: Ars., Carb-v., Mosch., Mur-ac., Nit-ac., Nux-m., Phos., Phos-ac., Rhus-t.

The mental symptoms are often of the greatest importance. Little particulars come out sometimes in mental symptoms that lead you to think of a remedy, not to give the remedy because of the keynote, but to sit down and meditate upon it for a few minutes, to ascertain whether or not it fits the whole case, whether the remedy that is calling attention to itself has all the rest of the symptoms. The mental symptoms are of great value, especially when the patient is in a state of semi-consciousness, when he is going down into a state of prostration. There are changes in his mind, in his manner of speech, and answering questions. If he looks as if he could answer correctly but does not, then such remedies as Carb-v., Hyos., Phos-ac., Phos., must be studied. When his answers do not fit the question, when they are irrelevant, when he answers a question that has not been asked, then Carb-v., Hyos., Nux-m., Phos-ac., Sul-ac., will be the remedies to consider. When he lies and looks at the physician but does not answer the question, he looks as if he could answer, but never says a word, Arn., Hell., Hyos., Nux-m., Phos., Phos-ac., Stram. must be thought of. He lies and looks into the physician's face and reflects a long time, and finally answers with great difficulty, it seems that he cannot get his mind to compass the idea, and he answers slowly, Cocc., Hell., Nux-m., Phos-ac., must be considered. In a general way, those having slow answers and slow speech, as if meditating before answering (the semi-conscious state), are Ars., Carb-v., Cocc., Hell., Nux-m., Phos., Phos-ac., Rhus-t. He answers correctly, but soon returns to a marked state of stupor, is found especially under Arn., Bapt., Hyos.

Again, his mental state becomes more active, and he

takes on delirium and rage, but more particularly wants to run away, wants to escape, wants to get out of the window, the following remedies must be examined: Ars., Bapt., Bry., Cocc., Hell., Hyos., Lach., Phos., Rhus-t., Stram., Zinc. There is sometimes one reason, and sometimes another, for his wanting to get up and escape. When the patient thinks he is away from home and wants to get up and get out of the window and go home, Bry., Hyos., Lach., Op., Rhus-t., Verat., must be thought of. If in his hallucinations the most frightful rage is observed, when he strikes, bites, cuts, seeks to kill, do mischief, destructive rage, Carb-v., Hyos., Laur., Lyc., Op., Phos., Phos-ac., Rhus-t., Stram., come in for a share of consideration. If on closing the eyes he screams out as if he saw horrible visions, Bry., Hell., Lach., Stram., are to be considered. Raving, wild delirium is often best covered by Hyos., Lyc., Nit-ac., Op., Phos., Secale, Stram., Sul-ac., Verat.

ADDRESS

VITAL ACTION AND REACTION

"A medicine is not too high to cure so long as it is capable of aggravating the symptoms belonging to the sickness, in the first hours in acute, and in the first days of a chronic, sickness.

—Hahnemann's Organon.

TWO DIFFERENT PRESENTATIONS

Some understand Homœopathy as a science presenting human sickness in forms to be perceived:

From center to circumference,

From head to feet,

From within out,

From highest to lowest,

From the vital centers to the periphery.

This may be said to be the vertex presentation whereby one thinks from things first to things last, perceiving the loves and the hates as the first and deepest of any sickness in man.

A sickness can be perceived in:

Perversion of the desires and aversions;

Perversion of the intelligence;

Disturbed memory;

Physical sensation perverted;

Disturbed functions or organs, with the attending circumstances;

Perverted sensations and sufferings of *parts*;

Tissue changes and pathological conditions;

Sensations and sufferings dependent upon the pathological conditions.

Causes that excite each of these are parallel to the perverted states themselves, in each sphere.

Any physician who can view a sick man in this way, from first to last, *will be able to secure evidence that will enable him to adjust materia medica so that order will certainly be re-established.*

This may be called birth by vertex-presentation.

Some physicians are utterly unable to perceive that the mental symptoms are first, will and understanding perverted, and are unable to perceive that the man himself has been unbalanced by heat, by cold, by light, and by electricity, in instances of excess, of defect or of perversion. They are utterly unable to perceive that the man as a whole, as of himself, may be perceived in a grasp collectively, and mentally analyzed by the measure of excess, defect, and perversion. Such men always see ultimate tissue-changes, pathology, as both cause and ultimate. I say see because they do not perceive.

The first-cited vision is to be perceived; the last can be seen and touched. This latter might be termed breech-presentation.

These two classes of men must always differ:

The first are philosophers and rational men; the others are materialists.

One class think from things first to things last, including all items in their places, and giving each its full value in relation to the whole; the other see the ultimates and give no value to the whole.

The first see sickness in its perversions:

Of the loves,

Of intelligence.

Of memory,

Of bodily sensations,

Of causes and

Of circumstance;

In greater and in lesser;

In general and in particular;

And these as they extend into ultimates.

The first are adherents of, and filled with, the doctrines; the second are not of, but against, the doctrines.

The second must see results of disease. They have no perception of causes and circumstance. When they see what they call causes they see only ultimates; they appear to lack ability to group the first conditions of disorder. They do not see *order in the phenomena of disorder, nor in the symptoms of sickness*. They see sickness only in its endings, or ultimates.

To heal the sick, man must perceive what in the body is in disorder, and he can perceive this only by viewing the phenomena of disorder. The phenomena that represent progress from cause to effect are often ignored until ultimates that can be seen and touched are present. This assumes that a thing can be a thing and at the same time the cause of itself.

DOSAGE

A fatal error prevails in many quarters: to suppose that increasing the size of the dose makes it more homœopathic. It is not yet clearly understood that the attenuation should be similar to the plane of the perversion, the

disorder, in the economy. Increasing the degree of the
potency may hasten the cure, but it often increases the
aggravation; diminishing the potency diminishes the
homœopathicity, and if the drug be increased in quantity
the relation departs from the similar to the dissimilar,
hence becomes not the curative power.

USE OF THE REPERTORY

As Homœopathy includes both science and art, Repertory Study must consist of science and art.

The scientific method is the mechanical method; taking all the symptoms and writing out all the associated
remedies with gradings, making a summary with grades
marked, at the end.

There is an artistic method that omits the mechanical,
and is better, but all are not prepared to use it. The artistic method demands that judgment be passed on all the
symptoms, after the case is most carefully taken. The
symptoms must be judged as to their value as characteristics, in relation to the patient; they must be passed in
review by the rational mind to determine those which are
strange, rare, and peculiar.

Symptoms most peculiar to the patient must be taken
first, then those less and less peculiar until the symptoms
that are common and not peculiar are reached, in order,
from first to last.

These must be valued in proportion as they relate to
the patient rather than to his parts, and used instead of
ultimates and symptoms pathognomonic.

Symptoms to be taken:

First—are those relating to the loves and hates, or
desires and aversions.

Next—are those belonging to the rational mind, so-
called intellectual mind.

Thirdly—those belonging to the memory.

These, the mental symptoms, must first be worked
out by the usual form until the remedies best suited to
his mental condition are determined, omitting all symptoms that relate to a pathological cause and all that are
common to disease and to people. When the sum of these
has been settled, a group of five or ten remedies, or as
many as appear, we are then prepared to compare them
and the remedies found related to the remaining symptoms of the case.

The symptoms that are next most important are those
related to the entire man and his entire body, or his blood
and fluids: *as sensitiveness to heat, to cold, to storm,
to rest, to night, to day, to time.* They include both symptoms and modalities.

As many of these as are found, also, in the first
group, the mental summary, are to be retained.

There is no need of writing out the remedies not in
the mental group or summary; these symptoms, relating
to the whole patient, cannot be omitted with any hope of
success.

We must next look over all the record to ascertain
which of that group are most similar to the particulars of
the regions of the body; of the organs of the body; of the
parts; and of the extremities.

Preference must be accorded to discharges from ulcers, from uterus during menstruation, from ears, and
from other parts, as those are very closely related to the
vital operation of the economy.

Next must be used the modalities of the parts affected,
and frequently these will be found to be the very opposite
of the modalities of the patient himself. A patient who
craves heat for himself, generally, and for his body, may
require cold to his head, to his stomach, or to the inflamed
parts, hence the same rubric will not fit him and his parts.
Hence to generalize by modalities of *isolated* particulars

leads to the incorrect remedy or confounds values placed upon certain remedies.

There are strange and rare symptoms, even in parts of the body, which the experienced physician learns are so guiding that they must be ranked in the higher and first classes.

These include some keynotes which may guide safely to a remedy or to the shaping of results, *provided that the mental and the physical generals do not stand contrary, as to their modalities, and therefore oppose the keynote-symptoms.*

Any remedy correctly worked out, when looked up in the materia medica, should be perceived to agree with, and to fit, the patient; his symptoms; his parts; and his modalities. It is quite possible for a remedy *not having the highest marking in the anemnesis* to be the most similar in image, as seen in the materia medica.

The artistic prescriber sees much in the proving that cannot be retained in the repertory, where everything must be sacrificed for the alphabetical system. The artistic prescriber must study materia medica long and earnestly to enable him to fix in his mind sick images, which, when needed, will infill the sick personalities of human beings. These are too numerous and too various to be named or classified. I have often known the intuitive prescriber to attempt to explain a so-called marvelous cure by saying: "I cannot quite say how I came to give that remedy but it resembled him."

We have heard this, and felt it, and seen it, but who can attempt to explain it? It is something that belongs not to the neophyte, but comes gradually to the experienced artistic prescriber. It is only the growth of art in the artistic mind: what is noticed in all artists. It belongs to all healing artists, but if carried too far it becomes a fatal

17

mistake, and must therefore be corrected by repertory-work done in even the most mechanical manner.

The more each one restrains the tendency to carelessness in prescribing and in method, the wiser he becomes in artistic effects and materia medica work. The two features of prescribing must go hand in hand, and must be kept in a high degree of balance, or loose methods and habits will come upon any good worker.

AN ADDRESS PRELIMINARY TO THE STUDY OF HOMŒOPATHICS

It is not an easy grade to the pinnacle of pure Homœopathy, or as it should be admissible to say, to Homœopathy. I know that the statement admits that there is a quality of Homœopathy prevailing not strictly pure, which is so true that argument opposing it is unnecessary.

The condition of medicine leading up to the new system nearly a century ago could scarcely be written or spoken of *forcibly enough* to impress the mind with the *gravity of the situation*, or to *portray* the injury to the human race. At that time medicine was in a state of chaos. Hardly can it be said that there was any good in it, and, as to its history, it was entirely traditional. It was composed of powerful and drastic measures, and its only claim to respect was that its measures were sure to *kill speedily* or to cure *lingeringly*. These measures were bleeding, cupping, leeching, vomiting, cathartics, sudorifics, soporifics, etc.

To what extent has medicine advanced? Have the numerous fads and fancies furnished the world with a better system of old medicine than then existed? Is the deadly administration of concentrated compounds, alkaloids and resinoids a better and safer system? Then, drugs in massive doses were hurled through, but now they are administered in such a form that they are diffused throughout the body, depressing the vital energy and ultimating disease forms. Then they used coarse forms of crude drugs and now they use the dangerous, concentrated forms of deadly drugs, and, as much now as then, *without law or principle.* Then the physician compounded his own medicines, now the chemist and pharmacist prepare the nostrums and inform the learned (?) doctor in regard to the fullest particulars and uses, in order that he may be prepared to administer these potent concentrates to the dying sick. These new agents come from the laboratories so rapidly that the druggist can no longer keep posted as to the names—much less the physician as to the properties of the medicines he uses. No sooner has a flooring of concentrates been threshed out than a new one comes, so that every year an entire Materia Medica, new and clean, is manufactured for the use of this highly learned profession.

How different is this from the remedies used by the New School! Remedies once proved and verified stand as a fixture, under the same specific indications, so long as man dwells upon the earth and needs aid for sickness. *The remedies discovered by Hahnemann will stand the test of experience for the ages to come, as they have grown stronger by use since their discovery.* Fifty years have built and confirmed the Homœopathic Materia Medica, while the Old School has had many new ones, and, like the shifting sands, no man can predict where the next one will come from, nor the ending of the one now in use.

Many changes have come over this system of traditional medicine. Its adherents, failing, by their methods, to obtain the respected results, and jagged by the thorn in the flesh—Homœopathy's success—have betaken themselves to profound research, which has been heralded by mighty leaders: Koch, Pasteur and others. The chaotic jumble now denominated scientific medicine is a stench in the nostrils of rational men, and ought to be patented for a modern medical kaleidoscope. *Such is the boasted medicine of experience.*

A microcephalic of Philadelphia some years ago offered one hundred dollars as a prize for the best essay exposing the fallacies of Homœopathy; so great is the task, he makes a great offer. But how inexpensive it would be to secure an essay on the fallacies of traditional medicine! So-called "regular medicine" has made many changes, as silly as they are numerous, because not based upon law. Its votaries speak of progress. What can they mean!— with no principles to conserve, no law to obey, and only speculation to offer as the foremost elephant of the advancing juggernaut? *It is the medicine of lawless experience and speculation. It is not a result of discoveries, but the opposition of disgusted patrons and Homoeopathic statistics, that has impelled the apparent industry in this so-called science.* It has not been for the love of the dear people whom they mock in the wards of public hospitals that they have changed, but the spur of comparative failure and chagrin following the useless experiments upon the sick *a la* Koch, Pasteur, etc.

The moderation observed in dosage has been so worthy of imitation that even the pseudo-homœopath finds consolation in the fact that he can hoodwink a confiding public with these deceptions—they so resemble homœopathic forms of medication from which they were taken. But the simple only are thereby deceived.

For the deceptions practised by pretenders in our own ranks there can be no need of apology. They and their faults are too well known, and the causes are:

First, The increasing demand for the genuine.

Second, The comparative infancy of the new system.

Third, The imperfection of the machinery of instruction.

Fourth, The imperfection of books.

Fifth, To generalize, want of opportunity, capacity and desire.

Allopathy concerns us very little; its way and that of Homœopathy have long since parted. Homœopathy has made grand strides. We recognize Hahnemann as a great master, a loving father and a God-fearing man.

In 1833 he finished his masterpiece, the ORGANON, of which there are many translations, it having gone through five editions, the first of which appeared in 1810. The growth and prosperity of this great system of medicine have gone on until thousands of physicians are practising it, and colleges, hospitals, dispensaries and journals are spreading it to the ends of the civilized world. The continued study of the doctrines of his new system is leading to better application, and the unsettled questions of the past are rapidly diminishing. Hundreds of practitioners now scattered over the land rise up to testify to the fullness of the law and the success following obedience to principle. Their testimony is a satisfactory demonstration that Homœpathy pure and simple is all that is desired in the cure of the sick, that the law is universal, and the failure must come from causes above enumerated. Obedience demonstrates that Homœopathy rests upon fixed principles —on a law—and not on a mere rule of practice, to be changed for something better, or when fancy dictates a new whim.   (ORGANON § 2.) As well say or suppose that the apple could do otherwise than fall to the earth when its stem is disconnected from its mother tree.

There can be but one great system of Homœopathy. Men who rise to the fullness of uses in its application have broken the fetters of prejudice, bigotry, intolerance and self conceit, and have followed on after the light— never faltering though often stumbling, never sneering though often doubting—until the full heat and light of the mid-day sun hold them spellbound in the knowledge and love of uses. These attainments are within the grasp of all who love knowledge for uses and not for selfish ends.

Homœopathy exists in varying degrees as to application, from the crude, with a mixture of traditional methods, up to the highest results of absolute obedience to known law. Every practitioner admits the value of the law by his efforts to follow it, inasmuch as he practices to the fullest extent of his knowledge and turns aside only where knowledge of law was defective. Then it follows that the degrees are only the shadings from ignorance to knowledge, and they are almost infinite in number from the kind-hearted mother with her family medicine case to the discriminating master, all honestly seeking the happiness of human kind or mercenarily grasping to sell relief of pain for filthy cash.

The inexperienced must be assisted and instructed in order to practice Homœopathy without resort to traditional medicine. *But assistance can be of use only when desired and appreciated.*

To acquire the knowledge necessary to conduct a practice without resort to doubtful methods demands arduous toil and constant application, while the mind is held in a receptive attitude and the longing of the heart is for truth *because it leads to what is good* and not to sell it for a price.

The doctrines of Homœopathy are elevating and simple to the mind that is right, and, when known, following their dictates is easy; for it is easier to follow well-marked paths than to flounder in the mire of traditional medicine. It is hardly necessary to affirm that one who knows how to be obedient to fixed principles has no incentive to, and will not, depart from them. It cannot be denied that many seek, and few discover, the pure doctrines of Homœopathy. That many would call the necessary labor too great a sacrifice cannot be disputed. That the Creator knows to whom to intrust His Sacred truths I have no doubt. That any man who seeks the elevation of man and will work earnestly shall receive his portion should not be disputed. It is impossible for him who is ignorant of the principles of Homœopathy to realize the great good to man that can come from a full knowledge and application of the *law of similars*.

They who are ignorant of the higher and fuller uses of Homœopathy assume that they are wise, or that knowledge of fixed principles does not exist, and declare that the use of anodynes is justifiable when the appropriate homœopathic remedy is not known. They often use such agents to the detriment of the patient and of the system which they profess to believe is founded on law. They are unable to see that obedience to law is liberty, and suppose that license to violate law can be granted by themselve

Obedience to principle must stand before the pocketbook, reputation or other selfish motives, or the physician cannot rise to the constant and perfect reliance upon law with the feeling of satisfaction, and that it is right and all that is good to do. In every instance where disobedience is urged, the impulse is ignorance and selfishness, to the end that man pays tribute in some way to the physician, instead of the physician serving the man. The question: "Why not rely on law?" has never been answered but in two ways: "I do not know," or "It is not profitable."

When we comprehend the wonderful work that Hahnemann performed and the magnitude of the ORGANON (which was so complete, as he left it, that no man has been able to add to it, nor, in spite of sneers, been able to take from it), can we refrain from reverence and the tacit belief that he was aided by all-wise Providence? When we consider how ably he opposed the pathological theories of his day (the pathological notions of a century ago, now abandoned, were advocated then with as much assurance and pertinacity as those now in vogue, as the Old School accepts and abandons theories as flippantly, and with as profound reason, as a siren, her lovers); when we realize the extent of his learning in all branches of science, the wonderful physical endurance that enabled him to remain every third night in reflection, and the love that, under all circumstances, he manifested toward the human race and God; and when it is known that the source of man's love is the fountain of inspiration; then may we comprehend the depth of truth in, and properly revere, his masterwork, the ORGANON OF HEALING.

Indeed, has it been said by all masters since its writing that new truths come out of it, after every reading, to suit the varying degrees of advancement in the progress of each faithful observer, no difference how old or how wise. The masters of these living doctrines and the materia medica have been constant readers of this great work. Not one of the prescribers has ever claimed a discovery not fully set forth in this work, but all in their greatest accomplishments have said that they based their successes upon the ORGANON. It is the first book for the student to read, and the last for the old and busiest physician to ponder over.

When Lippe, Wells and scores of others advocated a continuous reading of this book during their long careers, should we not similarly look upon it with a feeling of profound respect? Should we not crave the hidden truths that have made these faithful followers of law so successful? To whom would a rational man apply for light when desiring to follow law in healing the sick and measuring out uses to man? Naturally to Hahnemann and his faithful adherents, and not to those who smile at what they choose to consider the ravings of an aged man.

There are some professed homœopaths who, by words and actions, denounce Hahnemann as a theorist, a fanatic, and as visionary, but these have never cured sick people as Hahnemann did. Let all men learn of him until they can do as he did; for he was, and still is, the teacher above all others. He was the first advocate of Homœopathy, and we must look to him, and all deviation from his teachings should receive another name.

There should be no controversy with men when principles are the thing considered. The truth often cuts men deeply and urges to dispute, and wounds thus made seldom heal by first intention or without loss of blood. Controversy seldom teaches him who does not seek the truth. The rational man accepts the truth because he is prepared for it and because it is truth. The sick come in distress after all else has failed and they are in a receptive attitude; while the old and hardened follower of traditional methods comes in the attitude of rebellion, and his egotism and bigotry cannot be overcome. To him the sunlight is as dark as smoke.

Hahnemann formulated the principles of Homœopathic therapeutics. Isolated statements had been made previous to his labors, showing that glimmerings of truth had occasionally appeared, but not bright enough to permit the arrangement into doctrines. He so arranged the rules of practice in the ORGANON and CHRONIC DISEASES that the system of homœopathic therapeutics may be considered complete.

Homœopathy rests not upon theory nor opinion, but upon facts. Hypotheses and reasonings have no place in treatise on that upon which human life depends. It is, of course, impossible for the medical theorist to reflect upon medical facts, because he has no knowledge of facts to consider; hence he reasons that perhaps the vomiting is caused by a disordered brain, or by a congested liver, or is reflex from the uterus, and so on, indefinitely. This theorist is more likely than any other to think that an exact diagnosis is of great moment, and yet every hypothesis shows the shifting basis of his false conclusion.

The minds thus perverted by false reasoning are outnumbered only by fluctuating opinions, and with them there is no substantial way and roadbed because the wandering, the confusion and the mental fluctuation prevent settlement upon any course or path of continued operation. With them there is no *indicated remedy*, and a continuous whirl of medicaments comes before the mind. The sickroom is filled with bottles and the patient's stomach distended with things too numerous to mention: from home-made decoctions to an Irish stew.

The more accurate the diagnosis and the more substantial its basis, the more inaccurate the prescription that is based upon it. The diagnosticians are the poorest prescribers, yet, in spite of all this, no harm can come from the finest sagacity in naming diseases. *It must be understood, however, that the diagnosis does not reveal the nature of a disease in a manner to image a remedy.* The diagnosis is the name of ultimates and exteriors, while it is the interior nature that must be perceived through the peculiar, characterizing signs and symptoms, in order to discover the remedy that will cure. (ORGANON §§ 6-8.) The highest order of this peculiar insight leads to selection of remedies of the highest degree of similarity, hence, to the highest order of healing.

Medical opinions concerning a given sickness are as plentiful as doctors. Even in this day of medical sunlight, there prevail the lightning changes in medical opinions, as an afflicted mortal rambles over a large city among the medical luminaries; to receive their costly and worthless diagnoses. This might not appear so hazardous were it not a fact that treatment is supposed to rest upon the diagnosis. Fortunately, for the patient as for the doctor, the supposition is not criminal. Our own Chapman, with his prescription test case, has demonstrated that the simplest case cannot secure two similar prescriptions, even when the greatest minds in allopathy are consulted. The result was quite different with the New School, as all the physicians named the same remedy. The same test can never be repeated with similar results.

The epidemics in the last twenty-five years have revealed wonderful similarity of methods and remedies. The Yellow Fever Commission portrays the certainty of method and results, in the records forming the statistics for Memphis and New Orleans. These man had no connection with each other. They labored and gained results that demonstrate that they were inspired by principles, as the same remedies were used in the different cities for the same symptoms, and with similar results.

Exactitude of methods, and similar remedies for similar symptoms the world over, with the same good old materia medica which becomes better with age and use, should appeal to the minds of men in a way to secure a hearing.

In the practice of Homœopathy, a master, wherever he may be, has something on which to base a prescription. When else was this ever so marked as by Hahnemann, when, after his study of the cholera epidemic, and reference to the symptoms of the materia medica, he decided that Veratrum, Cuprum and Camphor were the remedies suited to the epidemic; yet he had never seen a case of cholera? When asked what remedies would correspond to this disease, he simply recalled the provings. The nature of the disease appeared similar to what he had seen in the provings of Camphor, Veratrum and Cuprum. He therefore concluded that these remedies ought to cure this sickness. They were thereupon successfully used. They are our sheet-anchors in cholera today, and they ever will be. This was no opinion of Hahnemann. No, he had simply obtained the symptoms of the provings, and compared them to those of the disease. From this he said that these would be the remedies. Homœopathists thus have a power that is not found elsewhere in medicine, viz., that of prevision.

Positive principles should govern every physician when he goes to the bed side of the sick. (ORGANON, §§ 1-2.) The sick have a right to it. Before the time of Hahnemann there was no such thing. The sick were villainously treated. Since the advent of this most beautiful and perfect system, the people have a right to demand exactitude in methods and knowledge. Better to do nothing than to do something useless. It is better to watch and wait than to do wrong. Every action in Homœopathy must be based on a positive principle. Every action of the physician using Homœopathy should be based upon the principles of the system. He should say: "Thus saith the principle, as doth the grammar in every word of your speech." Some say, "I do not believe;" but let it be known that belief has no place in the study of Homœopathy. The inductive method of Hahnemann gives no place for unbelief; hence it is that Hahnemann has formulated the first paragraph of the ORGANON:

The first and sole duty of the physician is to restore health to the sick. This is the true art of healing.

BIRTHDAY OF HAHNEMANN

It naturally comes into our minds to celebrate the birthday of Samuel Hahnemann on the eleventh day of April. Some will do this by a banquet, some by speeches, some by silent heart-throbs. Some will celebrate openly and outwardly, while in secret they administer tinctures in physiological doses and compound tablets, and alternate two medicines, neither of which is related to the sickness in hand. The silent, heartfelt thankfulness that Hahnemann was born and lived his life and left us the results of his discoveries in the ORGANON, CHRONIC DISEASES and MATERIA MEDICA PURA, is the best way to celebrate this wonderful man's birthday.

Hahnemann fulfilled his usefulness, and no man ever took his place. This is true of all great and useful men. Every man that does his utmost in useful work leaves no one to do his work. Every man must seek his own work and do it; men fail when they try to fulfill another man's work. Many great men have followed Hahnemann; each has done his own work. Men have become great in Homœopathy in following the principles laid down in Hahnemann's ORGANON, in teaching, translating, compiling, and prescribing, but not a single man has become noted by using tinctures, compound tablets, or ignoring the doctrines of potentization. Some of these have become noted politicians, but none of them have been noted teaching the Philosophy or the Materia Medica. The men who have been noted teachers in our Materia Medica have been men who have openly stood for the principles of potentization, the single remedy, the similar remedy, and all the principles found in the ORGANON. All such men will celebrate the birthday of Samuel Hahnemann; many others will make speeches, and eat and drink and be merry.

CLASS-ROOM TALKS

Chronic tendency to congestion of the head, when Bell. has been the remedy that gave relief to the acute expression of the disease, Calc. Now, I don't mean you to understand that during the attack Calc. would be the better remedy. Bell. corresponds more fully to the acute manifestation. Calc. would *agg.* too strongly; but after the attack a dose of Calc. will cure the tendency to repeated return of these congested conditions.

So when each time the patient takes a cold, he has swollen tonsils, tonsilitis, and has chronic induration of the tonsils—Bar-c.

Now, we do not mean that Bar-c. would be the best indicated remedy during the acute attack—many remedies may be better indicated—but that a dose of Bar-c. *after* the attack, *would be* indicated, and would cure the tendency to return.

Don't commence the treatment of any chronic disease during the exacerbations.

In epilepsy you will never cure unless you first find a remedy that covers and corresponds in every respect to the acute attack. Then follow with the complimentary or chronic as the curative.

In chills and fever a prescription before or during the paroxysm will *certainly* increase the violence of the paroxysm, and hinder, if not complicate, matters.

CLASS ROOM TALKS

Hahnemann has been accused of alternation, of saying that Bry. and Rhus. alternated.

Now, Hahnemann did not mean you were to put one remedy in one glass and one in another, giving first of one and then the other; Bry. and Rhus. are complements of one another, and Hahnemann meant just this: You have had the symptoms and given the similar, Bry., and you will often find that when Bry. has ceased its action the symptoms of Rhus. will begin to shadow forth. Now, wait a little; you will have a clear picture of Rhus. You give it, and after a little Rhus will have done its work. Again the symptoms of Bry. may appear, and so on until you have finished your case.

Arn., Rhus, and Calc. often follow one another *this*

way: A sprain in joint, bruised condition of muscles, would be well covered immediately by Arn. The injury does well for a time, but after a week or two there is still some weakness and pain. Now Rhus is also similar, but belongs to a later period. So Rhus takes up the case, carries him comfortably on for some months, when he suddenly finds its power over the condition gone, and that he has a rheumatic stiffness in the strained joint coming on after *cold, damp* weather.

Now Calc. is indicated and will finish the case.

Hahnemann has said that we would often find that certain of the remedies rotated, *i. e.*, Sulph., Calc., Lyc., one might say of that, as of alternation, to place each in a tumbler by the bedside, giving from first, second, and third in succession, etc.; but that is not the point. The great master intended you to know that many times (not always) the symptoms of sulph. would be followed by those of Calc., and those again by symptoms of Lyc., returning to Sulph. after Lyc., and so on until the case is completed.

It is well for you to know these things, that you may be watchful and prepared to solve the problems as they arise.

The better prescribers use the most profound reasoning in the study of their cases and in their search for a remedy. To show you how you must think and study out your symptoms—by a comparatively simple case—and how to prescribe when you seemingly have but one symptom:

A lady comes to my office with extreme restlessness of lower extremities. Well, I think that is Zinc., preeminently, and many, many others. Yet I do not stop there. I inquire further, and find that a few days before she has been out in the rain and got wet. "Where, your feet?" Oh! no! My feet were protected but my head got very wet. Why, think I, that sounds like Bell. I must see if Bell. has restlessness of the limbs. Sure enough, Bell. has it, and Bell, cures with no further return of symptoms.

CLASSIFICATION OF CONSTITUTIONS USELESS IN PRESCRIBING

Why should we attempt to classify constitutions as an aid in prescribing? Every individual is a constitution, and no two sick persons can be classified as of the same class to the satisfaction of any clear, observing, and thinking homœopathist. It is a fatal error to classify constitutions, as no two are sufficiently similar, when observed by a genuine homœopathician to form even a common class. Human beings are a thousand times more complex than the chess-board in the hands of most skillful players.

Every change in combination in mental or physical signs and symptoms brings a new view of the entire patient as observed collectively. Normal mental methods come to all thinkers in such diverse appearances as to justify the well-known statement that no two minds are alike. In similar manner, all abnormal minds appear to the alert physician as sick individuals. Mental abnormalties may be classified by their common manifestation by the alienist, but the classification is never useful to the homœopathist when searching for a remedy. The classification is made up from common symptoms of the mental-disease symptoms for the purpose of medical diagnosis, but *the peculiar symptoms in each and every morbid mental case must guide to the prescription,* and these prevent classification.

Nothing leads the physician to failure so certainly as classification. The physician who prescribes on a diagnosis is a failure, except for his chance shots. Individualization is the aim of every homœopathic physician. The symptoms that represent the *morbid* constitution or *disorder of the*

individual are the ones that the skillful prescriber always seeks. Symptoms that are uncommon in one constitution are common in another, because such uncommon symptoms are common to some diseases and uncommon to others.

Classification is necessary to the proper study of diseases, pathological conditions, and diagnosis, but every case of sickness in an individual is so dissimilar to another case that each and every patient must be examined and measured by the symptoms that represent his disordered economy, or prescribing will be followed by very ordinary results.

CORRESPONDENCE OF ORGANS, AND DIRECTION OF CURE

Hering first introduced the Law of Direction of Symptoms: from within out, from above downward, in reverse order of their appearance. It does not occur in Hahnemann's writing. It is spoken of as Hering's Law. There is scarcely anything of this law in the literature of Homœopathy, except the observation of symptoms going from above to the extremities, eruptions appearing on the skin and discharges from mucous membranes or ulcers appearing upon the legs as internal symptoms disappear. There is no specific assertion in literature except as given in the lectures in Philosophy at the Post-Graduate School.

The innermost of man consists of will, understanding, memory; and these are extended outward through the general physical organism. This idea belongs here in considering the direction of symptoms—from the innermost to the outermost. We meet patients in whom we make what we would not know would be a good prescription except for a comprehension of this relation of the innermost and the outermost. A patient returns after a prescription has been made, who, from his symptoms would think himself worse, yet he could not be so considered except by his reasoning

18

that something has appeared which he did not have before. Then the doctor would be tempted to change the remedy if he is not familiar with correspondence of organs. By his knowledge of correspondence of organs he is able to know whether the patient is better or worse.

The physical organs correspond to internal man; to the will and understanding. The intellectual faculties consider a proposition presented, weighing it in the light of things learned to determine whether it be false or true, partly false or partly true. The memory holds it while it is examined and considered, and the intellectual faculties digest what is received, separating truth from false, and appropriating the truth and rejecting the false.

The stomach receives food; it and the small intestines digest and assimilate that which is good for the body, and cast off that which is not suitable, that which is indigestible, false. These correspond to the intellectual part of man, doing for the body what the intellecual faculties do for man.

The kidneys perform similar work, separating the false from the true in the blood. The worn out part of the blood is manufactured into urea, urates and is carried off. The kidneys do for the blood what the intellectual faculties do for truth.

At first you may not perceive any relation in these things, but long observation and examination of these reveals much. When you are treating a patient insane in the intellectual faculties, stomach disorders or intestinal disorders appear as the patient improves, cramps and diarrhoea occur, the disorder extending through the intestinal canal. In another patient, kidney affection with albumin in the urine results, in the course of reaction from mental disorder. Pain in the back and albumin in the urine appear although the nurse says the patient is improving. When the reverse is true, it is deleterious. In the course of treatment of a patient with albumin in the urine, when mental disorders appear, the patient is growing worse. Others have observed stomach and kidney disorders improve while mental disturbances appear. When prescribing for stomach disorder patients, and mental disorders appear, antidote your prescription immediately. When the reverse occurs, it is in the order of cure. Reaction will soon follow, the stomach disorder or kidney disorder will soon pass; do not interfere. Thus we have from within *out*, or from without *in*. It is an infallible correspondence.

In the course from within *out*, according to law, we do not always have mental changes followed by skin symptoms—that is a more rapid development. It is slower and more gradual when stomach or kidneys are disordered. Then it goes through the series of organs; as the stomach improves, catarrh or eruptions appear. That patient will remain well.

Sometimes the intellectual faculties correspond to the lungs. The lungs do for the body what the intellect does for the man. When the patient is threatened or settled in phthisis, and following a prescription, the lungs, improve and the intellectual faculties are involved, that patient will die,—you cannot cure him. Whenever intellectual disorder is followed by catarrh of the lungs or bronchial tubes, by any lung, kidney, stomach or intestinal disorder, after your prescription; that patient is improving.

When an individual is sick in the will, when loves are turned to hatred, when he desires to destroy his own life, or flees from, or hates his own children, when a wife is averse to her husband, or the entire voluntary system is perverted; in this sort of insanity, what will occur? When a correct prescription is made, the heart or liver will become affected, these correspond to the voluntary system. Not stomach or kidney affections, but heart and liver disorders will occur when prescribing for will affections. If you have a heart affection improving on your prescription, and a desire to destroy life follows, you must antidote the prescription; the symptoms are taking the wrong direction. When rheumatic affections disappear from the extremities and go to the heart, and later the patient wants to destroy his life, the course is from without *in*.

The voluntary corresponds to heart and liver. There is enough to indicate that divine revelation and the letter of the Word are based on these correspondences, and no man knows it so well as the ancients knew it. Where love of God is referred to, we find the word heart in the Scriptures. The intellectual faculties are referred to when it says "binding up the loins," "the loins bound up with truth." In the word of God are found all these correspondences, and from these correspondences we learn the nature of man's life and body. Man's life, soul, mind, and will, correspond to the organs of the body.

Through familiarity with Swedenborg, I have found the correspondences wrought out from the Word of God harmonious with all I have learned in the past thirty years. Familiarity with them aids in determining the effect of prescriptions. A man, sick in his mind, does not appreciate how sick he is, and is not able to judge of his condition. He thinks he is worse when liver symptoms appear; he *says* he is worse. That is the course from within *out*; be not deceived. The threatened condition of the liver will pass away with the remedy selected for the mental disorder.

These things must be clear:—otherwise you must take a low plane in the homœopathic art:—otherwise you will interfere with your own work, meddling with good work accomplished. Without such knowledge, knowledge of Homœopathic Materia Medica is insufficient except for acute cases. Homœopathy is suited to old chronic, suppressed conditions: gonorrhœa, itch, eruptions, and syphilis. Hahnemann could not know these things and without them no man can do what Hahnemann said could not be done. He said effects of drugs are incurable, but he used only the 30th potency and could not do these things. You cannot handle suppressed conditions without this knowledge.

You have wondered at the work I have done. The work you have seen in my practice differs from that of others because of this knowledge. Those who do not have it, blunder and destroy the lives of human beings because they do not know what is taking place. Correspondences are only the outgrowth of observations. They are not available to the physician except by the law "Similia similibus curantur." Think on these things; meditate and profit by it; use it. Few know truth; the world is ignorant. The less a man knows the less responsibility he has. When you perceive truth, a duty accompanies it. You are a million times more responsible. When you come within range of eternal truth, law and order you take a tremendous responsibility upon yourself. What we hear at conventions is usually opinions of men; what we hear now is not opinions. You can see from your own knowledge that this must be true. I have no opinions and I avoid offering any until I perceive the stamp of eternal truth.

This is a beginning, but the same thing runs through the organism. Sexual organs usually are associated with the will. Women who suffer from sexual organs, uterus and ovaries, have both loves and intellect affected from suppression. Men who have sexual disturbances involving the sexual are predominantly affected in the intellectual organs.

DIPHTHERIA

This disease is generally looked upon with terror, and well it may be, as it demands more than ordinary knowledge to conduct its victims to safety. To say that Homœopathy is wanting at the bedside of these cases is far from true. It cures all cases where good vitality is present and where its remedies are wisely administered. To assume or admit that our lack of knowledge must be a common cause of so many failures is both true and untrue. It is true that more knowledge is required than the ordinary homœopath possesses, or he would not be compelled to admit the several deaths in his confessions and reports. But to say that our knowledge and Homœopathy in its present state of development could not be expected to do better is far from true. Our science is now developed to a high state of perfection, but individuals often fail to apply it in this disease with wisdom and judgment, and therefore lose many subjects.

The disease is not constantly with us, and when it comes it generally assumes a form unlike its previous appearances; and by the time the physician has carefully looked into the epidemic phases and remedial agents it has gone, leaving upon his hands severe and unfavorable terminations to cause regret and disappointment. The physician of studious habits and active practice, however, may so keep in touch with his principles and Materia Medica as to keep his death list remarkably small, but it must be observed that he does not prescribe for every symptom that shows itself on the instant of its appearance. I will venture to say that any physician's death list will be large if he hurries into bed chambers, looks at the tongue, takes the temperature, feels the pulse, looks into the throat, makes a culture, disinfects the house, washes the throat with antiseptics, etc. I will also venture to say that any physician's death list will be remarkably small if he goes to the sick room and observes all the symptoms of the patient, all the surroundings of the house and room, sees all the obstructions, and knows the full purport of all things there, waits and watches the development of the sickness until its every feature has been manifested, if he knows when that time has come, and then carefully compares all the symptoms of this sickness with the symptoms of the Homœopathic Materia Medica, and knows how to select the potency, how to administer it, and when not to give it.

How many of you can say all these things to yourself? How many of you do it in just this way. Do not most of you entertain the idea that you must make great haste to get medicine into that child's stomach or it will get worse? Do not the most of you fear that the people will turn you off and get another physician if you do not do something at once? Do you know of any other class of work that would not be jeopardized and ruined by such haste as all of you do at the bedside in one of these serious sicknesses? If you are not guilty of this charge then you are not hurt, but it is so true of so large a number of our best men that no harm can come from hearing about it. To go to the bedside with fear and trembling is death to the sufferer. To go to the bedside with confidence born of knowing and from having trusted our means of cure so long, means life to the patrons of Homœopathy. It is not that you are ignorant of your principles and your Materia Medica, but that these are not invoked at the time of greatest need. Through fear and haste you act and fail, whereas you should watch and wait and discover there is no hurry, and if the sickness has not yet shown what medicine this life stands in need of, wait even if you go and come repeatedly. Let it develop until its character is stamped upon the case so that no mistake can be made.

A mistake in the first remedy nearly always means death, or at least it masks the case. It would be strange if you, who know so much about the art of healing, could make a first prescription of a remedy so far from similar that it did not act. You know if it is similar at all it will make changes in that symptom image, and if it is similar enough it will cure; therefore you need not hope that if your first prescription did not cure it was so dissimilar it was harmless. You must expect to cure, or begin the cure with the first prescription; then all is easy, as the changes now observed are such as bring joy to the hearts of the family and to the doctor. You must, therefore, never prescribe on the first flitting evidences of the sickness, but according to the true saying: "First be sure you are right and then go ahead."

The first prescription, when correctly adjusted to the symptoms, will cause the membranes to fade out and all the characteristics of sickness with it.

The first prescription, when incorrectly chosen, will most likely change the symptoms, but the patient will go on from bad to worse and the next prescription must be a matter of guess-work, as the index has been spoiled, and hence the mortalities.

You know enough about your Materia Medica to do good work if you apply it properly. The Materia Medica is full and rich, and the Repertory points out the general and particular features. Guernsey's cards are most useful aids. They are correctly compiled and within the reach of all. It is not more Materia Medica that is needed, but a correction in the faults at the bedside. The careful follower of all Hahnemann's instructions in *taking the case* will avoid the errors I have mentioned, and save the necessity for a *kind and generous counsel* to say: "The treatment is just such as we would have given had we been here in the beginning!"

To find out which remedy to give is the important matter to be considered. The characteristics of a fatal case of this disease are as follows: 1st. No individualizing symptoms. 2nd. An ignorant physician, and this is the commonest cause of failure. The patient might as well be sick without symptoms as have plenty of symptoms and a doctor who knows not the meaning of symptoms.

A favorable prognosis may be made where there are plenty of symptoms to indicate a remedy and there is a doctor present who knows how to read these signs of nature. Always consider first that which is not commonly found in this disease and examine the remedies having such striking features.

The exudative inflammation in the throat, nose or larnyx, with the marked weakness and zymotic manifestations grouped as diphtheria, finds for remedies the following: *Acet. ac.*, Ail., *Am-c.*, Apis, *Ars.*, *Arum-t.*, Bapt., Brom., Bry., Canth., Caps., Carb-ac., *Crot-h.*, Elaps., Hep., Iod., Kali-Bi., Kali-chl., Kali-mang., Kali-ph., *Kreos.*, Lac-c., Lach., Lyc., *Merc.*, *Merc-c.*, *Merc-cy.*, Merc-i-f., Merc-i-r., *Mur. ac.*, *Nit-ac.*, *Phos.*, *Phyto.*, Rhus-t., *Secale*, *Sul-ac.*, Sulph., and no doubt many others.

It often happens that the nurses speak of the suffocation as soon as sleep comes, which is a symptom that often leads the neophyte to Lachesis, but this remedy may not cover the rest of the symptoms. The following remedies should be consulted, as they all have it as well as the general zymotic state, weakness and exudation: Am-c., Bry., Arum-t., Crot-h., Hepar., *Kali-bi.*, lac-c., LACH., Lyc., *Rhus-t.*, Secale, Sulph.

The constant picking at the lips and nose has often pointed to Arum-t.

A type of cases often observed where bleeding is an alarming sign; bleeding from nose, mouth and throat, when Bry., Crot-h., Lach., *Phos.*, Secale, Sulph-ac., would be the group to examine.

The odors from the mouth sometimes become important and lead to the study of remedies having putrid odors:

Apis, *Arum-t.*, Bapt., Bry., Carb-ac., *Crot-h.*, *Kali-bi.*, *Kali-chl.*, *Lach.*, *Lyc.*, Merc., *Merc-c.*, NIT-AC.,, PHYTO., *Rhus-t.*, Secale, Sulph.

The well-known mercury breath always leads to the examination of the various preparations of that remedy, such as MERC., Merc-c., Merc-cy., Merc-i-f., Merc-i-r.

The ropy, stringy mucus coming from the throat and air passages is often an important factor and the following remedies are to be examined: *Apis*, Arum-t., Carb-ac., KALI-BI., *Lach.*, Merc., Merc-c., Merc-i-f., PHYTO.

If white, Lach.

If Yellow, KALI-BI., Lach.

If the liquids which the patient attempts to swallow come out of the nose, consult ARUM-T., Canth., Carb-ac., KALI-BI., Kali-ma., *Lac-c.*, Lach., Lyc., *Merc.*, *Merc-c.*, *Merc-cy.*, *Phyto.*, *Sul-ac.*

The gangrenous aspect of the throat is found in: Ail., Am-c., ARS., *Arum-t.*, Bapt., Carb-ac., Crot-h., *Lach.*, Kali-ph., KREOS., *Mur-ac.*, Nit-ac., *Phyto.*, Secale, Sul-ac., Sulph.

When ulceration is notable: ARS., Arum-t., *Bapt.*, Chlor., *Hep.*, Iod., Kali-bi., *Lac-c.*, Merc., Merc-c., *Merc-cy.*, *Mur-ac.*, NIT-AC., *Phyto.*

When swelling of the external throat and cervical glands is a marked feature: Arum-t., *Lach.*, MERC., Merc-c., Nit-ac., RHUS-T.

The following remedies have the disposition to constant swallowing observed in some cases: Arum-t., Hep., *Lac-c.*, *Lach.*, *Lyc.*, Merc., Merc-i-f.

From a lump in the throat: LACH.

The difficult swallowing in this disease is so common it can scarcely be taken as a guiding feature. Yet sometimes empty swallowing is very painful when solids can be swal-

lowed easier and then the following should be inspected:
Crot-h., LACH., Lac-c., *Merc.*, Merc-i-f., *Merc-i-r.*

Pain when not swallowing or pain ameliorated by swallowing is often important. CAPS., IGN., Lac-c., Lach.

The marked distress in touching the throat is often a guiding feature and then Apis, Brom., Bry., Lac-c., LACH., PHYTO., become a group of importance.

The pain is marked in some cases when anything warm is brought in contact with the throat, warm drinks, etc.: Apis, Lach., Lyc., PHYTO.

When cold things aggravate: Ars., HEP., LYC., Sabad., Sulph. are to be considered.

The membrane has too many features to be examined in this short paper, and hence a repertory must be consulted. But when the exudation is predominantly on the right side: *Apis,* Ign., Lac-c., LYC., Merc-i-f., Phyto., Rhus-t.

When it extends to the left: Lac-c., LYC., Sulph.

When predominantly on the left: Brom., Crot-h., Lac-c., LACH., Merc-i-r.

Extending to the right: Lac-c., LACH.

When the exudate alternates sides, LAC-C, stands alone.

When the exudate is predominantly in the nose: Am-c., *Kali-bi.*, *Lyc.*, Merc-c., Merc-cy.

When it extends to the nose: Kali-bi., Merc., *Merc-c.*, *Nit-ac.*

When the larnyx is the locality affected the state is far more serious and the following remedies must be consulted: Am-c., Apis., Arum-t., BROM., Carb-ac., *Hep.*, *Iod.*, *Kali-bi.*, Kali-mang., *Lac-c.*, *Lach.*, Merc-cy., Merc-i-f., *Nit-ac.*, PHOS., Sang.

When extending into the trachea: Iod., KALI-BI., *Phos.*

DISTINCTION BETWEEN THE SIMILAR AND THE SIMILIMUM

There is one point worthy of consideration; we are trying to make a distinction between the *similar* and the similimum, with which I do not agree. I have not any doubt, from experience, that two medicines may be similar enough to the totality of symptoms, and either may be the similimum, each would be similar enough to cure it; and how can you say both of these are, or either of them, is, the similimum. If you go into degrees you may consider it in this way: The medicine may be so dissimilar, that in dynamic power it would have little or no effect upon the disease; it then approaches it in a degree of similarity by becoming more and more similar. As it approaches in similarity it sustains an inability to change the symptoms that exist. It may be sufficiently similar to spoil it, to change and not effect a cure, until you have not improved the patient, but only changed the symptoms. I have observed in the management of intermittent fevers more than in any other class of complaints, giving medicine that has a few characteristics in intermittents, but which does not correspond to the genus of the disease or patient, and immediately follow it with its complementary, and you may change it from time to time for five or six weeks; I have seen it in so many cases. Medicines may be similar enough to effect curative results in a patient, and improve the health of that patient, improve the general condition whether an acute or chronic disease. When that medicine has done all the curing it is capable of, then its complementary will take up the work and go on with it. This is a matter of experience fully established by the Organon and every man's experience, and it seems to me the paper does not call out anything new, for it is in keeping with every man's experience.

Where there is psora or acute miasm, you can have a medicine similar enough to spoil the case, or similar enough to have a curative action; or the similimum, which is the medicine that cures the symptoms present, eradicates them completely.

EMERGENCIES—EUTHANASIA.

Condems Marphive

I am frequently asked, what should be done in times of great suffering for immediate relief? To those who desire to obtain reliable information, and who wish to practice in accordance with our principles, I would say, take the symptoms of each individual case and select the remedy capable of producing similar symptoms. **In a** general way this is all that would be expected of me for an answer to the question, by those who are conversant with materia medica.

Consumptives often suffer greatly when left to themselves, and some medical practitioners, knowing no better way, give Morphine and other stupefying agents, thinking that they allay human suffering.

This kind of practice cannot be too strongly condemned. Firstly, it is an acknowledgment that our law is not all-embracing; secondly, it is the *poorest kind of relief to the patient*. But I would not deprive medical practitioners of all means of relief for their patients, without furnishing as good or better ones.

The consumptive, when going down the last grade, needs the comfort of a true *healing art*, and not the make-shifts of mongrelism of allopathy. The homœopathic remedy is all that he, who knows how to use it, needs to allay the severest distress. Every true homœopathist knows the value of these wonderful remedies.

A few hints may not be out of place.

When the hectic fever, that so rapidly burns the patient up, is in full blast; the hot afternoon skin, the night sweat, the constant burning thirst, the red spot on the cheek, the diarrhoea, the stool escapes when coughing, *the intense fever* P. M.; the constriction of the chest, suffocation; then should *Phos., very high,* be administered, but *never repeated.* An aggravation will follow, but it must not be meddled with, as it will soon pass off, leaving the patient free from fever, and he will go on till death, many times, comfortably. *It is regretable meddling that causes the dying man so much misery.*

The distressed suffocation and inward distress in chest and stomach, streaming perspiration, great sinking; must have the clothing away from the neck, chest, abdomen, gastly countenance, and choking, call for *Lachesis,* and it may be given as often as occasion requires, but to give satisfaction and prompt relief, not lower than two hundredth.

To this ghastly picture, if we add, he is covered with a cold sweat, and there is one on either side of the bed fanning him, and the abdomen is distended with flatus, and the breath is cold, *Carbo v.* in water every hour for six hours, and stopped, will give rest and beatitude with many thanks.

But the time is yet coming when even these remedies will not serve us.

The ghastliness of the picture has not changed, and to it we have added the pains of dying cells—death pains, the last suffering. Such pains come on when mortification begins. If it is in the abdomen, we may avert it by differentiating between *Arsenicum* and *Secale,* but if this pain comes in the last stage of consumptive changes, we are beyond these remedies. Much later there is a remedy, and it is *Tarantula cubensis.* It soothes the dying sufferer as I have never seen any other remedy do.

I have seen *Ars., Carbo v., Lyc., Lach.,* act kindly and quiet the last horrors, but *Tarantula cubensis* goes beyond these. I have lately administered it in the thirtieth cent. potency.

When death is inevitable, the first named remedies seem to be mostly indicated, but no longer act, and the friends say, "Doctor, can't you do something to relieve that horrible suffering?" the pain, the rattling in the chest, with no power to throw the mucus out; the patient has but a few hours to suffer, but he can be made as quiet as with the terrible Morphine in a very few minutes by the *Tarantula* thirtieth.

I believe that no physician would use a narcotic if he only knew a better way.

What is more inhuman than to leave the suffering patient in his last moments to writhe in the agonies of dissolution, surrounded by weeping friends? The true physician will embrace the opportunity to exercise his skill at these moments. It has come to pass that I am invited frequently to stand at the bed of *moribund* patients, whom I never attended during their curable ills, and as many times do I thank the Grand Master for the wonderful means of allaying the pangs of the flesh, without resort to the necessity of departing from that law which I have so many times pronounced universal; even in the last moments—a euthanasia.

GALL STONE OR KIDNEY COLIC DISCUSSION

In any case of gall-stone or kidney colic you cannot tell if there will be more stones. When the stone has been formed, it is separate from the patient. When the patient is under the influence of pain, it is the spasm from the stone in the ureter; clutching of the muscles. The remedy that fits the constitution has a tendency to prevent the manufacture of more stones and relieves the spasm that occasions the pain. After the remedy there may be an outpouring of stones, either renal or gall-stones. In one

case a teaspoonful of stones were discharged in one or
two days. The fibres were relaxed and the kidney was
emptied of stones. This the remedy does when aimed at
the patient. Often Belladonna is indicated; it is not deep
enough for the patient, but it is complemented frequently
by Calc-c. or Calc-ph. when the picture is of Bella., will
relieve the suffering but does not meet the condition.
Natrum sulph. will often fit the constitution and relieve
the acute trouble.

Natrum sul. or the constitutional remedy, whatever-it-
is, induces healthy bile formation. You cannot promise
there will be no more colic if you fit only the condition. So
long as stones are there, they may be passed. The constitutional remedy is the best thing for the patient. It
will set the kidneys to manufacturing healthy urine. There
is no more to say about it, but it takes time.

You will not cure all old liver and kidney cases. The
patient may be incurable, and such will continue to manufacture stones. They have too low a vitality. Sometimes
the carefully selected remedy will hold the patient but
ten days or so. Then the chances are against cure, and
the surgeon can do no better. If the remedy hold long in
a steady improvement and rouses reaction, he can be
cured. The reason cancer and consumption cannot be
cured in some patients is that the reaction does not
hold up.

HINT TO SPECIALISTS

A quasi-homœopathic gynæcologist once said to some
of our students; "If you undertake to cure these diseases
(displacements) with your homœopathic remedies you will
fail. I have tried remedies and have never found them
of any value. I now replace the uterus and adjust a pessary immediately." In such cases what has become of
the law? And yet some specialists cry out that the
specialties are not sustained. Shall the common average

physician sit down and worship such gynæcology, when he, though not pretending great skill, can do better than the specialist, taking his word for it. This is not to underrate him who uses all his means in the right place for the greatest good. There is room for all the specialties, but our specialists must do better than the common practitioner, or they must not complain of being scolded. We expect that the specialist shall not simply and only know the mechanical portion of his department, but that he shall also be expert in the materia medica of his department. It will do for the average doctor to say, "Oh, you materia medica fellows are experts; we are too busy to learn these fine things;" but it will not do for our specialists to be guilty of ignorance in this department. They must know how to cure with remedies, or they must not lay claim to special qualification. When I talk with a specialist I expect to learn of special indications for remedies, and I am generally disappointed. The specialist has the same pathogenesis to work out his case by that all have, but he generally relies on somebody's hard work, trying to make them fit his cases, and as a rule it does not apply. Every man who claims special excellence in any one department should search the provings for a therapeutics peculiar to his own demands and build for himself. Several years of hard study will reward his labors and he will know none the less of the accumulated experience of others in the application of these same pathogeneses recorded in works on therapeutics. The specialists stand accused of ignorance of the materia medica—indeed, they are their own accusers when they acknowledge the demand made upon mechanics for the majority of cases treated. Failure to cure by the materia medica should be the exception in all non-surgical diseases, and when other means are resorted to they should be looked upon as but palliative and not curative. There are instances when it is judicious to

19

palliate, but let no man call these means curative. The curse of Homœopathy is the too free use of palliatives, and this is because of the wide-spread ignorance of the philosophy of Homœopathy and the materia medica. Doctors use palliatives when thy do not know what else to do, as the surgeon cuts off the leg when it is the last resort; had he known how to prevent the disease-processes he would have saved the leg. It is a common practice to apply a support to hold in position a displaced uterus and then begin to build up by medicine. Who is wise enough to know what to administer after the symptoms, the only true expression of the disease, have been removed? Yet this is the way some of our specialists go about it, and then complain that "the law is a failure." There might be some reason in first taking the symptoms by which to select a remedy and then applying a pessary; but to the experienced the folly of this will appear, as it is so well known that the symptoms immediately disappear without mechanics. Support is not needed after the right remedy has been taken two days. Again, if a support be used, one has no evidence of good or bad selection.

The cure of these diseases is possible without support with pure medicinal treatment; the demonstrations are too numerous to deny; then let the specialist lay no claim to proficiency who is not able to do better than the average doctor. It matters not how often a woman is examined, only that she is safely, gently, and permanently cured. The question of frequent examinations is one to be laughed at. But the question arises, first of all, do you cure safely, quickly, and permanently? If the physician can make more out af a patient by making frequent observations, and his patient will stand that kind of business, it is well enough, and he must settle with his own conscience if he have such a thing; but he must not so interfere as to delay recovery which should be more or less rapid in most cases. I have the right to take exception, and to criticize, when women go to specialists and pay enormous sums for the treatment of diseases that should be cured with a few doses of a properly selected homœopathic remedy. These things have occurred, and not with our tyros, but those standing in the lead. I can produce the notes if any man dare dispute it, and the worst part of the whole business is that the greatest pretentions are cloaks to the most profound ignorance. These men are generally too wise (?) to be taught by an American author or teacher. They go on with their circumscribed armamentarium for local use, and the thimbleful of *materia medica*, which is all they have, serves the purpose of homœopathic show. If the representatives of the homœopathic school would learn the polychrests so that they could compare them throughout, the demand for mechanics and local slops would decrease. There should be no fashion in medicine; what was good fifty years ago in the hands of the masters should be just as good today, and the deviation comes out of departing from the methods of the early physician who had not the labor-saving and brain-saving machines. If the masters could cure such cases with simply great labor, how much better ought we do. The high degree of perfection will never come to our specialties so long as the specialists are content with the palliatives now in vogue. I am astonished at the amount of palliation that can come from some of these mechanical supports, but I am never astonished at any great skill in the use of remedies in the hands of our specialists, and I still fail to see any good reason for sending a non-surgical case to a specialist to be treated. When they arrange a family circle of their own to include the materia medica and correct philosophy, then and not until then can they claim patronage that naturally should fall to the specialist. I fail to see any good reason why a homœopathician should advise a patient to consult a pro-

fessed homœopathic specialist, whose principal means are
those developed and used by the allopathist. If there is
any reason to suppose a homœopathic physician can use
allopathic tools to a better advantage than the allopathist
himself, I fail to see it. If allopathic means are better
than ours, why uphold the law which is the *sine qua non*
of Homœopathy? If a combination of allopathic and
homœopathic means goes better, why not associate with
congenial spirits, the eclectics?

HOMŒOPATHY: ITS FUNDAMENTAL PRINCIPLES OUTLINED

As we were about to enter upon a discussion that may
lead beyond the probability of ready comprehension, and
as I may encounter, even at this center of Hahnemannism,
those who have not traveled beyond "*faith*" and "belief,"
permit me to ask my hearers to lay aside both, and with
me enter upon a line of thought and investigation, and
accept the outcome regardless of preconceived opinions,
belief, or faith. These have no part in a scientific discussion. One should proceed without opinion, without faith,
without prejudice to weigh the statements found in the
sixteenth section of the fifth and last edition of the
Organon of Samuel Hahnemann.

The doctrines contained in this section are the result
of many years of thought and classified experience, and
they conflict with the statements of accepted authority.
But if it be the foundation of truth, even in part, we must
explore its interior and bow to its revelations. Though
Draper and Carpenter have failed to discover these inner
precincts, they have not demonstrated that Hahnemann's
conclusions were illogical or impossible. With cell-forma-
tion they have ended; but life, the home of disease, is
unknown to them. The opponents of this doctrine, which
the followers of Hahnemann have accepted as a great

truth, may search in vain and quote authority without end, and the only result attained is: Not found, not demonstrated; unknown. These authors, being ignorant of this vital dynamis, deny its existence; they cannot see it; cannot manipulate it; and cannot demonstrate it by the common instruments in chemistry and physiology. Nevertheless, the time will come when physiology must deal with this question as a factor not in dispute; then will the great void in this science be filled with that which will make medical science to rest on firm foundations; while at present from old-school standpoint it has no foundation, and with the Hahnemannian school our foundation is disputed.

As it is probable that I shall be accused of extremism, let me say, by way of explanation, that not all so-called homœopathists admit the truth of the dynamic doctrine and choose to call it "dynamic theory." There are graded believers in Homœopathy as in religion. Some are born to position, others acquire it. To be born of Christian parentage does not make one a Christian. Yet believing in Christ and His teachings, without following His example or obeying His commands, will distinguish him from the Jew. In like manner believing in the *Law of Cure* makes a homœopathist. But like the followers of Christ, it is only possible to be an exemplary one by close relation at the throne of grace, or measuring every action by the principles under the law. Therefore it will be observed that to be an exemplary follower of the master-healer, it is necessary to be near him, and follow after him in all his steps that the highest degree of wisdom may appear in our methods. Not that I would blindly follow a leader who has been extensively courted; but that after discovering Hahnemann to have been the greatest living healer it behoves that we study him in all his intricate philosophy to ascertain, if possible, wherein rested his great powers as a physician, and then see whether as a healer he is worthy of followers. If we have discovered that he was an original thinker and philosopher, and his teachings are as he declared them to be, viz.: the only true method of curing the sick, let us follow as far as he has gone, not wavering a hair's breadth, until we have arrived at the point where the master left us and his great philosophy. They who practice on a part of Hahnemann's teachings and fill the great void with "results of experience," do so with methods that the master unequivocally condemned; and while it may not be thought kindly of, the statement is true; they are not the homœopathists who have followed in the footsteps of the master. They have not lived closely to the law, and are not Hahnemannians. Hahnemann said to a friend of his in Paris, who was complimenting him on the great number of his followers. Says Hahnemann: "Yes, there are a great many homœopathic doctors, but all my true followers can be counted on the ends of my fingers."

It is as an exponent of the philosophy of Hahnemann that I speak to *you*, his professed followers. It is because I have learned that the Central New York Society desires to live close to the master and learn of him, as far as he had advanced, that I traveled so far to address you on this occult subject.

While some of the enemies of Homœopathy, and some professed followers of the Law of Cure, have said that this great master was visionary, and many other harsh things, it may be well to observe that he never ceased to think with strength; his very last thoughts are to be fully appreciated before we attempt to walk alone, or build a philosophy out of other material.

Before entering upon a fuller discussion of the statements which contain the master's conclusion, let us look into the life of this great man, and see what manner of man was he, and how he was led to such a conclusion relating to the invisible vital dynamis. We want to know whether he reasoned it out by a pure mental effort, or arrived at it after the use of potentized medicines—as a result of experience.

Burnett says: "Of Hahnemann's father sufficient is known to be sure that he was no ordinary man, inasmuch as he taught the young Samuel to think for himself—for which purpose he is said to have shut him up alone and given him a theme to think out."

If Ameke's history be read it will be seen at once that Hahnemann displayed wonderful energy in securing his primary training, as his father was a man of limited means.

Everywhere facts confirm the historian, wherein he states that Hahnemann never admired metaphysical speculations: he always concluded on facts, never on theory or speculation. I refer you to his essay on the "Speculative System of Medicine," *Lesser Writings*, p. 567, wherein a masterly handling of the subject was done, showing a wonderful mind and a complete knowledge of the medicine of his time, which he manipulated so iconoclastically.

In 1792 he challenged the physicians to justify themselves for the treatment administered Emperor Leopold II. Even thus early the master-mind saw the perniciousness of the practice in vogue. Neither was he wanting in knowledge of many sciences.

He was the first to make the proving of drugs a system. From 1790 he continued the proving of drugs, and throughout his writings, he recommended the use of drugs only whose effects are accurately known, which knowledge is to be discovered only by proving upon the healthy; and this is in keeping with his manners and acts—everywhere we find exactitude of thought and method.

While translating Cullen's *Materia Medica,* in 1790, he

met the latter's explanation of the action of Cinchona bark in curing chills and fever. Cullen attributes the curative influence to a "strengthening power it exerts over the stomach." Hahnemann refuses to accept this explanation, and cites the following: 'Substances, such as strong coffee, pepper, arnica, ignatia, and arsenic, which cause a kind of fever, extinguish the periodicity of fevers." "For the sake of experiment, I took, for several days, four drachms of good Cinchona bark twice a day." The results are too well known to be recalled here; but it will be observed that Hahnemann did not refuse to accept Cullen's explanation without a reason on definite information, while Cullen's opinion was a mere speculation, such as men feel compelled to offer when expected to say something. From facts, Hahnemann was led to remark that Ipecac must produce certain forms of artificial fever in order to cure intermittent fever. Gradually was he advancing by deduction to the great discovery of the Law of Cure. Up to this time, while he had seen the evidence, he had not formulated the *similia similibus curantur*, in fact, nothing is seen of it until 1796, in an essay which appeared in *Hufeland's Journal*, and is a part of the *Lesser Writings*, p. 295—"Essays on a New Principle for Discovering the Curative Power of Drugs." In this paper he advises medicines in crude, but small doses. "In a dose just strong enough to produce scarcely perceptible indication of the expected artificial disease." At this time he had not discovered the nature of the vital dynamis.

In 1801 he wrote a paper, "Cure and Prevention of Scarlet Fever" (*Lesser Writings*, p. 369), wherein he recommended tinct. Opium, one part to five hundred of alcohol, and one drop of this to be shaken with five hundred of alcohol, the patient to take one drop of this preparation at a dose.

It was after 1801 that his centesimal scale was

brought into use. In this year he used Bell. and Cham. in about the third or fourth dilution.

Very soon he discovered that "the diminution of the action of the drug was not proportionate to the diminution of its quantity." Also the astounding fact became evident that "medicines could be so diluted that neither physics nor chemistry could discover any medicinal matter in them, and yet they possessed great healing power."

Hufeland says Hahnemann was the greatest chemist of his day, therefore was not in ignorance of the actual inability of the science to measure the quantity of medicine in his newly discovered healing agencies. His enemies have said he was highly educated in physics, botany, chemistry, geology, astronomy, pharmacy, etc. His greatest and last attainment was his discovery of dynamism, which has distinguished him from all men and established a Hahnemannism that will stand as long as the world stands.

They may run away with Homœopathy and befoul it into a modern nastiness, a mongrelism, and by virtue of the might and numbers vote it to mean anything they chose, but they have no power to change Hahnemannism, which stands and must forever stand as a living truth wherever men love truth and are not afraid to speak their true convictions. I do not favor isms; but, Mr. President, in this case our only safety is to stand by this one for the simple reason that when any other name has become popular it will be stolen as the honored name of Homœopathy has been stolen, and is no longer an expression of the doctrines of Hahnemann and its most conspicious representatives who do not make use of his methods. If an inquiring allopath seek information of one of these modern representatives, he will learn nothing of the teachings of Hahnemann. Why is this? Simply because the colleges have not taught the sixteenth section of the *Primer*. They have not taken neophytes up through the primary work, but have placed them at work with the advanced course, which is never learned without the primer. Where have we such a parallel in other sciences? One of the conditions necessary to the successful perpetuation of this science is a knowledge of its first principles and how to teach them.

Let us now proceed to inspect the various editions of this *Organon*, and we see what a careful man our author was. He was not a man to adopt a theory of others before having thoroughly tested it and having observed the facts upon which the theory was based. Everywhere we see originality of thought, firmness, great power of observation, comparison, and most wonderful reasoning. Metaphysical speculation was repulsive to him, which he carefully avoided in the first edition of the *Organon*, which was published in 1810. He was eminently practical in all that he said and did. Thus, you will search in vain in all the first four editions of the *Organon* for the term and idea of the vital force. He only spoke of the interior of the organism.

In the seventh section of the first edition: "There must exist in the medicine a healing principle; the understanding has a presentation of it, but its essence is not recognizable by us in any way, only its utterances and actions can be known by experience."

Twenty-three years later, when seventy-eight years old, in the fifth edition, published in 1833, in the ninth and tenth sections, he distinctly calls a unit of action in the whole organism of the vital force. From this it is evident Hahnemann arrived at this conclusion after a long and practical experience, inasmuch as he was led up to it by his early perception of the similar vital principle contained in the medicine (see first ed., fifth section), which is only recognized by its action upon the organism. I have shown you that it was not metaphysical speculation that led the master to the idea of the vital dynamis, but a long series of practical and experimental research.

If we would think for ourselves, let us inspect some of the facts that relate to general medicine and see if we can answer some of the questions that are propounded, and then revert to the vital dynamis. We read in the time-honored text-books that there is such a condition of the human body known as *diathesis*— in fact, several of them; again, that these diatheses are hereditary and predispose to disease. What is this diathesis out of which grow so many diseases? In one subject comes cancer; in another insanity; in another tuberculosis; and in another epilepsy, or Bright's disease, or Hodgekin's disease. What is the stromous diathesis? What is this state of bad feeling that precedes any fixed organic change that locates in an organ? Can it be that this latent wrong in the vital power is not worthy of consideration? Can it be that the kidney can take on structural change and become waxy without cause? You must say, No! What is the cause of this lesion, and why do not these named exciting causes always produce the same results, and why does not every person subjected to these exciting causes become afflicted with waxed kidneys? You answer because there is a predisposing, determing influence at work. Yes, the diathesis. But the diathesis has no foundation in fact, only a thing of imagination. A convenient explanation of unknown things; a figure-head in the text-books, out of which we have had no benefit, and learned no lesson from the old school, whose literature has so wisely furnished us with a meaningless lot of terms.

We read of the weakness, of the dropsy, etc., etc., coming from Bright's disease, but we do not read of the pre-historic symptoms; are they of no value? Are they not present? Yes, they are present. Then what are they? We read of exciting and predisposing cases but we do not

read why a similar combination of exciting and predisposing causes is not always followed by Bright's disease.
We have a right to ask this of a system of medicine that
claims scientific attention and public patronage. Another
example, if you please, we read of a self-limited disease
called scarlatina (scarlet fever). Any allopathist will
warm up in opposition if you tell him that scarlet fever
is not a self-limited disease. If it be a self-limited disease
it must result in resolution or death; the child must recover by statute of limitation, or—die. They do not all
die; some are left even under old-school treatment to tell
the tale. From these we learn that ear-discharges are the
result of scarlatina. This otorrhœa is not a part of
scarlatina—as according to accepted teaching—the disease
is self-limited. The child was a picture of health before
the scarlatina: then, what is this new trouble? Specialists
treat the otorrhœa as if it were a new disease *per se*; if
so, whence has it come and what is the nature of it? A
novice can tell you a long name and affirm that it is catarrhal; but that is not satisfactory. Where did it come
from? Did it come spontaneously, or was it the result of
some latent wrong in the vital dynamis? I say in the
dynamis, as there was no tissue change before, and the
scarlatina has long gone. We do not know that this new
trouble is essentially chronic; and that in scarlet fever there
is no chronic element. Now, has this sore ear simply developed this, a propitious time? Has the scarlatina so
weakened the mucous membrane of the aural tubes that
they become the favorite sites for the expression of a
something that the disease when badly treated has aroused
into action? I say when badly treated, because when the
disease is properly treated, otorrhœa does not follow. I
no longer see such troubles, and have not had them since
I have been able to recognize their true nature. What is
this something that may exist for years in a latent state—

be handed down from generation to generation, and come to view at any time and cause chronic troubles to follow self-limited diseases? We have a right to a civil answer to a question of this kind. If a vital wrong is capable of existing for years in an invisible state outside of the tissues, there must be some invisible precinct that stores it or it does not exist. Can it now be doubted that a disease may exist for years with or without a morbid anatomy? Rokitensky says scrofula has no morbid anatomy. To be logical, according to the material school, there is no scrofula and no stroma; that scrofulous manifestations have no cause, and consequently no reality. Why do not all injuries of the synovial membranes of the ilio-femoral articulation result in hip-joint disease? Why do some abscesses close with the evacuation of pus, and others form sinuses and fistulæ? Look where you may in literature other than Hahnemannian, and you will find mere speculation, theory, and no practical deduction.

Hahnemann describes three constitutional miasms that may exist in latency, that develop and progress in the vital "dynamis without" changing the tissues that may spring into destructive activity and attack organs and give shape to countless lesions called disease; that these miasms should be recognized as primary wrongs out of which grow incurable maladies, and all structural changes. Shall we learn a lesson from these reflections, or shall we pass them as mere theories? Hahnemann teaches the nature of these miasms; it is not my province to discuss them, but to simply call them up as the essentials to the complete study of the sixteenth section. The questions to be answered from all these are:

First. Have we such a condition as an invisible immaterial disease?

Second. If so, are all diseases of the same nature, and

Third.　Is it rational to attempt to nullify a disease of immaterial nature by material substances.

Hahnemann's early deduction was that disease, being of an immaterial nature, could develop only on a similar basis or in a similar sphere, when in contact with a similar quality of force; and to again reach it curatively, a force must be found equally as immaterial.

The mystery of the vital force for all practical purposes in the healing art has been solved by the immortal Hahnemann, and named the vital dynamis. His deductions are summed up in the sixteenth section. This section furnished the keystone to the doctrines of Hahnemannism, and without which the great arch must flatten and collapse; without this finishing doctrine his followers would be where all are who have rejected it—floundering in the mire of uncertainty and floating in the swift and muddy rivers of guesswork and disappointment. The study of the sixteenth section clearly sums up what the great philosopher believed disease to be. Let us enter this wilderness and see where we are directed. If we accept the teachings we must admit that (the results of disease) lesions, tissue changes, cannot be considered as primary expressions of disease, but as a consequence. The molecular vibrations or vital activities, are a warning that a continuance of the expressions of wrong life must mean progressive death. To consider life in the sense that Hahnemann looked upon it, as normal activities within the organism, and we must then look upon these normal activities changed by cause to be the abnormal, which is disease. The only evidence of disease are the definite expressions that deviate from the normal, which we choose to denominate the language of the vital wrong (section 7), "Hence, the totality of these symptoms, *this outwardly reflected image of the inner nature of the disease, i., e., of the suffering vital force.* Localization is at all times a secondary state or the result of disease, while changed feelings are the primary manifestations. The primary or changed feeling often escapes observation, as in a gonorrhœa; but the disease has been pervading the economy for a period of eight days, and the localization finally appears as a discharge. The same is true of all contagious diseases, and as far as is known, of every disease. If we look upon disease with any other view and consider it *per se* when it localizes itself, and then search for a name to fit it, by virtue of its morbid anatomy, or its location, we trace it to its observable beginning, and as though it had no cause, and study it in relation to changed cells as a something with only an ending but with no beginning. But when looking at all tissue changes as the result of disease, we are in position to inquire: What is the disease proper? This guides into the pre-historic state when there were no tissue changes, and yet there will be found ample expressions to convince us that all was not perfect in the invisible vital kingdom, and the scalpel has not been directed. Then it is with this pre-historic state, these vital activities, that we have to deal. Before the change of tissue has occurred there must have been a cause of morbid vibrations—a condition of morbid vital activities, or cell-changes could not have been wrought. What is the nature of that state or condition that existed before the tissues and cells changed their shape? There must be two, the right and the wrong; the former the correct life function known by the absence of all subjective sensations— a feeling of bodily comfort and ease; and the latter by the presence of subjective morbid feelings. The former is known as health, and the latter as sickness or disease. These cannot be measured as a quantitative influence, as the cause is only qualitative in itself, and its results are but a perversion of a proper force. It will be as difficult to demonstrate that quantitative influence is necessary to produce vital changes as to demonstrate that there is a measurable quantity in noxious forces so hurtful to man. Therefore, we may conclude that causes purely qualitative act destructively. We now have the right to assume that all vital changes primarily are only qualitative in the sense of misapplied force, and that these morbid vibrations are the disease, and all there is of disease *per se*.

Now, we may assume that life is a dynamis capable of perpetuating its own identity when the medium through which it acts if not destroyed or impaired. Again, to act upon the dynamis and not disturb the medium there must be force brought in relation with the vital force equally as qualitative and as free from quantitative consideration. It hardly needs further demonstration to show that this vital perversion is possible, but we observe daily the wrong feelings that have been known to exist for years without quantitative changes or localization. Thus have we arrived at Hahnemann's conclusion. But now we glean that if an equally subtle dynamis is necessary to cause disease and disturb the harmonious relations of the vital activities—and it is admitted that the Law of Similars expresses the curative relation and the only law of the kind known to man—must we not conclude that this curative power or force, to be a corrective principle, must be equally qualitative and subtle with the life-principle, with the disease cause, with the disease itself? The vital affinity cannot appear between forces of foreign relations; they must be *similar* in quality and devoid of quantity. Power used in the sense of overpowering an antagonist has no place in the science of homœopathics, but it is a consideration of a given force deranged or perverted to be simply harmonized and restored to equilibrium.

It will at once be observed that a surplus of force is impossible only as a surplus in a qualitative relation which has no part in the similitude of a purely qualitative problem. To attain the highest degree of similitude, not the quantity of a given power, is the aim. The similar is quality with similar expressions of activity in the *sine qua non*, as we have demonstrated, that there is no quantity necessary in the consideration. Therefore, if this be only a spirit-like dynamis—and I believe the demonstration is clear—all of the quantity taken or made use of must be that much more than similar—therefore, unlike—and that much more than the demand to restore equilibrium; in other words, contrary and in no relation curative. Not in any sense restorative, but, on the contrary, retarding the return to normal vibration by impairing the medium through which the vital dynamis must operate. In relation to cure, it has so often been said by the master there was yet too much medicine to cure. The dose is yet too large to cure. The use of the term quantity conveys the idea of strength, which has no part in any homœopathic sense as related to a curative agency. To reduce remedial agents to primitive identity of a qualitative character only that they may act through the new medium, is the aim of the true healer. Not until they are divested of their own media can they be quickly corrective or be active in any sense as similar agencies.

This view may appear to oppose some statements of Hahnemann. In section 45, "The stronger disease will overcome the weaker one." This is only apparent. The two diseases, being partially similar, overcome each other only in part; but the part of the one overcome only in part reproduces itself and runs its course unmolested." In section 34, "For it is by virtue of the similitude, combined with greater intensity." This statement may be correct; but I believe it to be only apparent, and that the similitude is the only necessary demand for the destruction of both, or, rather, the correction of the wrong in the dynamis or spirit-like vital force. There being no entity, there can

20

be nothing to overpower—only a perverted effort to be corrected. Any disease will subside apparently by natural decline when met by a noxious influence of similar dynamis of sick-making possibilities, regardless of intensity. This view strengthens the Law of Similars and is in harmony with immaterial activities. It is not adding a new force, but applying a force to correct a perverted life-principle.

The noxious, disease-producing influences have nothing in common with material agencies. When so crude that they can be seen and manipulated, they are feeble sick-making agencies. (The skeptical experimenters, in provings made with attenuations, forgot that a special predisposition is frequently necessary for contagion, and that this predisposition cannot be made to order, but must be utilized when found, which affords a propitious opportunity for the pure experiment through which we discover the sick-making power of drugs). (Section 31). The dangerous and most noxious agencies are of the unknown. The most astute have failed to find the cholera or yellow fever causes. The cause of small-pox is yet unknown. The subtle influence that in one stroke swoops down upon a village is not measurable by our crude senses. The small-pox poison, when attenuated with millions of volumes of atmospheric air, comes to the surface through the mails and through old clothing by inhalation and the slightest contact. The impression wrought upon this spirit-like dynamis accumulates until the medium is threatened with destruction—all from a simple perverted life-force.

In this sixteenth section: "Neither can the physician free the vital force from any of these morbid disturbances." No, because the life force being an immaterial force like electricity, there is nothing to purge out, but a simple vital perversion to be corrected, and as the wrong is essentially immaterial, nothing but an immaterial something can be similar enough to it to act upon it as a curative. A material substance may change the organism and thereby suppress or suspend an immaterial wrong, but the latter will return so soon as the former, its medium, resumes its normal conductivity.

It will be observed at once that the essentials of cure do not exist in operations upon the organisms, and as material substances operate largely through the organisms, the true disease is not reached. The object then must be to avoid operating upon the organism and essentially through the vital impulses by correcting the perverted vital activities. The causes of disease existing in a highly attenuated form are similar in equality to the vital dynamis; hence the affinity or susceptibility. This same affinity must be acquired by a drug substance. The attenuation must be carried on until a correspondence of spheres has been reached, or until resistance is no longer possible. The point of the highest degree of similitude in quality between two activities is variable, as it is in a degree observable in a very wide range of attenuation, as many quick cures are observed from low attenuations, but, more commonly, the high and highest attenuations furnish the most striking examples. That low potencies cure, nobody disputes; and this does not refute the doctrine; but it must be admitted that it is by virtue of the inherent dynamic principle that it is curative, though more feebly curative in the low than when the drug it attenuated to a quality equal to the quality of the attenuated disease cure and the qualitative vital dynamis. The striking changes sometimes observed from low attenuations are the results of primary action on the organism which Hahnemann seeks to avoid. To bring about such results medicines must be repeated, while a single dose of the attenuated medicine would prove curative, and not influence the organism primarily. From a practical standpoint let us look upon the results of obeying the instructions of the master, who was always guided in his later years by the doctrine of the sixteenth section, and contrast them with the result of those who disobey this teaching.

The former class has followed closely the master's teachings, accepting the dynamic doctrine, and in this line have they made their cures, with the same evidence claimed by the other class, simply the patients recover. They have not felt the need of other methods than those taught by Hahnemann. They have not gone backwards, but, on the contrary, they have made some progress. How have they progressed? Let us see. If you will consult section 41 of the *Organon* you will see. Here we see that Hahnemann declares it almost impossible to eradicate some diseases because they had been complicated with drugs having no relation to the disease. He says that his remedies were always capable of curing effectually all simple diseases. Hahnemann then used but thirtieth cent. potency when this section was written with few exceptions. What have his faithful followers to say as proof of the truth of the doctrine and as proof of progress? That many of these most complicated diseases can be wiped out. That the drug symptoms can be subdued by very high attenuations, leaving the simple original disease to manifest itself through the natural medium, when it can be cured by the thirtieth potency of the master. They who have rejected this doctrine as a dogma have never seen this work and they never will. Yes, we shall progress if we observe facts, and unflinchingly cling to the doctrines of the immortal Hahnemann. Let us look at the contrast. What can be said of this class? Their cures are only a deception. Had they really cured their cases they would not need to resort to the latest whim of an empirical profession. They have abandoned the teaching of the sixteenth section, and what is the result? They know that they cannot cure the sick and they even refuse to believe that anyone else can. You never dispute a cure where it is in keeping with your daily observations. They say that ague must have Quinine, when the follower of the master cures all his cases with the attenuated appropriate remedy. The materia medica that has been found so satisfactory in the hands of Hahnemann and his followers has been a failure and it needs revising. There must be something wrong and we want no greater evidence of their failure than that the chief defamer, J. P. Dake, requires in his practice a large stock of Warner's sugar-coated pills, composed of crude medicines. If this be true of the chief, what in the name of heaven must the lesser lights need. who must, of course, be less skilled? They have declared that any one who simply selects his remedy under the *Law* of Similars is as high as he can attain in the art of healing; and he may thereafter cover his patients with mustard, and apply all the local measures he chooses. Even they say that the local treatment is assisted by the internal remedy.

The first departure from the dynamic doctrine is dangerous and leads toward non-success, and careless method is the outcome. Safety comes from simply not following the law of selection, but also the teaching of the sixteenth section must be heeded. Look at the alternation departure, and see the laziness of his thoughts. Examine the prescription file in any drug store of a large city. What do you find? Simply a lot of prescriptions called homœopathic whose only element of Homœopathy is the signature of a long professed homœopathic practitioner.

Hahnemann regarded this vital dynamis as a unit of force (see section 15), and the departure from health as a unit of force. We cannot study the sixteenth section and ignore this portion of the dynamic doctrine. How absurd must it appear to one who has a clear comprehension of

#272

these truths to consider for one moment the problem of alternation which the master has so unequivocally condemned in section 272, and its note. Take a mental state that clearly indicates Nux vomica, and associate it with a Pulsatilla menstrual condition, with menses too late, scanty, and pale. In the former Pulsatilla is contra-indicated by the crabbed temper; in the latter Nux is contra-indicated by the conditions of the menstrual flow. The two, therefore, are contra-indicated, neither of them corresponding to the unit of force known by the totality of symptoms. Can it be possible that by combining them it will make either or both homœopathic to the demand of this unit? Hahnemann everywhere speaks of using only such medicines as are accurately understood by having been proved on the healthy human body. Here we have a compound about which little is known. Can it appear rational to suppose, or assume, that with a compound unknown, composed of elements neither of which is homœopathic to this unit of force, that they can act uniformly curatively? These departures, wherein the doctrine of the sixteenth section is not heeded, are the foundation of all ill-success; of the cry for a revised materia medica, and of so-called modern Homœopathy. I must say again, that modern Homœopathy is built out of the departures from the doctrines of the immortal Hahnemann. These men have found the materia medica so inadaptable to their wants, that a majority of their prescriptions are composed of crude drugs. These departurists have so departed from the methods of Hahnemann that the homœopathic profession as a mass is to-day but a caricature, having violated every principle of the philosophy that has anything distinctive.

They may find momentary comfort in it, but every true man must feel like uttering, "Father, forgive them, they know not what they do."

HOW SYMPTOMS CHANGE.

EDITORS HOMOEOPATHIC PHYSICIAN:—For the interest of the members of the Rochester Hahnemannian Society, I desire to comment on the case related by Dr. Grant to the Society, and published in HOMOEOPATHIC PHYSICIAN, October, page 538, last line, where the Doctor gave Stannum. He notes that the patient came back and stated that the sputa had changed in the taste to "salty." Stannum has the salty taste as well as sweetish, and it is very common for a drug to convert one symptom into another within its own sphere in curing. If it converts a symptom into one not within its own sphere the cure will be slow or prove to be not a cure.

When a patient returns and reports symptoms worse or changed, it is proper to look to see if the new symptoms are found under the medicine taken. If they are found there the prescription is a good one and the physician may say to himself, *Sac. lac.* If the new symptoms are not found in the search into the same proving there are two conclusions to be settled by waiting:

I. The case may need another remedy.

II. If the cases goes on to quick recovery it will be found that the new symptom or symptoms will some day belong to the pathogenetic symptoms.

The cultivation of this watchfulness leads to great accuracy in prescribing, as much will be gleaned that comes under useful knowledge. The field is a very large one, and the field of high potencies is especially a fertile one. Observing what develops in the aggravation of high potencies and the direction of symptoms is the grandest study in the materia medica.

HOW TO STUDY THE REPERTORY.

After all the symptoms of a patient have been written out the *Repertory* should be taken up. The beginner should not attempt to abbreviate the anemnesis, but should write out the *full general rubric* for exercise, if nothing more. If *melancholy* be the word, the remedies set to the word should be written down with all the graduations. If the *melancholy* appear only *before* the menses let a sub-rubric be placed in a manner to show at a glance the number of remedies of the *general class* having the *special* period of aggravation. Many of the most brilliant cures are made

from the *general rubric* when the *special* does not help, and, in careful notes of ten years, would bring down many of the *general rubric* symptoms, and furnish the best of clinical verifications. The longer this is done the more can the busy doctor abbreviate his case-notes.

The special aggravation is a great help, but such observations are often wanting, and the general rubric must be pressed into service.

Again, we have to work by *analogy*. In this method Boenninghausen's *Pocket Repertory* is of the greatest service.

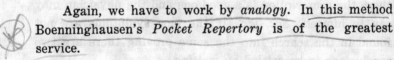

Take Minton's most excellent work, and we find menstrual agonies are ameliorated by heat, peculiar to Ars. and Nux., and by moist heat, to Nux-m. But the symptoms of one case are not like either of these remedies, and we must go farther into the materia medica. We can there form the *anemnesis* by analogy and make use of the *general rubric*, taking all the remedies known to be generally ameliorated by heat and warmth applied.

To be methodical, the general rubric should appear in the notes of the prescriber and the special below it. If this plan be carefully carried out, a comparison of ten years' work would be a most instructive perusal. What is true of a remedy generally may often be true in particular, especially so in the absence of a *contra-indicating exception*, well established.

If this plan be followed by beginners, always reading

up the *Materia Medica* with the *anemnesis*, by the time business becomes plenty the work becomes easy and rapid. A young man can prescribe for a few patients a day and make careful homœopathic cures, and he can gain speed enough to prescribe for twenty or thirty a day after a few years. Any man who desires to avoid *this careful method should not pretend* to be a *homoeopathic physician, as the right way is not in him,* as the desire must precede the act.

The patient does not always express the symptom in the language that would best indicate the *real nature* of the symptom. Then it is that judgment is required, that the physician may *gain a correct appreciation* of the symptoms. So often is this true that the young man and often the old is led from the true expressions of nature, and he will make an inappropriate prescription. The task of taking symptoms is often a most difficult one. It is sometimes possible to abbreviate the *anemnesis* by selecting one symptom that is very peculiar containing the key to the case. A young man cannot often detect this peculiarity, and he should seldom attempt it. It is often convenient to abbreviate by taking a group of three or four essentials in a given case, making a summary of these, and eliminating all remedies not found in all the essential symptoms. A man with considerable experience may cut short the work in this way. I have frequently known young men to mistake a modality for a symptom. This is fatal to a correct result. The symptom is the sensation or condition, and the modality is only a modification. The symptom often becomes *peculiar* or *characteristic* through its modality.

When a sensation is looked up in the *Repertory*, all the remedies belonging to it should be written out, and individualization began by modalities.

I am frequently asked what is understood by *peculiar*

as applied to a case. A little thought should lead each man to the solution.

A high temperature, a fever *without thirst,* is in a measure *peculiar.* A hard chill with thirst for cold water is peculiar. Thirst with a fever, with the heat, is not peculiar, because you can safely say it is common to find *heat with thirst,* and uncommon to find heat without thirst. That which is common to any given disease is never *peculiar.* This may seem too simple to demand an explanation, but let him who knows it go to the next page. Pathognomonic symptoms are not used to individualize by, and are never peculiar in the sense asked for.

I am asked what I mean when I say to beginners, *treat the patient and not the disease.* My answer always is about as follows: The symptom that is seldom found in a given disease is one not peculiar to the disease, but peculiar to the patient, therefore the peculiarities of the patient have made the disease differ from all the members of its class and from all others in the class, and make this disease, as affecting this patient, an individuality by itself, and can only be treated as an individual. This individuality in the patient manifests itself by *peculiar* symptoms nearly always prominent, and always looked for by the true healer. The man who gives Acon. for fever knows nothing of the spirit of the law or the duties of the physician. The same is true of *Colocynth* for colic, Arsenicum for chill, etc.

"What shall we do when we find several peculiarities in the same patient and one remedy does not cover them all?" Here is where the astute physician will pick up his *Repertory* and commence the search for a remedy most similar to all, and if he has been a student for a few years he need not go about asking foolish questions. The lazy man has spent his days in the folly of pleasures, and the man of limited belief has shot out so many valu-

able things that he is constantly up in public asking
foolish questions and reporting cases with symptoms so
badly taken that he reveals the whereabouts of his past
life. He has not made use of the *Repertory*, and shows
a complete ignorance of the *rubrics* and the usual form-
ality of taking symptoms as taught by Hahnemann. It
is a blessed thing that they are not responsible for all their
ignorance. Where shall the responsibility rest, and who
shall "throw the first stone?"

It is so easy to wink at the sins that we ourselves are
guilty of that is seems impossible to find judge or jury
before whom to arraign the first law-breaker.

The cry for liberty has been a grievous error, as
liberty is and has been most shamefully abused. It means
a license to violate law, and only a modest elasticity is
necessary and full eclecticism is the product. It is liberty
that has driven out of use, or limited the use of, the
Repertory that all the old healers so much consulted. If
Bœnninghausen used a *Repertory* with the limited remedies there proved, how much more do we need to consult it.

HOW TO USE THE REPERTORY

Ever since the appearance of my Repertory in print
many of my friends who use it have urged me to
write out my own method of using a repertory. I realize
that it is a most difficult undertaking, but shall attempt
to explain my method. I doubt not but most careful prescribers will find that they are working in a similar manner.

The use of the repertory in homœopathic practice is a
necessity if one is to do careful work. Our Materia Medica
is so cumbersome without a repertory that the best prescriber must meet with only indifferent results.

After the case has been *properly taken* according to
Hahnemann's rules it is ready for study. I do not intend

to offer in this manner the ordinary rubrics, because all
know them so well. A case that is well taken and ordinarily full will show morbid manifestations in sensitive
ness to many surroundings, such as weather, heat and cold,
also in the desires and aversions, mental symptoms and the
various regions of the body.

When I take up a full case for study I single out all
the expressions that describe the general state, such as
the aggravations and ameliorations of the general state
of the patient or of many of his symptoms. I next consider carefully all his longings, mental and physical, all
the desires and aversion, antipathies, fears, dreads, etc.
Next I look for all the intellectual perversions, methods
of reasoning, memory, causes of mental disturbances, etc.
All these I arrange in form together, in order to set opposite each one all remedies in corresponding rubrics as found
in the repertory. By the cancellation process it will soon
be seen that only a few remedies run through all these
symptoms, and therefore only a few are to be carefully
compared in order to ascertain which one of all these is
most like the particular symptoms not yet lined up to be
considered as the first ones have been considered. Hahnemann teaches in the 153rd paragraph that we are to give
particular attention to such symptoms as are peculiar and
characteristic. He teaches also that the physician must
pay his earnest attention to the patient. Now if these
two things are duly considered, it will be seen that Hahnemann's idea was that a characteristic symptom is one that
is not common to disease but one that characterizes the
patient. All the first lot of symptoms singled out for a
more comprehensive view are such, as characterize the
patient, and are predicated of the patient himself. By
treating a portion of the symptoms in this way we have
reduced the list of possible remedies to a few or perhaps
only one. As it is necessary to consider the totality of the

symptoms for a basis of the homœopathic prescription, it is now necessary to examine all the rest of the symptoms in order to ascertain how these few remedies correspond with all the particulars.

It may be said that the above is only routine work and everybody does it just that way. True, but after so much has been accepted the more intricate problems come up. To work out a well-rounded case is the simplest part of repertory work, but when one-sided cases appear and when the patient states his symptoms in language that cannot be found in provings the case is fâr different. The record of the patient should stand as nearly as possible in his own language. From an extensive correspondence and many years of teaching graduates, I have come to the conclusion that it is a difficult matter for many to know when the record of symptoms contains the possibilities of a curative prescription. Many cases are presented with no generals and no mental symptoms—absolutely no characterizing symptoms—only the symptoms common to sickness. When a successful prescription is made on such symptoms it is scarcely more than a "lucky hit." It cannot be classed as scientific prescribing. Many records are presented with pages of vague description and one keynote that has served as a disgraceful "stool pigeon" to call forth a failure from many doctors.

Unless the symptoms that characterize the patient are brought out in the record the physician should not be surprised at a failure. The remedy must be similar to the symptoms of the patient as well as the pathognomonic symptoms of his disease in order to cure.

To show something about the requirements of repertory work, I will try to bring out hyopthetical groups of symptoms such as come to every man. In a well-rounded case, or as an isolated group, we frequently meet with what is called "writer's cramp." This must be divided

into many elements before it can be properly put on paper
as a work out case or fragment of a case. If we should
take "writer's cramp" and say no more about it, we would
have only a limited number of remedies to look to for
cure. But our resources are unlimited, as will be seen.
"Writer's cramp," when examined into, will be found to
mean cramp in fingers, hand or arms, or all three. Sometimes numbness and tingling of one or all three; sometimes sensation of paralysis in one or all three; sometimes
tingling of fingers and hand, and all of these conditions
from writing or worse while writing.

Cramp in fingers while writing; Brach., cocc.. cycl.,
trill., mag.-ph. stann.

Cramp in hand while writing: *Anac.*, euph., mag.-p.,
nat. p., sil.

Numbness in fingers while writing: Carl.

Numbness in hand while writing: Agar. *zinc.*

Paralytic feeling in hand while writing: Acon., agar.,
chel., cocc.

Cramp in wrist while writing: Amyl.-n., brach.

The above brings out about all that can be found in
the Materia Medica on this subject, and failure often follows owing to the scanty clinical and pathogenetic records
to which we have access; but we have just begun to consider that vexatious group of symptoms. It is true that
sometimes the above scanty showing presents just the
remedy required. But oftener it does not, and then we
may proceed as follows:

Cramp in the fingers, hand and wrist or such parts
as are affected: Use the general group on Page 938 of my
Repertory—a long list.

Numbness of fingers and hand: Pages 999 and 1000,
using also the general group.

Sensation of paralysis of hand and fingers: Use the
general groups, pages 1118 and 1119.

After these have been carefully written out, turn to
the general rubric in Generalities, on page 1287, "Exertion," and write out such of these remedies as are found
in the complex symptoms from exertion. Writing is nothing else but prolonged exertion. When this simple lesson
is learned the physician will see at once that the same process will show the remedy in those who have lost the
power of the hand and fingers, or have cramps, etc., from
playing stringed instruments or playing the piano or the
prolonged use of any tool or instrument. It is using in
proper manner a general rubric.

Furthermore, after cures have been made with remedies selected in this way, such remedies may be added to
the scanty list of particulars first referred to, and in this
manner will our repertory grow into usefulness. This is
the legitimate use of clinical symptoms. It is the proper
application of the general rubric to the end that our
scanty particulars may be built up. The new Repertory
is the only one ever found that provides a vacant space for
annotating just such information. If the large number
of correct prescribers in the world would join in this ex-
ension, we could soon have a repertory of comparatively
extensive particulars. Our generals were well worked out
by Bœnninghausen and much overdone, as he generalized
many rubrics that were purely particulars, the use of which
as generals is misleading and ends in failure. The success
coming from Bœnninghausen's Pocket-book is due to the
arrangement whereby generals can be quickly made use of
to furnish modalities for individual symptoms, whether
general or particular. This feature is preserved in my
repertory, as all know who use it. But it is the generals that can be used this way. A large rubric made up
of promiscuous particulars, none of which are predicated
of the patient is a "hit or miss" when applied in general
and usually a miss. For example, "aggravation from writ-

ing" is a rubric of particulars. In no instance is there one wherein the patient himself is worse from writing, but the eyes, the head, the hands, the back (from stooping) etc., make up this rubric. It is useless to resort to aggravation from writing when a headache is the symptom and find the remedy refers to a complaint in some other part wholly unlike headache. To make use of this modality for mental symptoms when it is applied to complaints of the hand is perverting the uses of circumstances. Aggravation from writing should be limited to the symptoms that are worse from writing and kept with them, as it is not a general. It is so done in my repertory. This is wholly different in the great rubric "motion." If we study Bryonia from that rubric, and from the Materia Medica we will see that such a large number of particular symptoms is aggravated by that remedy that it appears that the very patient himself is worse from motion.

Hence, it will be seen that motion is a rubric that must show the extent of aggravation in relation to the general bodily state by general and particular, and it must be retained in the generals. Any rubric that modifies so many particulars that the very patient himself seems to be so modified must be classed as general. Many wonderful cures have been made from the use of Bœnninghausen and many wonderful failures have followed, and it is from the above cause. The new repertory is produced to show forth all the particulars, each symptom with the circumstance connected with it. It is in infancy and may remain so very long, unless all who use it unite to preserve their experience in well-kept records and furnish the author with such. The author is devoting his life to the growth and infilling and perfecting of this work, and begs all true workers will co-operate by noting errors and omissions and, above all, noting such modalities of particulars as have come from generals and been observed in cures.

IDIOSYNCRASY

This term has been used in allopathic nomenclature, to define a condition supposed to be a special hypersensitive state always present in a particular patient. It is well known that some patients have an increased irritability for certain drugs. This susceptibility has been called, for want of a better explanation, an idiosyncrasy. It is a peculiarity of many people, so supposed; but, as a matter of fact, every person has some idiosyncrasy or pecular susceptibility to something. Cases are on record of most striking susceptibility to certain poisons and noxious gases. In California, a child four years old was poisoned with four single drops of Laudanum. I have seen dangerous symptoms follow a single drop of Aconite in an adult. I know a large robust woman who becomes stiff and rigid in her joints whenever she inhales sewer gas or air from a common country closet vault. A man lately reported a case to me for advice, a traveling man, who stated that whenever he slept in a room where persian insect powder had been used he broke out with patulous eruptions and became a great sufferer. I once knew a man who would suffer greatly from the mere trace of camphor that he would accidently inhale in spite of himself in his ordinary travels. I am acquainted with a physician who dare not take a teaspoonful of custard, or he will have diarrhoea in less than two hours.

A practicing physician told me years ago that he could not carry Rhubarb in his saddle-bags, as it always gave him a diarrhoea soon after inhaling it, we have people among us who are made sick by the commonest articles of the dinner table. I presume every person has observed this peculiar idiosyncrasy. Why did not some wise man in allopathic medicine explain this, and not leave it for Hahnemann to solve by the law of similars? How simple

21

that the similar power or force should create within the body such a turmoil. Were there no idiosyncrasy there would be no disease. This susceptibility being present, the noxious agent, though a million times too small for the microscope to reveal, will do its work and bring on disease, and even death, and the wonderfully wise pathologist has not solved the etiology or the method of this active destruction upon its medicine.

In drug proving we find a single dose of a drug exerting its power upon one prover, and the others escape until after having taken many doses or taken it many days. The highest potencies affect some provers, and large doses of the tincture are required to influence others.

Homœopathicity is almost, if not quite identical with idiosyncrasy. A patient of mine said I must not give him anything with Strychnia in it, because the smallest doses of that drug made him worse, but his remedy was Nux vomica, which he detected in the second potency and declared it was Strychnia. It cured him permanently. It is fortunately a fact that our crude prescribers seldom make a close selection, or they would do a world of harm. The sensitiveness of a sick nerve to a homœopathic agency is wonderful, while the subject may bear a great amount of inappropriate crude drugging without apparent distress. It is more than likely that the four-year old child that was poisoned with four drops of Laudanum would have found its remedy in potentized Opium in a single pellet. This idiosyncrasy can be produced by medicinal substances; thus, the provers of Thuja may get a diarrhœa after onions; the provers of Colch, are made sick by the smell of eggs; Plumbum provers cannot eat fish; Lycop. provers cannot eat oysters; while Ignatia provers are made sick by eating sugar and sweets; not that all suffer in this way, but many. These peculiar idiosyncrasies are also cured by the corresponding remedy. Many times I have cured with Thuja the peculiar diarrhoea brought on every time the patient eats onions. What explanation has our learned pathologist for this state? Can he by his wisdom cure it. No, his good patients go on suffering from their peculiar constitutional wrongs, and the good old doctor consoles him or her by soothing words or a dose of Opium or chalk mixture.

All there is of medicine that can permanently benefit man has come through the philosophy of Hahnemann; and this great stumbling-block of regular physicians (?), the idiosyncrasy, has become a keynote of scientific medicine, and explains itself when the philosophy of Hahnemann is understood.

The marked idiosyncrasy is not always observed for the crude materials, as is well known to all Hahnemann-ians, an instance of which is observed where crude common salt will not produce the slighest disturbance, al-though the patient craves and takes it largely in food, but the higher potencies produce the sharpest aggravation. The same may be observed with lime salts when there is a marked bone-salt inanition. Therefore, in cases where Lime is the remedy and Lime-water is ministered, not the slightest medicinal effect is produced; but the higher potencies act curatively, after which the corresponding saline is appropriated from the natural source, the food eaten.

This extreme susceptibility, called idiosyncrasy for want of a name to describe an unknown something, is clearly an underlying pathological relation of curative drug action, and is manifested by the over action of this cura-tive drug in many instances.

The richest field of drug proving is found in provers with the peculiar idiosyncrasy for certain drugs. Hence the value of potentized drugs for proving although only a few of our large numbers of provers bring out symptoms.

The continued taking of potentized drugs develops a
susceptibility to certain drugs, and such provers become
better after several attempts. I have observed that patients become more sensitive to the homœopathic remedy
after several years continuing to take purely potentized
medicines, while the taking of crude substances so phleg-
matize the system that no fine symptoms will be evolved
or felt. I have patients with whom I can develop the curative antagonism by the single dose of the highest hand-
made potency, who, if more medicine were given, would
become sick of the over-drug action. Then it is plainly
to be seen that chronic and acute idiosyncrasies are present in the subject, and instead of a fault to be regretted
in a patient, should be studied comprehensively in its
relation to its expressions, viz., symptomatology. This is
the beautiful and pleasant work of the Hahnemannian. We
are not baffled but encouraged by the existence of this
so-called idiosyncrasy, as by finding it we have gained a
strong hold, in the way of information, upon the constitution of our patient. It may be his or her peculiarity and
the guiding symptom to a curative selection.

LANDMARKS OF HOMŒOPATHY

It is a source of much astonishment that so many apparently
good homoeopathic physicians depart from the law and order methods
of practice and adopt faith-cure, Christian science, hypnotism, mind-
cure, osteopathy, etc. It is undoubtedly because of a lack of knowledge of the science of Homoeopathy. The Art has been studied,
but the Science of the Art has been neglected.

Homœopathy demands that the prescriber shall use
for curing a substance that is capable of producing similar
symptoms upon the healthy. If we must accept the cures
of the hypnotist we must accept the cures from all sources.

The hypnotist does not know the quality or form
of the force that he uses. He does not know the symptoms
it will produce upon the healthy. He does not pretend to
use it against symptoms similar to those which it will pro-

duce. If this is true why should the homœopathist think of using it?

I believe it to be in the interest of Homœopathy and of the patient to stand upon our ground—to stand by the Law of Similars.

The symptoms produced by hypnotism are mostly observed on the sick and feeble, hence are doubtful.

No human being should be deprived of his freedom nor have the latter in constraint.

It is a fundamental principle in Homœopathy that cures are changes in the condition of order from center to circumference. This is not true of any of the isms, pathies and fads now bidding for patronage in the healing world. It is familiar to all who know the doctrines of Homœopathy that removal of symptoms from place to place, on the surface or from the surface, never benefits the patient but often proves harmful to him.

Results are often brought forward exhibited as cures, yet no law has been confirmed, no symptoms have been verified, no directions have been observed in the changes. If we are to accept such results as cures, we must admit the cures of traditional medicine. If we are to accept the opinions of men we have no line between Homœopathy and Old School.

It is the old story of placing experience prior to the *law*. It is the same as observed in the numerous followers of the early educators: Hering, Lippe, etc. They followed experience and not the doctrines. All who were able to follow the doctrines were saved from the fall.

We have only to think a moment to conclude. Think of the many who listened to the teachings of Hering and how many of them now practice as he taught? All were taught experience; when they saw Hering's cures they were convinced. When they went out for themselves they had forgotten the teaching, they could not see through Hering's spectacles and their results were different.

The Art of Healing must not be taught first. The Science must be taught first, and the Art next—the law first and experience following.

To convince pupils by the clinic is incorrect teaching.

The proper method is to teach first the Science and convince the mind that the doctrines are true; then the Art may be taught by Clinics.

This method will end in permanent education. Men who have fallen, were such as had observed the Art and the results and thereby believed, but lacked the knowledge to do the work and hence fell away and denied. It is time that our faithful practitioners opened their eyes to this important fact.

There is nothing simpler! Why does a man fail? Simply because he does not know. His belief may be all right, but he does not know how. The knowing how consists of knowledges and these have been neglected. No one possessed of these knowledges ever went wandering into hypnotism, Christian science, faith-healing, osteopathy or employing crude drugs.

All who possess these knowledges are busy healers of the sick. They are the successful ones, and unless personally objectionable to the public, are prosperous. The truth saves men from the hypothetical allurements of medical practices.

To know what and how physicians of the world practice appears to be the knowledge mostly sought but to know why would more probably lead to successful methods. What does it signify what is practiced in medicine if there is no good reason for the doings?

A student leaves his preceptor to enter practice for himself. He applies the remedies as he thinks his preceptor did but without the same results. The conclusion is that he was not using the preceptor's reasons for such practice. It must be concluded that a successful man is one who has worked out the reason for his doings. Again all who would imitate his application without his knowledges will fail and fall away from strict methods of practice.

There is another ism that destroys Hahnemann's teaching, viz., the misunderstood keynote system. This system appeals to the memory only. It does not train the mind to *know the character of the remedies*. It makes the memory hold only a few fragments of the remedy. It omits the nature of the remedy or the image of the patient, which was the soul of Hahnemann's teaching. If we omit from our thoughts this soul, this image, we omit all upon which a homœopathic prescription rests, viz., *the totality*.

I believe it to be the duty of every true man to oppose the fragmentary short-cut to prescription-making. The publication of small books circulated to make prescribing easy is sure to make homœopathic prescriptions impossible to those who use them. The author has watched the passing of some of these short-cuts but he does not expect to live to see easy prescribing. The *basis of a homoeopathic prescription is the totality of the symptoms*, which must be meditated upon until the image appears to the perception.

Full records of the cases must be kept.

Great care in keeping potencies must be observed.

The study of potency as related to persons is important.

Science of Homœopathy must be dwelt upon more, and the Art no less, in order that our honest men be not confused over faith-cures, hypnotism, osteopathy and other isms too numerous to mention.

Homœopathy is making wonderful strides in curing chronic miasms but they are upon the lines laid down by Hahnemann. The author has no discovery of his own to introduce to the world. He has learned to be faithful to, and contented with what has been handed down.

The Law of Similars will direct to curative remedies for all that are curable and comfort such as are incurable, if we can keep our selfish ends in subjection.

MALARIA FEVERS—THERAPEUTICS

By "malaria fevers" I mean such as are mixed, and not distinctly intermittent, generally denominated typho-malaria; exclusive of the variety which has, as a class, a clear apyrexia; such as are especially met in this city. This paper is intended to apply to the class of mixed fevers confined to St. Louis, to the cases blending from the complicated intermittent to the complicated typhoid. It is known that some of them take on a predominance of typhoid symptoms, and some of them a predominance of symptoms found in complicated intermittents. It is this hybrid state that causes us so much vexation. I have undertaken the task of furnishing the best guide to remedies for our own circumscribed work. I have not mentioned many remedies generally thought of great importance, because I have not found the symptoms indicating them. Should I go into remedies so seldom indicated, this paper might extend beyond endurance. Hence the remedies are those most useful.

Antimonium crudum.—The gastric derangement, nausea, and vomiting, great exhaustion, white tongue, and thirstlessness, constipation, or diarrhoea, must guide to this remedy. The concomitants, few or many, can seldom do away with indications for this remedy.

Arnica.—This is a frequently used remedy. The sore bruised feeling all over the body; the patient complains of the "hard bed" and the aching, sore feeling in the whole body, the soreness compels him to move and he turns upon the other side, which in turn becomes sore and bruised and compels him again to move. There is thirst and moaning; he cries for relief "or he will die." There is great exhaustion and pain in the stomach and bowels, pressing and cutting pains in the stomach with nausea and vomiting; very often eructation, tasting like spoiled eggs, with bad taste in mouth, diarrhœa of a blackish water with bits of bloody, mucous stool; repugnance to food, milk, broth and meat; coldness in the stomach, and if there is a chill, it is preceded by great thirst.

Arsenicum alb.—Prostration, anxiety, and fear of death; extreme exhaustion, with thirst for water, little and often, for cold water, which causes nausea and vomiting; diarrhoea, stools scanty, dark, watery, offensive, with tenesmus, and the patient is covered with a cold sweat and blue spots. The tongue is dry and cracked, and the mouth and throat are parched and he wants only water enough to moisten the dry, mucous surface. In the beginning he goes from bed to bed, and is not relieved by the motion (unlike Rhus), yet his anxiety and restlessness compel him to move. The after midnight aggravation of fever and anxiety are especially guiding. The relief from warmth in general and warm drinks is also important. The burning in the stomach, bowels, mucous membranes, and skin, so common in many cases, is happily met by Arsenicum.

The involuntary stools generally point to Ars., but Arn. and Phos. have sometimes been indicated. The latter I have not often found indicated; occasionally the following symptoms have been present, indicating Phos. The dry, burning mouth and tongue, with constant thirst for large quantities of ice-cold water, which is vomited when becoming warm in the stomach, or gurgling from the stomach down through the abdomen, causing an involuntary stool from a relaxed ani; hot head, desire to be magnetized, with overpowering fears; thinks he will see some thing coming from the corner of the room; bleeding from the nose, and septic exudation about the teeth (sordes); the face is blue, bloated, and Hippocratic; the terrible dryness is not relieved from drinking, and he wants a stream of cold water poured down his throat, there are stupor and delirium, and he slides down toward the foot of the bed (like Phos. ac. and Rhus). He answers no questions or gives wrong answers to questions; great indifference.

Baptisia.—The peculiar sodden condition of the patient, with his besotted countenance, the face discolored and dusky, and the mental disquietude; his body he thinks is scattered over the bed and he is striving to arrange the scattered members; he thinks his limbs are talking to each other, his answers are irregular, as if he were intoxicated; he seems to comprehend the question and makes an effort to answer, but falls to sleep, or into a stupor in the midst of the sentence; the tongue is foul and the mouth fetid; the delirium is greatest during the night the functions are all sluggish, and the fever never runs very high; the pulse is often weak and compressible, sometimes the surface is cold.

In diphtheria the mucous membrane is dark and looks as if it might slough, and the exudation is dark; the surface is tumid and threatens to become gangrenous; finally dark, ragged, putrid and ulcers form and the patient is too stupid to complain of pain; the tongue may be coated white or yellowish, white at first, but soon becomes dirty and brown and feels as if burnt or scalded and cracks; dark blood exudes. There is seldom much thirst, although if water be presented he will drink a large quantity and relapse into stupor. The typhoid abdomen and stool can be found under this remedy yellow, mushy, and pasty, or bloody and very fetid, stools of pure blood or bloody mucus, exhausting and excoriating; involuntary stools. The tenderness and tympany of the abdomen are well marked, Baptisia is not a specific for typhoid fever, yet will cure promptly if given when the above symptoms are present. It is the remedy to begin as well as finish the case, Arn., Hyos., Lach., Mur-ac., Opium, are especially related to it.

The Arnica patient forgets the word while speaking, but he does not begin his answer and fall into a profound sleep without finishing. Baptisia has the sore, bruised feeling of Arnica, but not the restlessness attending the soreness. The sensitiveness to pain is marked in Arnica and nearly lost in Baptisia. These remedies cannot be distinguished by the stools in many instances; both have dark, profuse, watery, fetid stools, and great soreness of the soft tissues as if bruised. The mental state and the besotted condition may be the only symptoms to base a choice upon.

A patient of mine was violently attacked with a chill; he moaned with pain and declared he would die; he purged almost involuntarily, a fetid dark, watery stool; he would not answer me civilly, but said he was sore as if bruised. Between the violent abdominal pains he was stupid, as if drunk; when aroused he was snappish and his words did not express his probable intention.

The stool made me think of Baptisia, but Arn. has the same, also the mental state, hence it must be the most appropriate remedy. It broke his chill. The violence of the attack led me to anticipate a congestive chill, but the remedy quieted him very speedily.

Baptisia is often given, I find, where Hyoscyamus would be a more appropriate remedy. In the latter the patient has a profound stupor, but when aroused he will answer correctly; the tongue is dry, black and stiff, but there is not the tumid appearance of mucous membrane as if sloughing would soon appear, or as if they would become gangrenous; Baptisia has involuntary stool, but not stools and urine like Hyoscyamus, nor does she attempt to expose the genitals in her delirium.

Arsenicum produces stools that cannot always be dis
tinguished from those of Baptisia, but the thirst, so sel
dom in the latter, the extreme prostration and restlessness
will enable one to select the appropriate remedy. Arseni
cum has the tendency to gangrene, but not the tumid
semi-transparent condition with the blueness. It has th
bluish, or dusky aspect of the skin, but it is attended with
a pinched condition of the countenance. Baptisia has
bluish, bloated condition of the face that is not so œde
matous as that of Arsenicum. It is the result af venou
stasis, not transudative, like that of the latter. Baptisi
has not the heat of Arsenicum; both have involuntar
stools, but Arsenicum has involuntary stools and urine
both have burning pain in the stomach, but Arsenicun
has marked nausea, not found in Baptisia. Baptisia cause
vomiting but without much nausea or effort. Baptisia sel
dom has much thirst, but when it is present, it is for
large quantity of cold water. It is not the important fac
tor of the Arsenicum thirst.

The Arsenicum delirium is a busy one; the Baptisi
is passive. He will sometimes lie all day without movin
if not disturbed; in the former, he is moving and is al
ways in a hurry; the latter will do as advised, if he can
the former is irritable and wants his own way, and he i
full of strange imaginations of vermin and burglars, an
he has many fears.

Hyoscyamus corresponds to the most continued typ
in an advanced state; the tongue is dark or black, dry an
stiff; he is unable to put it out, the lips are dry and bleed
ing, the urine is passed in bed unconsciously, and there i
much delirium. The patient answers questions correctl
and lapses into stupor, (Arn. has the same; Baptisia goe
into stupor in the midst of his attempted answer) Hyos
cyamus has cured cases when the patient has passed int
the state where it was impossible to arouse him. The pro
found stupor, pinched countenance involuntary urine an

stool, sliding down in the bed, picking at the bed-covers, picking the finger, mark the case as a Hyoscyamus state when taken in connection with his having gone through the first symptoms mentioned.

Muriatic acid is one of the neglected remedies, yet one of the most valuable.

The clinical symptoms: Clean, dry, red tongue, sometimes bluish, is an important guiding symptom (not the slick, and shining tongue of Lach, and Kali bich.) There may be unconsciousness, moaning, and restlessness; thirst for acids and wine are also important; stool dark and mushy; urine passed involuntary; loud moaning, lower jaw dropped, tongue shrunken and dry like leather; haemorrhage from the bowels. This remedy stands between Rhus. and Bryonia. The patient is not made better from motion, like Rhus, and not worse from motion, like Bryonia. It controls the septic process and blood changes as well as Bry. or Rhus.

Gelsemium—The heaviness of the limbs and thirstlessness; the bright eyes and contracted pupils; the active delirium; the extreme sinking feeling, paralytic weakness and fear of death; loquacity, talking in sleep. On the other hand the face is pale and sallow and the pupils are dilated, yet the heaviness is always present. The mind symptoms and nervous prostration are most marked; the septic symptoms are not marked as in Ars., Bap., Arn., and Phos. The tongue trembles and is coated yellow. The many symptoms pointing to cerebral hyperaemia, point to Gels. and seldom to Bell. in these fevers. The sleeplessness is as prominent as any feature of these fevers, and Gels. is most generally its remedy. He is wide awake all night. "Not one wink of sleep last night" is the common answer (Op., Coff.) There is often pain running up and back, with contraction of dorsal muscles and stiffness, as if there were some meningeal complication; pain from spine to head and shoulders.

Lycopus Virginicus—This remedy has been of great service to me. It is the remedy when the patient is stupid, will not answer questions, is waxy, cold and has a pulse very low, yet full and large, soft and compressible; hæmorrhage brown bowels, heavily loaded, tawny, expressionless face; if he has a fever it is not high, and he chokes and swallows; his eyes are expressionless; the veins are full and the face is bloated; the eyes seem to project from their sockets.

Rhus-tox, is one of the most important remedies. The restlessness, better from motion, great thirst, dry tongue, sordes; reddish, watery, frothy stools in the morning, have been the symptoms calling for Rhus. The chilliness, like being dashed with cold water, and like cold water coursing through the veins, fever continues without sweat, and the restless aching, are often met. The patient, often moves for relief; he finds a new place, and because he is completely exhausted he thinks he can rest; but soon the horrible aching and restlessness come on and he is compelled to move and find a new place, and this is continued night and day, and there is no rest and no sleep; there is a dry cough.

Bryonia is the remedy to be contrasted with Rhus. The pains may be severe, yet they are made worse by the slightest motion; he wants cold water in large quantity, but only occcasionally; there is the dry, brown tongue, and the bowels are generally constipated; the stool is dry and hard as if burnt; the bowels are tympanitic and there is a foul, bitter taste in the mouth; bleeding from the nose is common; there is often a dry cough and the right lung is often involved; there is delirium; he is busy and wants to be taken home; the fever and delirium are worse from nine o'clock till midnight. In Rhus the fever and delirium have been worse during the whole night and often continues all day. I see, by comparing my note-book, that several of my cases cured by Rhus had aggravation of mental and febrile symptoms at 5 a. m. and p. m. Bry. seldom has the twitching of muscles so common to Rhus, and of the two, urticaria, commonly in the beginning of some fevers, can only be found under the latter. The general aggravation from cold is characteristic of Rhus, but Bry. is oftener ameliorated by cold.

The long-lasting severe pain in the head is found, in my Bryonia cases, in the temples and eyes; improved by cold; eyes were turgesced and the face was bloated and blue.

Colchicum was given in one case where the patient had an extreme disgust at the sight or smell of food, with marked benefit.

Natrum sulphuricum is a very important remedy. The patient says he has not been well for a long time; his sleep has not rested him, and his mouth, has for a long time had a bad taste and his tongue is covered with a thick, yellow, pasty fur and tastes bitter. He now vomits bile and slime and has pain in the back of his head and his bones ache; the chill comes on and he runs into a quasi-continued fever, with chills occasionally; he has no appetite, his skin is yellow, and he has a yellow diarrhoea mixed with green slime.

Ipecac.—The aching in the back, thirstlessness, constant nausea, vomiting of green slime, red and pointed tongue, bitter taste; the case abused by quinine, Ipecac, is the remedy.

In the third and fourth week, some cases become very low; the tongue is sometimes red and slick, the papillæ all absorbed, and a smooth, slick glossy surface on the tongue, and there is much vomiting of viscid, stringy mucus and bile. The patient is listless and delirious alternately.

Eupatorium perf. has improved cases when there was a bitter taste in the mouth, aching in the bones as if they would break, yellow skin, violent headache, day and night, worse during the scanty sweat, if there should be such a moisture; in many cases there is no perspiration, but great dryness of the skin and vomiting of bile.

When searching for remedies that correspond most faithfully to the fevers with absent sweating stage; Ars., Bapt., Bell., Bry., Cham., Colch., Eup.-perf., Gels., Hyos., Ign., Ipec., Kali-bi., Lach., Lyc., Merc., Nit-ac., Nux-v., Opium., Phos., Phos-ac., Rhus, and Sulph. may be consulted.

It will be found mostly that we are curing our patient from this list of remedies. When the exhaustion is the most marked feature, Arn., Ars., Bapt., China, Gels., Hyos., Lach., Lycopus, Phos., Phos-acid., and Rhus have been most useful.

When the congested symptoms have been prominent, Arn. has been the remedy. It will be observed that I have not mentioned many of our so-called sheet anchors, as I have not found them of much service. Acon., Bell., and China have not been indicated in any of my cases. I have made use of bathing and inunction of lard in some protracted cases with great benefit, but never cathartics, stimulants, or quinine.

The single remedy is my reliance. I give the selected remedy every four hours in these fevers, night and day, until improvement begins, and then I repeat cautiously.

MANAGEMENT OF DISPLACEMENTS WITHOUT MECHANICAL SUPPORT

It should be stated in other than the Hahnemannian Association that the displacements of the uterus could be cured, or palliated even, without mechanical support, the advocate would find few believers, either in his statement or in his plan of action. But it is expected that the law of cure is universal; therefore it is almost needless to assert that our materia medica is ripe enough (which we all know) to manage these conditions without mechanical support.

Any physician in active practice among women must find a large percentage of his cases belonging to this category. The various classification resorted to in text books for pathological study have very little value in the matter of cure; the wilderness of symptomatology furnishes us the only hope of taking these cases to a successful termination, which is a permanent and radical cure. The Hahnemannian finds no place in his practice for mechanical support; he relies always upon the indicated remedy. There can be no proof like actual cures. This method is successful or it is attended with failure; living witnesses must testify to its usefulness. The report of a few cases would seem quite useful as an explanation of what must be done and how the work must be carried out to avoid the use of mechanical support in displacements.

Whenever a patient presents herself to a Hahnemannian physician for relief for the complexity of symptoms belonging to displacements, not only the symptoms of the displacement but all the symptoms of the case, from childhood to the present time, must be accurately written down as it is possible to obtain them, after the method directed by the *Organon*. The fullest detail of general symptoms must be taken, as it is quite probable that the symptom image will be made up or strengthened by what would be considered as concomitant symptoms. An examination such as is generally given is of the smallest importance in the case, and reveals none of the peculiar characteristics upon which the physician must rely for his symptom image. Many of these cases appear wearing the mechanical support of the last physician in attendance. Under these circumstances, the symptoms of most value do not appear. With the support, she is relieved and permitted to walk,

22

stand and perform her family duties with out much suffering. The mechanical support must be removed at once by the physician or the patient, if she be so instructed. She must be immediately placed upon Sac. lac., and at least a week permitted to pass before a full symptom image will be found; it sometimes requires a month before the symptoms appear that were present before she was tampered with by mechanical support.

The patient will usually remark to the physician, "I cannot walk if my supporter be removed." Now this is what becomes necessary, and is usually what I want to hear her say. I immediately ask the question, "Why can you not walk, if this supporter be removed?" The answer brings the symptoms that I write down, and with the others the image becomes complete after she has rested a sufficient time to permit the symptoms, that have been removed by the pessary to return, so that finally the fullest expression of the symptom image is made out. Sometimes she may be able to relate with greatest fullness all the symptoms that were there before the pessary was used, and even the symptoms that will come back after the removal of the support, because she has become so familiar with them that she can relate them in full. Others have given little attention to the real symptoms of the case, having worn their pessary so long, and been subjected to such extensive local treatment.

It matters not how soon the symptoms are gathered, only so they are gathered in completeness as the honest expression of nature, and not the misrepresentations, such as must come in many cases where the mechanical support has completely changed the surrounding parts. If these details are not carried out in fullness, no physician need undertake to make a homœopathic prescription. The symptoms that have been removed—no matter how removed are the outward expressions of the inner nature of the disease to be cured. If they are not present, they must be permitted to return in order to appeal to the intelligent physician, as all diseases do, by signs and symptoms, and so long as they do not appeal to him by signs and symptoms they are incurable. When all support has been sufficiently removed, the rule is that these diseases do appeal to the intelligent physician by natural signs and symptoms.

It has been said that mechanical support is necessary in aged women. This is seldom true, if ever, as the indicated remedy will remove the displacements in feeble and broken-down women. For an example, let us look at the following case:

A woman sixty-five years of age consulted me for procidentia. She was compelled to wear a bandage whenever she walked; lying down gave her some relief; bloody, watery leucorrhœa which was offensive. She was greatly emaciated, waxy, bloodless, scrawny. Skin very dry and shrivelled. Toes becoming dark with gangrenous patches. Occasional attacks of bloody diarrhœa. Great weakness. Believed herself near the end. Had suffered from this extensive displacement for more than twenty years. Had on numerous occasions attempted to wear mechanical supports, always failing because of the soreness of the parts. Secale cured in a very short time, and the woman has gained flesh, strength and color, and is in excellent spirits. In such instances, if cure can be performed where mechanical support can not be tolerated, why not in cases most suitable to mechanical contrivances? This remedy would be seldom thought of by routinists for displacement, but it corresponded to the peculiarities of the patient.

Another case wherein a remedy was administered that would seldom be thought of, if aimed at prolapsus, was as follows:

A tall woman suffered many years from extreme prolapsus. Great bearing down in the pelvis. When at stool, numerous hemorrhoidal tumors protruded, which seemed full of sticking pains; much burning, and often attended with hemorrhage. Extreme pain, aching, bruised, through sacrum and hips when walking; pain extending down the thigh. The only comfortable position was lying in bed; Aesculus cured that patient promptly. When she appeared for treatment she wore a horseshoe pessary, which was removed in the usual manner by the patient, and the symptoms of the prolapsus permitted to appear.

Another important application of a remedy: A middle-aged woman, mother of several grown daughters, appeared with what seemed to be a most important, peculiar mental symptom, which was explained by her husband. She only desired to be relieved of her mental anxiety at first, saying nothing about any displacement from which she had long suffered. The anxiety was of the nature of fear in the absence of her husband, fear that he would never return to her, fear that he would die, fear that he would be run over by the cars. It had grown so much upon her that she would weep during his entire absence; even attended him at his place of business to be with him. She had no desire to mention that fact that she was then suffering from a displacement, and was then wearing a pessary, not thinking that her displacement had any relation to her mental anxiety. But in the search for symptoms, it was ascertained that she had been treated extensively for a displacement, and was then wearing a pessary. She knew so little about Homœopathy that she supposed it possible to continue with her specialist for the displacement and had simply consulted me because she had heard of some case in the management of mental cases. The removal of the pessary was insisted upon, which was carried out. She then informed me why it had been necessary, and the nature of the displacement, which had been carefully diagnosed by her attending physician. The other symptoms of the case, as they developed, were copious menstrual flow, which was black and clotted; extreme sensitiveness of the genital organs, which prevented wearing the usual napkin during her monthly indisposition. These completed the symptom image which was so like Platina, that a beginner should not make a mistake. This remedy was quite sufficient to remove not only the mental symptoms, but the necessity for the continuation of any mechanical support.

It is not necessary to continue the further report of cases. Remedies having a reputation, when indicated, for curing such conditions are Bell., Lil-t., Murx., Nux-v., Pod., Puls., Sepia. The indication for these medicines should certainly be very simple; they are in all the text books; they are open to the study of any physician who desires to follow the law. It is no secret method that the Hahnemannian physician employs in the management of these cases. "He who runs may read."

If the patient presents the vascular fullness, the bearing down pains in the pelvis, as if the uterus would escape through the vagina; the extreme sensitiveness to the jar of a wagon or a street car; the marked heat of the menstrual flow, whihch is generally copious, clotted, black, mixed with bright red blood; the instinctive demand to press the external genitalia with the hand or with a napkin to prevent the protrusion of inner parts. With symptoms, who could help thinking of Belladonna?

With the same dragging down and the same desire for external pressure over the parts, we should add the awful sense of hunger in the stomach, even after eating, which has an emptiness, a goneness, a sinking; lingering constipation with a sexual instinct that drives her frantic. Who could help but think of Murex?

Then slightly deflect the picture with an overpowering sleepiness, so that during the entire day she can scarcely keep awake—who would not think of Nux moschata?

Then consider the extreme snappishness of temper with intestinal pains, with much pain and urging to stool, which is not successful; continued urging to urinate; who would not think of Nux vomica?

With all these bearing-down pains at every stool; with prolapsus of the rectum; alternating of diarrhoea and constipation; after the diarrhoea, which completely empties out the colon with gushing stool, the awful emptiness of the abdominal cavity which amounts to a deathly goneness, as if she must sink—who could help but think of Podophyllum?

It may next be asked how rapidly are these cases cured. To a great extent this depends upon how much the symptoms have been disturbed by previous inappropriate treatment, and how much the constitution of the patient has been broken down by overwork, and the tenacity of the primitive miasm against which remedies must be directed. For instance, when Belladonna has been the medicine that has given the immediate relief, it will naturally be followed by its chronic. No case should be abandoned after the mere removal of the symptoms of displacement. Deep acting medicines become indicated as the final remedies in the case when the first remedy has only laid the foundation for cure. In my experience two remedies have usually been sufficient to cure, and the time required has been from six months to a year. In extremely broken-down constitutions the time is much extended. The percentage of failures should be very small. Indeed, no more manageable class of condition, come under the observation of a careful prescriber. No more could I say to emphasize this than that thus far I have met with no failures; all that have appeared have never desired, nor felt the necessity for mechanical support.

MUREX-SEPIA.

Editor Medical Advance:

Please ask Dr. Kent where he got the symptoms of *Murex.* p. 478 of Advance, "pains in *Murex* aggravated while lying down." If he is right I must rectify Murex in my *Therapeutics.* p. 972, where it reads, "ameliorated by eating and lying down." According to Dunham, *Hom. Review* iv., p. 405—the mental symptoms are greater when sitting than when walking; when walking they cease and reappear again when sitting down. Page 406, Hering's patient was obliged to go to bed and lie there. The excessive fatigue and debility in the lumbar region lead more to relief from lying down, and still there is that mental symptom. Perhaps Dr. Kent will kindly clear up the point as it seems he copied that symptom from Minton, p. 227. "all pains come while lying down." and which can only be taken from Hering's second case, where she felt no comfort in any position. Another question is whether *Sepia* has relief from lying down. Minton gives under *Sepia*, amelioration *on or after* rising from bed or from a seat, which may lead to aggravation during sitting and lying. In the study of symptoms we cannot be too critical." S. Lilienthal.

The "empty, all-gone" feeling in the stomach is relieved by lying down, but that is not in harmony with the general conditions of Murex. In Sep. this symptom is relieved by moving about, and aggravated by the smell of food.

The flushes of heat in Sep. are brought on by motion (Hg). In most remedies we have opposite conditions. In Sep. some complaints disappear during violent exercise, and others are better by rest. (Allen Encyclop. p. 649.) "She felt best when at rest, and while lying."

In Murex the flushes come on in bed, as well as when moving. The headache of Sep. is made better in the open air if it is pleasant, and by *violent* motion.

Murex: "A sensation as of the creeping of a snake over the entire region of the short ribs, upon the left side; Great depression of spirits; it seemed to her that she was hopelessly ill. *She was obliged to go to bed and lie there*" Dunham, Science *Therapts.*, page 384.

These are not the *uterine pains* so fully brought out and cured by Murex, but a myalgia unlike the cutting pains in the uterus that come on when in bed, and are relieved by sitting and walking, until fatigue comes on when she must lie down for relief, and the cutting pains in the uterus come on again, going through and up diagonally, compelling her to get up and walk. I have seen Murex 200, produce this state and when I find it in practice, I am sure that Murex and Murex only is the remedy.

With the pains there is not the restlessness of Rhus. It is the pain not the restlessness that compels motion by walking. In one of my provers; "The cutting pains in my lower belly waken me in the night and compel me to get up and walk. When walking the bearing down comes on which makes me want to hold myself with my hand."

This prover would lie down to get relief from the sensation that her uterus would issue from the vagina, and after lying awhile her pains would begin to come on. This, I have many times verified in practice. But I never saw it expressed until I examined *Minton*, page 227. In *Allen, Vol.* VI, Murex. General Symptoms; "*pains worse when sitting* than when walking; and those which I cease to feel while stirring about return almost immediately on sitting still." Under *Inferior Extremities.*—"Pains in hips and loins—but that of hips still continues even when not

lying down." I interpret that to read, worse when lying
down and better from walking although not entirely relieved by walking. The aches and pains of Sep.—the
headache is worse from shaking the head, but better from
violent exercise. So with many of the pains of the body,
but the distressing bearing down pains are better from
lying in bed. The dragging down of Sep. which is so much
like Murex that I am unable to distinguish between them,
is relieved lying down; comes on while standing;
is relieved by sitting and crossing the limbs and goes off
while lying down. Again Sepia has apparently the opposite—page 624, *Allen's Encyclop.* near the bottom of
page. "At 8 a. m. the dragging and pressing sensation in
the abdomen returned; *pressure as though the contents
would issue through the genital organs.* The pelvic distress was noticeable the whole night at waking intervals,
and relief only momentary by lying on either side with the
legs flexed on the thighs and the thighs on the abdomen. I
waked this morning without the distress, but it returned
on stirring." . . . I cannot but conclude that generally
Sep. is better by lying down. Except some of the rheumatic, aching pains which are first made worse (by slow motion but finally made better by violent walking. Clinically,
whenever I have been able to observe, Sep. cures the prolapsus that has the horrible bearing down as if parts
would come out if it is accompanied by the "all-gone" sensation in the stomach, a lump in the rectum with constipation, the patient wants to hold the vulva with a napkin and the dragging down is relieved by crossing the
limbs, sitting and lying. These are the symptoms as they
are found, and Sep. cures not once in awhile, but always,
if not given too low.

See *Dunham's Science Therapeutics,* page 365,
"Whereas on the other hand, the Sep. pains are worse from
9 a. m. to noon, and are relieved by repose, being aggravated by motion and repose." This refers to the prolapsus

pains in his (Dunham's) contrasting it with Lil.-t., which
grows worse during repose like Murex, page 319. "The
pains are dull; pain like paralysis is predominant, amelioration from *warmth and violent* motion. Aggravation by
repose and at night." This shows that Dunham fully comprehended the two kinds of pain or distress produced and
cured by Sep. Dunham says that the majority of pains
produced by Sep. are aggravated by repose, but plainly
state that the uterine suffering is ameliorated by repose.

OBSERVATIONS REGARDING THE SELECTION OF THE POTENCY

I must apologize to the association for not having
written a paper, but I have been too tired and too ill to
prepare one; I made the mistake of putting its preparation off too long, until when College closed I had a little
break-down, and since I have not been able to write a
paper, I will, however, make a verbal report.

The question of what is the best potency for a given
case and the question of what is the potency that is best
for habitual use is a broad subject. When I was a boy, I
played with chickens' feet when they were being prepared
for the family dinner and it was my first study in anatomy. I found that by pulling certain tendons or strings
as I called them, that the corresponding toes would double
up. Every one of the toes could be made to contract by
pulling certain strings but it was a very clumsy motion
compared with the natural orderly movements of the
toes when they were on the chicken. This leads me to
jump a long way, to say that I have been in the office
of many homœopathic physicians who have in their
armamentarium nothing but tinctures, and I think that that
is clumsier than pulling the strings to make the chicken's
toes move.

I have been in other physicians' offices where nothing

could be found but CM's. In my opinion, that too was a
somewhat arbitrary selection; it showed a partiality for
a certain potency that was too arbitrary and not sufficiently based upon judgment. There is a wonderful lati-
tude between the tinctures and the CMs and in my judgment the selection of the best potency is a matter of experience and observation and not as yet a matter of law.
There is an almost endless field here for speculation and
observation, ranging from the tinctures to the highest
potencies, with the possibility of bringing out some useful rules for the guidance of others. The various potencies
are all more or less related to individuals and it is the individual that we should study. We might well begin with
Hahnemann's statement that the 30 is low enough or
strong enough to begin with. For many years I have
found it strong enough to begin with. Individualization,
in regard to potencies as in other branches of homœopathic
work, furnishes us with an additional element of accuracy
and success, enabling us to reach certain cases that we
otherwise could not reach. Some patients are very sensitive to the highest potencies and are cured mildly and
permanently by the use of the 200th or 1000th. There
are other individuals who are torn to pieces by the use
of the highest potencies. The indiscriminate use of only
one potency is very likely to bring reproach upon our art.
They all, from the 30th to the millionth, have their
place, but no single potency is equal to the demands made
made upon it by the diseases of different individuals. Then
the nature of the disease makes a difference; patients
who have heart disease, or who are suffering from phthisis
are apt to have their sufferings increased and the end
hastened by the highest potencies; they do better under
the 30th or 200th. Some times very sensitive patients will
do well on a high potency if they have been prepared for
it by the use of a lower one. I have frequently seen pa-

tients recover from their symptoms for a while under the 1000th and then the remedy would cease to act. A repetition of it would be followed by no effect. The 10,000th would then produce a very beneficial effect and make the cure permanent. Give the necessary doses at long intervals until the repetition brings no effect; then if you are sure that it is the similimum give it in a higher potency until that ceases to act and finally the highest. In this way we can put a patient upon a series of potencies and keep up a prolonged curative action lasting for several years.

The prolonged action is sometimes necessary in very chronic deep-seated diseases. A few months would exhaust the action of a drug if only one potency was used. Any potency, no matter what it is, high or low, will cease to act after a time. That shows at once the usefulness of knowing about more than one single potency of a medicine. Hahnemann gave us an axiom in this respect; it was "when the remedy ceases to act, give a single dose of sulphur to awaken the susceptibility." This would not be so often necessary if the potency was properly varied. It was also more necessary with the earlier practitioners of homœopathy because they had a limited number of medicines to handle compared to us. I have not used sulphur as an intercurrent for a long time because the indicated remedy will not so often cease to have a curative effect if the potency is properly varied. I have been told by many homœopathic physicians that they have used the 3rd, 6th or 12th, and obtained a fair result and then it ceased to act at all. Such prescribers have no range of potency and they fail to make a complete cure. Several times I have seen patients on repeated doses of the right remedy in a low potency make no improvement, simply because their susceptibility to that potency—not to that remedy by any means—had been exhausted. I have taken such patients and without changing the remedy but simply the potency got a curative result.

When a patient returns and upon examination you find the old symptoms still there although the patient says that he or she feels much better, that is not the time for repeating the dose. It is only a question of time when a cure will result. When a patient returns and says that he is losing ground, then it is the remedy that has ceased to act, not the potency. Now you need to hunt up another remedy and not a change of potency. Remember that these things are not as yet matters of law but simply the results of some observation. I have always been interested in experiments and observations upon this question, and there is a great deal of work for all of us to do in this field.

Of course it is only the men who hew close to the line that can furnish observations of value. I am always willing and glad to listen to such a man's experience with the greatest interest. One of the important uses of a society like this is to bring out the experience and observation of trained men such as make up the bulk of its members.

POTENCIES DISCUSSION

Question: What is the explanation of antidoting high potencies by using low ones? In tuberculosis, for instance, Sulphur is occasionally too deep-acting, and a less similar remedy may work up to a stronger totality so that better results may be possible.

Kent: The correspondence doctrine of series and degrees comes near to mastering the question of using potentization. The crude drug and the potentized remedy are opposite in action.

In proving a remedy, of one of the elements that exists in the body (Sulphur, for instance, helps make up the body), the prover takes crude Sulphur until it produces a proving. He is unable then to appropriate it from the food to build up the body, being cloyed with it. The symptoms of the Sulphur patient indicate that she needs it, but she is not able to appropriate it from the food. Each resembles the other.

Give the patient with symptoms of Sulphur the potency; if you give it cruder than it is in the natural body, etc., it only makes her worse. The higher potency of Sulphur restores order and she appropriates it from the food, not being fed enough to poison her.

There are distinct degrees from the potency to the **crude form**; according to the excitability of the patient, she reacts to the 200, 500, 1000, and so on, these being only illustrative. If a given remedy will make an individual react and appropriate that which is needed and help to appropriate from the blood that which is taken, the reaction may be to 5m, and though not eaten it is in the blood.

Degrees are in sevens, as in octaves of music. If you strike too high she is not sensitive, it is not sufficient. Keep to the mild potency so long as it works. It is not well to jump too many degrees. From the crude to 10m there is a range of degrees in the ordinary person. You do not go from the first to the last, in music, it does not preserve the chord, you take the thirds and fifths. You can repeat the series, beginning with the lower potencies, and do good work.

The patient will recognize these series. Too high a potency gives an unnecessary aggravation, and then will not perform the best curative action.

The best action is the slight aggravation, as in the first few hours in the acute disorders.

The ideal is the one that gives no aggravation but amelioration. We do not seek to produce an aggravation, that is not the best, not the longest curative effect.

No law is established for aggravations and ameliorations. Only by study of records in practical experience, can we see the best action in patients.

Question.—Can you give too deep-acting potency to be curative; would a less similar give safer results?

Kent:—The cruder approaches the opposite and antidotes; the low potencies approach in degrees to the higher potencies. In the Sulph. patient who needed Sulphur ten or twenty years ago, and today it would kill her; Nux, Pulsatilla, Senega, palliate but cure. I have seen Sulph. and Phos. act so strongly that I have regretted it. In lung cases, consider whether she has lung space enough to make recovery probable. If she can bear it, give it in a low potency, but do not give it if there is not lung space enough to warrant it.

Question.—I have a mentally deficient child, whose mind becomes clearer every time I advance in the plane. She has had BARIUM SULPH. It is an unusual case. Would you go to the bottom, and recommend the series, or higher to mm?

Kent:—There you may be going into trouble and confusion. One patient may run up safely, but ninety-nine cases would not have any action in those high potencies. The object is to keep the patient under the influence of the remedy the longest time possible; to follow up with just enough difference to react, to reach the best-acting plane.

From experience, I am led to use of a series from 1m to Dm (5cm) including 10m, somewhere near 50m, and cm.

Other potencies are given, to observe what action is forthcoming. You encourage the patient to become oversensitive by using the highest potencies, instead of going low to begin again.

As a rule, two doses (sometimes three) in the same plane give the best results. It has become almost routine, as the records indicate that the third dose in the same potency gives no effect.

It is a mistake to mix degrees and the different makes. If Allen, Ehrhart, or Kents has been started, stick to the same series and the same scale.

PURE HOMŒOPATHY DEFENDED

"What can be more astonishing than that professed homœopathic physicians should deny the efficacy of their own remedies?"

"What greater evidence can the public ask of ignorance of the system they profess to make use of to cure the sick?"

It has been known to many witnesses that I have not needed anything but homœopathic remedies in incurables.

I have been giving unusual attention to incurables, in private and hospital practice, where cancer and phthisis pains have been present, where morphine had, in other hands, entirely failed, and in all cases has the homœopathic remedy, when properly selected, been all that was needed.

Argument will fail to convince some physicians, for the reason that they cannot cure and they cannot be made to believe that any one else can. They do not know how to palliate and they do not believe that any one else knows. If they cannot cure, how then can they be expected to palliate or *vice versa*. You may freely say that for years I have offered to show that the severest sufferings from phthisis and cancer, can be subdued with potentized homœopathic remedies. You may say that my students all do it, and say openly that we do not need anodynes. Let any man select cases of cancer or phthisis and bring them to the Woman's Homœopathic Hospital, and bring his own judges, and we will teach him to palliate the most painful cases with the indicated remedy. We challenge the world to this very test. I might report cases and they would not be accepted, but there is the hospital that treats these cases and here is the place to see it done. We have now many cases of phthisis and some of cancer. A patient under my care who is being cured of a fibroid of the uterus, a tumor as large as her head, and she (the patient) is returning to health.

It is astonishing that physicians will not listen to men who know how to cure. I offer the wards of our hospital to show the work, and our work will sustain the position of the physicians in Rochester that have resigned. The post-graduate pupils under my tutelage have been trained in the art of healing, and I will guarantee that each one of them can do this work. If this be true, what a pity it is for the professed Homœopaths of your city to claim anodynes as needed means of relief.

Be sure to make this point emphatic, that I make, viz: I do not select my remedy any differently in curable and incurable cases. I am firmly convinced that a doctor who cannot select medicine closely enough to cure curable cases, should be trusted in no class of cases. The homœopathic physician does not know that his cases are incurable, and he selects the remedy, and that remedy palliates the sufferings of the patient in incurable cases and cures the patient in curable ones. The physician is a Homœopath or he is not.

REPLY TO DR. HUGHES

MESSRS. EDITORS: The foot-note on Page 400 of your November (1887) issue, leads me to make the following remarks:

While treating a rheumatic subject for slight pains, I was hastily called to her bedside. It was about ten p. m. That morning I had given her Bryonia 1m. She greeted me with the following words: "Doctor, the first dose of

23

your medicine gave me pain in the side of my head and
temple; every dose increased the pain, until now I cannot
stand it.   Every time I turn on the right side the pain
goes to that side; If I turn on the other side the pain
is there."

Thus far *Puls.* and Phos-acid were the only remedies
known to me for *pain in the head going to the side lain on.*

Is this Bry. or is there a new feature coming up?
The Bry. was stopped and the pains soon stopped. In the
morning I satisfied my curiosity by calling at the house,
and found her well. She has had no more rheumatism
and never had such a headache before or since. Several
times have I given Bry. when nearer the general symptoms than Puls. or Phos-ac., for pain going to the side lain
on, and have thereby verified these symptoms as belonging
to the pathogenesis of Bryonia. It would be unwise for
me to report this symptom to Dr. Hughes as a pathogenetic symptom. Why? It would be rejected as coming from
the 1m potency, *"not reliable."* Also must I refuse to report thousands of other symptoms procured in like manner and standing the test of verification in the hands of
hundreds of able and faithful men. This "empirical" practice is not based upon the *"Cyclopedia,"* (?) and why is
a Cyclopedia thus entitled to a name that omits the best
symptoms to practice on? Time will show forth the merit
of the great *opus.* It must stand or fall for itself, and
so will the methods based upon one corner of the philosophy of Homœopathy and rejecting the means whereby
the law can be made universal. I mean plainly and simply
attentuations above the 12th. I have but the highest
regard for Dr. Hughes as a professional gentleman, but
must openly protest against the rules for compiling pathogenetic symptoms—for the *Enclopoedia of drug Pathogenesy*—only the crudest image of the drug being observed.
If this one-sided drug image can furnish a basis for cor-

rect prescribing it remains to be observed in the distant future, while the evidence of the past stands out in bold condemnation.

The supporters of the crude system have never exhibited anything but a desire to create a very poor materia medica, poor enough to fit the slovenly methods of their practice. The crudest medicines and the crudest methods have marched by the side of grumbling materia medica men.

Does it not seem rather singular that these sticklers for crude drugs, are mostly alternationists, Quinine palationists, cathartic givers, local applicationists and so on? They acknowledge their own inability to use the materia medica to cure the sick, and do not believe that any one else can use it for that purpose. Will they do better after the *Cyclopoedia* is handed them? If not, of what good is this great work? It is to be hoped that they will greatly improve, become more scientific (!) and that the dear people will be the ones benefited. As to my "published lectures," I have but a few words to say. They must be quite imperfect, as they are off-hand, class-room talks, and mostly go to the press with scarcely a glance at the reporter's notes; at best they are only journal reading, but with all of these shortcomings they go into the race for the clinical test, to be measured by the first paragraph of the Organon of Samuel Hahneman. "The sole duty of the physician is to restore health to the sick." The objects of the *Clycopoedia* seem not to sustain this paragraph, but to make complication of bobtailed drug-effects overthronged into a chaotic jumble. Individualization would be quite impossible if compelled to rely upon pathogenetic symptoms as found in this work, but it is named a *"cyclopoedia,"* and therefore presumed to contain the complete knowledge of the provings on the healthy man. But it is not a *cyclopoedia.* Then what is it? It is a garbled toxicology, made to show the strength of the majority and the remedy most certainly will be administered by the hand of time when the dusty unworn pages are found upon the unfrequented shelves in the library of lazy doctors and in the dingy corners of second-hand book-stands. As a toxicology it would be of service but as a pathogenesy it is a travesty.

SERIES IN DEGREES

This opens up the consideration of Series of Degrees, which is to become one of the most important subjects in the treatment of chronic diseases. It will lead to the development of a distinct class of prescribers in our school, if it has not already done so. Its recognition is a distinctive feature in the practice of my pupils, many of whom have expressed their wonder that this doctrine of Hahnemann is so meagerly understood and so rarely used in the treatment of chronic diseases.

It has often been forced upon my attention, when observing the work of even careful prescribers, that they stop after making a most careful selection, and fail to do more than to start the cure in the right direction. The patient improves so long as the one potency will act curatively, and then the cure stops; yet the same remedy is indicated, known from the fact that the symptoms have returned and are the same as when the remedy was first given. I have noticed many times, in patients coming to me from physicians who always give a low potency that some curative action was observed, and then the remedy was changed, and again other changes were made. When the correct remedy was given again, in a higher potency, the cure began again. It is the same when the physician has given a high potency, and it has done all it can do, and will no longer act; another remedy has been selected which failed because it was not indicated. The one that was indicated has failed only because it has done all it can do in that one potency. The physician must learn that he cannot practice Homœopathy on one potency of each drug.

Many men always give a low potency; others always use the 30th, others the 200th; others always use some one of the very high potencies. It is to show a better way that this paper has been prepared.

Whatever potency a physician uses, that one potency is not sufficient for chronic diseases. It will generally do for acute sickness. Many chronic sicknesses are cured by keeping the patient under the influence of the one indicated remedy for two or more years. But this cannot be done, with continuous curative action, unless the doctrine of series in degrees is fully understood and used.

As there are "octaves" of musical tones, so there are octaves in the simple substance, through which, severally, it is possible to correspond with the various planes of the interior organism of the animal cells. If I take Nat-c. in crude form until I am sick, and have all or many of the symptoms that belong to it and are found in its pathogenesis, I there rest. Now, if Mr. Jones comes to me with symptoms precisely resembling those in the pathogenesis of Nat-c., and I give him Nat-c. in the same crude form that made me sick, it will make him worse. It will not cure him quickly and gently, but will aggravate his disorder and suffering. However, if I have learned that all drugs have precisely an opposite action when much diluted from that they have when used in crude form, I will give him Nat-c. in a diluted form to secure the very opposite of curative action, against the toxic action of the crude drug. This is but the crudest illustration of the changes denoting the first, the lowest or outermost, degrees.

Now I affirm that there are more striking effects of degrees as we go higher in the scale of potencies. I have

observed many thousand times that all potencies act when
the remedy is indicated;

that any potency will act two or more doses at long
intervals;

that then a change must be made; and

my experience has led me to go upward in the scale,
instead of downward.

Many times my patients have been able to specify the
powder that had their medicine in it.

After a given potency has acted curatively the usual
time, and then no longer helps, and the symptoms return
calling for the same remedy, I go higher; then my patient
tells me that that was the "same" remedy I had given in
the first place. What better test can we have that a remedy is acting? I always know my remedy is curing when
my patient returns and tells me she is feeling so much
better, herself.

I have often had physicians tell me that it was due
to suggestion that my medicines acted so well; but my answer to this is, that I suggest just as strongly with the
wrong remedy as with the right one, and my patients improve only when they have received the similar or correct
remedy.

After thirty years of active practice as a homœopath,
I find that I require all deep-acting remedies in the 30th,
200th, 1000th, 10m, 50m and 100m, and often need the dm
and mm. I am able to discover a vast difference in the
action of these various potencies.

I once used potencies that ranged nearer to each
other, but repeatedly found that the degrees must be far
enough apart to represent an octave, or failure followed.
I observed that after the good action of a 200th, after
waiting until it was no longer active, although I gave the
300, 500 and 800, the 1m acted much more strongly; and
the 300 or 500 generally failed. After much experience I

settled upon the degrees that I have mentioned. About twenty years ago I found myself in possession of nearly a full set of Fincke potencies, including the 45m and cm, many between these numbers. Frequently I gave the 45m with excellent results; but after it had done all it would, I would give an 80m, or a 73m, or a 60m, with failure—but nearly always the cm would work as the 45m had done, and my patients often said that the cm worked as did the 45m, of course not knowing the remedy nor the potency. The remark expressed the patient's measure of the action.

Many times I used to give first a cm, but found that when then going lower the action was seldom so strong as when climbing upward. Again, I often observed sharp aggravation when beginning the cm, but seldom observed aggravation when beginning low in relation to the sensitiveness of my patient's nature. Of late years, I always begin lower and gradually go higher, and thereby avoid shocking even the very sensitive women and children. An extremely sensitive woman will receive in the beginning, for a chronic condition, the 30th or 200th, then followed by higher potencies, while those not so sensitive receive the 10m to begin, and then the higher, as the case progresses toward recovery.

After long observation in the range of potencies, going up and going down, I have settled upon the octaves in the series of degrees as—30th, 200th, 1m, 10m, 50m, cm, Dm, and mm. Many of my patients' records indicate that the patient has steadily improved after each potency, to the highest, with symptoms becoming fainter, and he himself growing stronger, mentally and physically.

It is not an uncommon recital in the record that the patient continues to improve on each potency for three or four months. Any physician who learns the use of these degrees in chronic diseases possesses untold advantages over the physician with his one potency.

SYCOSIS

In the further study of the miasms we now take up sycosis, which is named from one of its symptoms, a disposition to throw out figwarts.

You may wonder why you have heard so little about sycosis. The fact is that little is generally known about this miasm. Hahnemann and Boenninghausen started the subject; its further discussion must go on, and the subject will finally be developed.

You will now and then see or hear a remark that indicates that some modern physician has seen a shadow, but the real object has seldom been observed. With one exception, as far as I know, in old-school medicine, there exists a complete darkness. This exception is Dr. Noeggerath, who thinks that latent gonorrhoea may be communicated to a woman by her husband, who has been cured (?) of this disease, which, in his opinion, is never eradicated from the system. It is the source of continual malaise, frequently the cause of early death, and often produces sterility. Diseases consequent on this are acute and chronic perimetritis, metritis, oophoritis, etc. If impregnation occurs, abortion follows, or only one child is born to that woman; exceptionally, two or three. Of eighty-one women, thirty-one became pregnant and only twenty-three went to full time. Without knowing it he has corroborated the doctrine of Hahnemann and his followers. Boenninghausen laid the foundation.

You naturally ask, how have we found out anything about sycosis, and how we know that there is such a miasm?

Out of a large volume of cases that I have gathered

together, I can give but a few because of our limited time.
I will mention from memory.

Years ago a man came to me with a sickly, greenish-gray countenance—a countenance even more appalling than found in chlorosis. He had enlarged glands in the groin, he had lost much in weight, he was stiff in the joints, and the soles of his feet were very sore. Years before he had had the gonorrhœa, which had been treated with injections, and the discharge had disappeared. Since then he had been taking tonics, but with no effect.

This was my first really recognized case of gonorrhoeal rheumatism. I commenced to read upon the subject, but my reading was very unsatisfactory. I could find but little information. It is not necessary to say that I did not succeed in that case. That man stood before me as he stands today. I saw him again on crutches. His face, which stamped the picture of the miasm indelibly on my memory, still haunts me. Sickly in extreme, I see him now as he walked in and out of my office with my vague advice and prescriptions. His sallow skin and stooping frame, his hollow, wandering eyes, pleading for help, and of me, who professed to be a physician. To be sure, he had sinned, and hence the contagion, but what of his sin in comparison to that of the ignorant man who suppressed his discharge, and of the profession that fosters such ignorance, bigotry, and unbelief, in all of which we see elements that retard investigation and honest thinking?

The next investigation that stands up before me is that of a young baker. He had been obliged to give up his business and go to the hospital. When he was sick eighteen months, unable to work, his former employer came and asked me to do something for the poor, forsaken young man. I found him walking on his knees. The soles of his feet were so sore that he could not stand on them.

His hip-joints were stiff, he was full of rheumatic symp
toms, and broken down completely. These symptoms had
all come on after the suppression of a gonorrhoea. I cured
that young man. Some time after he was put under
homœopathic treatment his gonorrhoea came back; and
when the gonorrhoea was cured he had no further trouble.

A man with a most troublesome nasal catarrh, that had
existed with increasing violence for eleven years, received
Calcarea very high, and was converted to Homœopathy
by the rapid cure of the catarrhal discharge, but it was
not more than a month later that he reported that he
had a discharge from the urethra, declaring that he had
not been exposed to infection. He admitted that twelve
years ago he had suffered from a gonorrhoea, but supposed
that it was cured, as very strong injections has been used.

Dr. Wesselhoeft reports an exceedingly interesting
case of a man who had been troubled with vertigo for
six years. Dr. Wesselhoeft prescribed for him, and the
vertigo disappeared, but behold! a gonorrhoea which had
been suppressed for many years reappeared on the patient.

These and similar cases which I could relate give us
some understanding of the beginning of that gigantic
miasm which we call sycosis.

Let us start out by saying that sycosis is a constitutional and contagious disease, which sometimes, though
not always, is manifested in the beginning by gonorrhoea.

There are two especial kinds of urethritic discharges.
One is sycosis and the other is not. They seem alike, but
you may abuse the one and not produce sycosis, while just
so sure as you stop the other without curing, you have the
constitutional miasm. It seems that the only relief that
nature has is from the discharge, and just as soon as the
discharge is stopped trouble begins.

Rheumatism is only the first shadow of the miasm,
which is often observed as soon as the discharge is sup-

pressed, but sometimes not for months after. One of my cases, where suppressed discharge was instantly followed by pains in the back and sciatics, was a great sufferer. This man writhed with double sciatics and neuralgic pains, rending in character, all over him. Constant motion relieved his pains; quiet was impossible. For many days he suffered before I found his remedy. This kind of rheumatic neuralgia is seldom attended with much swelling, the pain seems to be drawing and rending, and seems to belong largely to the nerve sheaths and tendons. Figwarts and bleeding excrescences are particularly characteristic of its later expressions. I have cured gonorrhœal rheumatism and have seen no figwarts, but in other conditions further advanced I have seen figwarts.

A man came to me with asthma. I gave him remedies which seemed to help him for a time, but I could not cure him. For a whole year I worked on that case. I knew that he had had gonorrhœa, but saw no relation between the gonorrhœa and the asthma. I did not understand the nature of the disease at that time. Finally I prescribed Natrum sulph. because it seemed suited to his symptoms. It wiped out the asthma completely, but in a short time figwarts began to appear about the genitals. Experience has shown that whenever these figwarts are burned off, deep-seated constitutional diseases invariably follow. I did not burn them. I gave him Thuja, which is complementary to Natrum sulph., and suited to the case. The figwarts disappeared and his old gonorrhœa discharge came back, which was, as these cases usually are, most difficult to cure.

The returning discharge is often unmanageable, and may resist treatment for years, because the miasm has become deep seated, and the discharge should exist until this miasm has been cured. Treating the discharge as a gleet is a most dangerous and unhomœopathic management.

Can you see anything in these facts in the light of what I have taught you, and do you see the relation of all these facts to each other.

Had I stopped that discharge by suppression, his old asthma would have come back. I would not have known why, and no one would have blamed me. Many such things have I seen. I practiced that way before I knew better, and I know whereof I speak. I have related to you some points that show you how I first saw a glimmering of the truth, but the great field is yet to be explored by you.

The manifestations of sycosis are often much like those of syphilis and psora, when each is in its latency or suppressed. You have aches and pains in the beginning of all three of the miasms, that resemble each other very much. Later, after the results of the disease have become evident through tissue changes, each miasm stands out in bold relief.

In syphilis, when its surface eruptions are driven back, it finally attacks the nerve centres, bone cells and periosteum. Psora is more general in its nature. It attacks the skin and all parts of the body.

Today I believe that sycosis is as deep a miasm as syphilis, with just as destructive a blood disorganization; therefore the anæmic aspect, waxy, greasy skin, red, smooth warts on mucous margins of anus and genitals, loose teeth, extreme nervous tension, phthisical condition, catarrhs wherever there are mucous membranes, epithelioma, and emaciation.

Some one says that if sycosis is so deep a miasm, would it not be a good thing to take the gonorrhœal virus and prove its effect upon the human system, in order to bring out the disease where we can study it? This has been done.

Medorrhinum is such a substance, and students who

have access to my office know that I have quite a volume of provings of Medorrhinum through the favor of Dr. Swan. It would seem that provers had nearly sacrificed their lives to bring out the action of this miasm.

This proving of Medorrhinum brings out the rheumatic states, the soreness in the bottoms of the feet, headaches in day-time, periodical headaches, restlessness, pains from sunrise to sunset, which are so characteristic of sycosis (syphilis has pains at night, from sunset to sunrise), and many deeper symptoms which are found in sycotic diseases. This proving confirms everything that I have told you about sycosis—all that we learn from the study of the disease itself.

Many severe cases of asthma, the result of suppressed gonorrhœa, are speedily cured by Medorrhinum and the symptoms of sycosis are brought out. Medorrhinum develops the suppressed miasm, so that its symptoms are harmonious and consistent. It does not cure the miasm. It does not cure gonorrhœa. It acts as a developing remedy, as does Psorinum and Syphilinum in the other miasms.

Deep rheumatic attacks are often due to gonorrhœa, though this is not always recognized.

Children may be born sycotic, where one or both parents are afflicted with gonorrhœa. Such children are likely to have cholera infantum, marasmus—pining children. I have watched these cases and have often found Medorrhinum the only medicine which will save the lives of these little ones.

As Psorinum has many times brought about a vital reaction after a typhoid fever when all energies were suspended, and when psora was at the bottom of the trouble, so will Syphilinum cause the same vital reaction if it be syphilis that is the cause of the suspended energy when convalescence is prevented; and so also will Medorrhinum cause a reaction when the sycotic miasm is the cause of slow convalescence. A careful study of the provings and ample clinical experience lead me to state these things with assurance.

Psorinum does not cure psora, and Syphilinum does not cure syphilis, nor does Medorrhinum cure sycosis.

I have traced epithelioma, red phthisis, cauliflower excrescences, sterility, and erosions to a sycotic origin. Pernicious anæmia often has gonorrhœa as its base.

This led me to the discovery of Picric acid as a sycotic medicine through its relations to pernicious anæmia. It even cures figwarts and gonorrhœa—of course, when indicated.

Iritis is supposed to belong almost exclusively to syphilis; syphilis when not suppressed may produce iritis. Gonorrhœa produces it only when suppressed.

One, two, or all three miasms may exist in the system at the same time. They may complicate each other. Let a patient start out with psora, then let syphilis ravage his system, finally the gonorrhœal miasm is added, while all the time he is being filled and overpowered with drugs. Just think what a complication we have to deal with.

Hahnemann recognizes the alteration of one miasm with another. He gives Merc. for syphilis, perhaps then psora comes uppermost and he finds Sulph. indicated, then sycosis comes and alternates with one or the other, and so on.

Make note of what you see in the backward course of disease (i. e., when it is getting well), and you will see more and more the relation of these things. Do not make haste to prescribe for old symptoms that come back. Be sure that the symptom is going to stay, for you will have flitting images. Old symptoms come and go and need no further repetition of the medicine.

If you give a new remedy when not needed, you spoil your case. Never prescribe for a moving image, wait till it rests. 'Tis your duty to understand your business before you attempt to do anything.

Miasms are the foundation of all chronic diseases. He who sees in Bright's disease nothing but Bright's disease, not the deep miasm back of it, sees not the whole disease but only the finishing of a long course of symptoms which have been developing for many years.

If you go at it like a common tinker you may cure acute sickness, but on your life, do not tamper with these chronic diseases. With your best endeavor you will make mistakes, but make them as few as you can. Do you see the necessity of going to the foundation of these things?

SYPHILIS AS A MIASM

Notes from an Extemporaneous Lecture

It is difficult to know where to begin and where to end the discussion of syphilis—how much to say, or what to leave unsaid. Volumes have been written about syphilis. Some are worth reading, others are not.

It doesn't help you to cure your patient or to understand the nature of the disease to go back and try to discover the first case of syphilis. You will gain nothing by supposing that it originated among the North American Indians, that it was a product of the French Revolution, or that it has been transmitted through many generations to ours from the remotest ages. It is sufficient to know that the disease exists. It is not in my department to give you its history or its diagnostic relations, but only to consider it as a miasm.

One important drawback to the study of syphilis is the fact that the disease as it comes to us through the books is always under allopathic treatment. Fox has given us some good points. Bumstead was no doubt a great syphilographer.

These writers have described the beginning, the

course, and what they consider as the end of syphilis; but
a large number of their cases were under allopathic treat
ment, and the result is that they have reported what they
call relapses which are studied as relapses, *i. e.*, returns of
the old disease.

The study of cases *without treatment* is what we need
But of such we have very few. Allopathy modifies the
disease in that it suppresses its manifestations. Study
Bumstead, and you will find pictured there its worst forms
and complications, but you will not find the correct form
The view is biased. There is no work in allopathy or
Homœopathy to-day that gives a correct view!

In allopathy, as soon as the chancre appears, it is
cauterized, then the glands are affected, and buboes fol
low; maculæ appear; ulcers appear in the throat, and these
are immediately cauterized, after which the hair falls out

What would be the result if the chancre were let
alone? Then we could see the true nature of the disease
We could see whether it tends to run a certain course and
recover, and to what extent this lifelong miasm is due to
suppression; whether it is altogether the result of sup
pression. Syphilis must run a certain course.

It often begins with chills and bone pains. After the
fifteenth day the chancre appears. This is the first effort
of nature to cure. This eruption is suppressed by allo
pathic treatment just as the psoric eruption is suppressed,
and miasm is the result. Thus syphilis, being a constitu
tional disease, is made, I may say, ten times more con
stitutional by suppression. The disease is thrown back
on the nervous system, the nerve force is perverted, and
a vicarious expenditure takes place. Often with the
chancre comes the buboes. These are treated with Iodine
and various ointments. Does this tend to throw out the
disease? No! It aggravates it tenfold.

Next come eruptions on the skin. Local applications
are immediately resorted to to suppress them.

Are they treated scientifically? I say No! *Hahnemann* says No!

Then come ulcers in the throat. Are they treated with an idea of their cause? Are they allowed to evolve themselves? No! They are immediately driven back. At every place the disease is refused its own expressions!

When the hair falls out, lotions are applied to the head to stimulate the hair follicles to hold their sprouts.

This is the course of treatment we find laid out in allopathic literature.

Under homœopathic treatment the course is very different. A patient comes to you with a chancre. Instead of cauterizing it let it alone. But the patient says, "It must be cauterized—it is the old way." Do not do it.

What if it increases and remains for two or three months? All right, that is what you expect. You are afraid the young man will go off and leave you? That has not been my experience.

The sore is painless. Tell him that if you cauterize it you will only make his condition worse. If you do not cauterize it, in the course of a few months you can restore him to health; he will be cured and will transmit no taint to his children. If some leave you others will not, and you will have enough remain to be cured.

Study the totality of symptoms and select your remedy.

Under the action of this proper remedy the sore becomes soft and commences to discharge enormously, instead of getting harder.

The standard authorities state that the bubo has little tendency to suppurate; but under homœopathic treatment it often suppurates, as this is the easiest way for nature to rid the system of this disease.

Thus Homœopathy changes the entire aspect of the disease from its beginning. Now the eruptions come to

24

the skin, and you will probably have to change your remedy. Then, by the right prescription, you cure the disease from within. The eruption is less though the stage goes on. You overcome the cause. You use no local applications, no washes or unguents. The sore which first appears is the last to heal. By this (which is in accordance with the law that, "diseases get well in reverse order of their coming") you know that the patient is getting well.

Now watch; the sore throat will appear. If you don't see the remedy the first day, have him call again in a few days. Watch his condition, the course the ulcer is taking, its color and direction. For a remedy to conform to all these things you must go to the *Materia Medica*. Again in the throat, the first patch that comes is the last to heal. The day you give the right remedy that day the ulcer ceases to enlarge, molecular death stops. When the last ulcer is gone it will return no more as long as he lives.

The next stage is the falling of the hair. Notice where it commences, and get the entire list of remedies that have falling of the hair, also a list of syphilitic remedies, and compare; but most of all the entire range of proved remedies. Use no Fowler's solution, no cantharis, no colognes.

Now, what do we see? It is a strange fact that the sooner one stage is cured, the sooner the next one comes on. In six months you may carry the patient through all the stages and cure him. The shadow of all the stages will present the guiding images for you to select your remedies from. Destroy no symptoms.

Hahnemann made the mistake, and many homœopaths have done likewise, of not distinguishing between chancroid and chancre, which fact accounts for some of his reports of cases cured very speedily with Merc. 30. The distinction between chancroid and chancre had not

een made in Hahnemann's day. The cures with a dose
f Mercury are not cures of the syphilitic miasm.

If you take syphilis, as abused by allopathic treatment, and attempt to adjust homœopathic therapeutics
o it, you will fail. Hence the bugbear that syphilis has
een to homœopaths. This should not be so.

There is a peculiar fact about the contagion of syph-
lis (it is true of sycosis also) that you will not find in
ccepted literature. 'Tis that the person infected takes
he disease in the stage which it is in at the time of in-
ection. He does not go back and have the disease from
he beginning, but finishes it from the stage which was
resent in the person who spread the infection.

A young girl was betrothed to a young man who
was suffering from a relapse. He had ulcers in his mouth,
econdary form of syphilis. One day she happened to
at out of the same spoon which this young man had
eon using. The result was that she took the disease,
nd came out with ulcers in mouth and throat. Her lover,
ery much alarmed, came and told me the circumstances.
watched that case, and saw her pass through the sympoms of secondary syphilis with ulcers in the throat, and
nally lose her hair. But she never had a chancre or a
ubo or eruption on the skin. I have seen several similar
ases which proved to me this principle of contagion.

The general course of syphilis is:

I. Primary Stage. { 1st. Chancre.
                     2nd. Buboes.

I. Secondary Stage. { 3rd. Skin affections, maculae, and
                        other eruptions.
                       4th. Ulcers in the throat.
                       5th. Loss of hair.

I. Tertiary.—Nerve and bone affections.

The disease may be supressed in the first stage and
emain latent for some time.

A young man came to me who had been sickly for eighteen months. His symptoms called for Kali-iod. I put him on Kali-iod., and in a short time he broke out with a syphilitic eruption.

I knew there was nothing in *Kali-iod.* which would produce such an eruption as that, and on closer investigation of the case, I found that he had had a chancre which had been suppressed by large doses of Merc., and the resulting syphilitic miasm was what had been making him sick. The Iodide of Potassium had antidoted the Mercury and the miasm had come out.

Any miasm may be suppressed and held latent and not show itself as such; but *when the miasm does not appear in symptoms* the person is sickly. In such cases it is often difficult to get the symptoms to prescribe on. The lazy doctor will not be able to find any; but by *close investigation* you can generally find some symptoms. If he really has no symptoms his case is generally incurable, since curable disease express themselves by signs and symptoms.

If he is really incurable, the symptoms of the disease have been driven back so deep that he has only an undefined sense of feeling badly. In the last stages, when the patient has "been the rounds" of allopathic suppression, he returns from the Hot Springs and comes to you, perhaps too late. He suffers from the category of nerve syphilis. He has bi-parietal pains, exostosis, thickening of the periosteum. We do not know that we would have such forms if it were not for suppression.

Under homœopathic treatment, although the patient taken in the primary stage does not get well without a shadowing at least of the secondary stage, yet of the tertiary forms the shadow is so slight that we cannot really say that they exist at all.

When syphilis attacks the nerve centres, we have

softening of the brain, brain tumors, and death. How much of the nerve disease is due to suppression we cannot now determine. These tertiary forms never get well unless you can bring them back into the secondary stages.

A patient who had been under allopathic care for many years, who had taken Iodine, Bromide, Corrosive sublimate, Iodide of Potassium, etc., in large quantities, came to me in the last stages of syphilis with agonizing head pains. I prescribed for him, he became weak minded, but the pains all left him. In the further treatment of the case what condition did I find next? What could we expect to find according to the law of direction? Loss of hair and then ulcers in the throat—sure enough, such was the case. The loss of hair and the ulcers worried him so much, that he went away and left me.

The case is none the less valuable, however, since it serves to illustrate the manner in which the disease may get well even when in the last stages.

You can see now the nature of the disease.

Under homœopathic treatment, though I have had many cases, I have *never seen a relapse*; while allopaths report relapses in a large percent of their cases.

You ask me to outline the treatment, which would necessitate my going into the numerous forms and groups of skin symptoms and nerve manifestations of this miasm. Volumes might be written on this subject and in the end you could be directed to study well the *Materia Medica,* and treasure up no names to arrange medicine for. Take the case as though you had never heard of such a set of symptoms in a sick man, but were perfectly acquainted with such symptoms in provings, remembering that the pathognomonic symptoms are not the ones you shall need the likeness of, but uncommon ones. Destroy no symptoms that nature has sent out to guide you to your remedies. Some patients will leave you, but if you are acquainted with the art of healing, you will have all you can attend to among the faithful and intelligent members of your cities and villages.

TAKING OF THE CASE IN DISCUSSION OF A PAPER.

This is one of the greatest tasks with which a phycian has to deal. One of the most common causes of failure and of the making of mongrels, is just like this taking of the case. We should examine a case in exactly the same way as we would examine a prover for the image expressed in the provings. When we have the full symptom picture of the case, we shall be able to see the patient in all his peculiarities, and shall also see how far he has deviated from his normal self.

The greatest mistake a young man can make in the beginning of his practice is carelessness, and even Dr. Dever's Colocynth case should have been recorded, and for this reason, not because he would not have known a Colocynthis case of colic again when he saw it, but if we have a record of all conditions and sicknesses that a patient has been subjected to in the course of his life, and in years after he comes to us again, our memory of the peculiarities of his constitution, forms a picture in our mind, of the action of disease in this case. These are true sick images, which we never get in any other way, and which the study of books can never teach.

I have thousands of records with opinions and prognostications, which, even if they fail, will teach me something. It is important, that only the general questions may be so put that they can be answered by yes or no, as, have you distress in the head, stomach, etc., but even that may be avoided by suggesting that they have neglected this or that organ, or that function. If a man says he has headache, there is nothing to prescribe upon, you do not care for that, but when he says with this or that modality, then you have a symptom to record. Questions must be so framed as to bring out explanations. Many patients will return to us with the question. "Doctor what did you expect after that medicine?" It is an easy matter to ask what they have observed, and when you have learned, of course you expected it. Many patients ask for a diagnosis, for your opinion as to what is the matter with them. The answer, of course, will be, "you have told me all your deviations from health, all the disturbances of which you are aware?" "Yes." "Well, this record is what is the matter with you."

The structural changes of course will be noted, and told them if advisable, but they are always a result of sickness, and not the true image of disease. In phthisis, granular disease of the kidneys, etc., you see such results but not the image of the sickness; therefore not the symptoms for prescription. Hahnemann never discouraged the study of pathology, anatomy, or the sciences, but constantly holds up to us the images of the sickness that leads to these results, and advises us not to make the mistake of prescribing upon other than symptoms.

No man can ever become great who has not the ability to see this nature of disease in the sickness around him. I consider myself the center around which my patients move in their orbits, the inner circle of which are very near to me indeed. These are the most intelligent, the most appreciative, the most teachable of our great truths, and the dearest of all with whom I have to deal. I am their trusted friend; they love me, and I love them. We enjoy each other. Outside of this is another circle, still a little farther removed, a little less intelligent, for whom I can do a little less. Back still farther is another, and another and still another; until the outer circle, that of ignorance, is reached, for whom I can do less than for all the rest; but even now, more than the old school, better than any other method. It is never among these that we make our brilliant cures, that we do the work of the master. It is in the inner circle nearest to our own intelligence in which these great things are done. I tell you gentlemen with the practice of Homœopathy such as we are aiming at, we have the power to change the whole moral nature of the man, to relieve and give control of passions, to prevent the development of evil in the young, and to restore the diseased nature of comparative health.

One more point and I have done. You can readily see how when one is continually running off after new remedies, remedies that have but few symptoms proven and recorded, and neglect the many remedies of which we have more exact knowledge through our own records and provings, that one would become more and more dissatisfied with his work every day, and necessarily resort to doubtful methods and finally mongrelism; so beg your young men to take their cases carefully, and record their progress conscientiously and in time they will become what all are striving to be, master prescribers.

Dr. D.: I would not go on record as opposing Hahnemann, but only instance cases in which such particularity did not seem necessary.

Dr. Kent: If in one prescription you had given Colocynth and in another for the same patient Cuprum, and still another something else, we begin to see the relation of remedies. How did the older homœopaths preserve the facts of one remedy following another well, or of their being inimical to one another, except by the most careful records and prescriptions.

TEMPERAMENTS

We see many absurd statements in our homoeopathic literature. Many of these statements are the ex-cathedra statements of our ablest men. These are quoted and handed down as accepted and demonstrated wisdom. Our clinical reports are full of these traditional whims. The clinician reports a case that is clear and strong in the reasons for the use of the remedy that cured, but he ends his reasoning by saying that, in addition to the symptoms, he favored the remedy because her hair was auburn, or blond, or dark, according to the remedy selected, which is fully approved by the guiding symptoms.

A man who is given to asking questions will naturally desire to know if Pulsatilla ever produced light-colored hair, or has ever changed dark hair to blond. If the former, then it is pathogenetically related to the case; if the latter, it is clinically related to the case. If neither, then why give such reasons for selecting the remedy.

If Pulsatilla has cured fifty consecutive cases in blondes, when the symptoms were such as were produced in healthy people, is that an iota of proof that it will not cure just as speedily in brunettes? And if it is not a reason that it will not cure in brunettes when the symptoms call for it, does it appear a fallacy to give Pulsatilla to a woman because she is a blonde?

If dark hair is not a symptom of disease, how can any physician use it as even one symptom in any given prescription? If it is a natural condition, why think of it as one of the elements to be considered in making a prescription If the hair must be red to be a distinguishing symptom in any given case, how red must it be to make the remedy clearly indicated; or if only slightly red what other remedies would shade in because of this slight difference in the color of the hair?

The true basis of a homoeopathic remedy is the collection of signs and symptoms, and these must be morbid, has been the teaching of Hahnemann and his ablest followers. And such teaching is the only teaching that conforms to law.

What benefit is it to pursue the study of biology to discover the difference in the natural constitutions of human beings, when it must be the sick (*morbid*) condition in the constitutions of human beings that must be fully and extensively evolved to guide the physician in healing sick people?

The color of the hair and eyes, the form or shape, the
tall or short, are not generally considered morbid, nor do
they take any part whatever in the sick image of any
given totality of symptoms. The bilious temperament
is too vague and too variable, even when morbid, to guide
to a remedy; for he may be better or worse from motion,
cold air, warm air, changes of weather, exertion, and
so on to the end of our modalities. No two observers
mean the same thing when they speak of a bilious condition or temperament.

If the mental predominates, it would mean half the
remedies in our Materia Medica, even if he is morbid in
the mental make-up. The motive temperament is found
in a large number of our most active and steady workers
in both mental and physical employment. The sanguine
temperament is found in many who are sound in body
and mind, and the words do not recall a single proving.
Temperaments are not caused by provings, and are not
changed in any manner by our remedies, however well indicated by symptoms found in persons of marked tempera-
mental make-up. To twist these temperaments into our
pathogenesis, symptomatology, or pathology is but a mis-
understanding of our homœopathic principles.

One who knows how to find a homœopathic remedy for
sick people does not pause long to take the measure of the
normal constitution of his patient, who has changed from
the normal to the abnormal constitution. This morbid
condition of body or mind, or both, is composed of signs
and symptoms not belonging to the health of the patient,
no matter how recent or long-standing they may be. The
study of general and particular symptoms so clearly de-
fines and outlines this morbid constitution that the study,
from first to last, becomes a positive and scientific problem. It is not something fanciful, but can be demonstrated
at the bedside as a positive and certain procedure from

beginning to ending, and it is entirely based upon facts, omitting all opinions and theories.

THE ACTION OF DRUGS AS OPPOSED BY THE VITAL FORCE

Perhaps all homœopaths will remember the very valuable paper published by Dr. Dunham, in his treatise on the science of Homœopathy, entitled, "The Primary and Secondary Symptoms of Drugs as Guides in Determining the Dose." Perhaps all will remember a similar treatise by Dr. Hale upon his imaginary law for selecting the potency. Also, that since these papers have been before the public, the homœopathic mind has been frequently directed toward the paragraphs in which this doctrine is treated of in Hahnemann's Organon, namely, §§ 63 and 64, coupled with § 115, which is as important in its bearing on the subject as the two sections named.

The sixty-fifth section should be studied, because it furnishes examples of action and reaction illustrating the doctrine taught in these sections.

As. Dr. Dunham's main idea was to refute the doctrine of Dr. Hale, that the primary and secondary symptoms furnish a sufficient guide for the dose, and as that is not particularly the aim of this paper, we may advance to a different view of these sections and the doctrine therein taught, believing that Dr. Dunham has left a sufficient argument against the folly aimed at.

§ 62. On the one hand, the pernicious results of the palliative or antipathic treatment; and on the other hand, on the contrary, the happy effects which the homœopathic method produces, can be explained by the following considerations, which have been deduced from numerous facts, which nobody had discovered before myself, although they had been, so to speak, within grasp, so that they might have been perfectly evident and of infinite benefit to medicine.

§ 63. Every medicine and every power which acts upon life deranges more or less the vital force, and produces in the individual a certain change, which may last for a longer or shorter time. This change is called the *primitive effect*. Although produced by the medicinal force and the vital force at the same time, it belongs chiefly to the power whose action is exerted upon us. But our vital force always tends to unfold its energies against this influence; the effects which are the result of this action, and which are inherent in our vital power for preservation, and which depend upon its automatic activity, bear the name of *secondary effect*, or *reaction*.

§ 64. As long as the primitive effect of the artificial morbific (medicinal) power lasts upon the healthy body, the vital force appears to play a purely passive part, as if it were obliged to submit to the influence of the power acting on it from without, and to allow itself to be modified by it. But after a while it seems in some way to become aroused. Then, if there can exist a state directly contrary to the primitive effect or impression which it had received, it manifests a tendency to produce it (secondary action, reaction) which is proportioned both to its own individual energy and to the degree of the influence exercised by the artificial morbid, or medicinal power; but, if there can not exist in nature a condition opposite to this primitive effect, then it seeks to establish its preponderance by effacing the change which had been worked upon it by the force from without (that of the medicine), and by substituting for it its own individual normal state (*secondary action*, curative action.)

§ 115. Among the primitive effects of certain medicines are found many symptoms which, in part, or under certain accessory conditions, at least, are the reverse of some other symptoms that appeared either earlier or later. Properly speaking, however, this circumstance is not sufficient to make us consider them as consecutive effects, or as the actual result of the reaction of the vital force. They constitute an alternating action of the different paroxyms of the primitive action only; and are called *alternating effects*.

After due consideration of these sections, I have come

to the conclusion that there is but one action of drugs, which is always to make sick. That which has been considered the secondary action is the action of the vital force, which always tends to cure. If we limit, as Dunham did, the basis of a prescription to the primitive effects, so stated, it becomes necessary to qualify our knowledge by an understanding of what is known or considered the primitive effects.

This involves a study of symptoms that occur after the prescription has been made and the remedy has acted. It also involves a study of symptoms that appear a long time after a proving has been made upon the healthy subject. These reactive symptoms often indicate what is going on, and indicate whether the patient is curable or not; often indicate when the action of the remedy is inimical to the cure. From the old teaching the so-called secondary symptoms never call for a prescription. This is true in fact, but to understand the full application of this statement, an extensive study of action and reaction must be had. The symption picture to be prescribed for must be made out of the sick feelings that endanger life or health, and reaction the evidence of repair of the vital force; hence the importance of knowing the full power of these curative energies.

In some instances, large doses of potent drugs produce violent effects, making deeper and longer lasting actions, such as are observed more particularly with potentized drugs. What are often mistaken for secondary symptoms are simply such symptoms as would come from highly potentized drugs as primitive effects or direct effects of the drugs in use. The more dynamical effects last longer and appear to be secondary to the more toxicoligical effects, but it is only an appearance. For example, one who has long been using Arsenic takes on the continuous appearance of the poison, in which we see the true drug action. So long as the drug is continued. the stimulating action of the crude Arsenic appears to keep up the nervous force of the subject; but as soon as the drug is withheld, the awful crisis comes. This is where reaction, if there be any reaction, must show itself, but often the vital force has been completely subdued by the toxic habituated influence of the Arsenic. Nothing but more Arsenic will save life.

In like manner we see the toxic habituating influence of Opium and other drugs. After the continued use of Opium, such a depression of the vital force comes that the discontinuance of the drug is followed by a fatal diarrhea, which necessitates more Opium being given. In such instances it would seem that the drug dynamis actually usurps the place of the vital force.

Under the action of small doses, we see the order of symptoms reversed. Some provers of Opium become constipated; others have loose stools, so that what would appear to be primary in one, would seem to be secondary in another case. One family under my observation always has a diarrhea—every member—after taking a small dose of opium; while it is common for most subjects in proving opium to have a constipation as what appears to be the primitive action of the drug.

The vital force attempts to oppose the primitive disturbance produced by outward forces, hence the reactive manifestations seem to be opposite in many instances. Hence, if opium begins the attack by a diarrhea, it will end by constipation. This must furnish us, in some cases at least, a wonderful example upon which to reason.

Now, if we attempt to measure the reactive energies in the state of health by our observation, we will see that the reactive energy is always greater than the primitive shock, as will be observed by reading the 65th section.

§ 65. Examples of (a) (primitive effect) are before the eyes of everyone. A hand that has been bathed in hot water has, at first, a much greater share of heat than the other that has not undergone the immersion (primitive effect); but shortly after it is withdrawn from the water, and well dried, it becomes cold again, and in the end much colder than that on the opposite side (secondary effect). The great degree of heat that accrues from violent exercise (primitive effect) is followed by shivering and cold (secondary effect). A man who has overheated himself by drinking copiously of wine (primitive effect) finds, on the next day, even the slightest current of air too cold for him (secondary effect). An arm that has been immersed for any length of time in freezing water is at first much paler and colder than the other (primitive effect); but let it be withdrawn from the water and carefully dried, it will not only become warmer than the other, but even burning hot, red, inflamed (secondary effect). Strong coffee in the first instance stimulates the faculties (primitive effect), but it leaves behind a sensation of heaviness and drowsiness (secondary effect), which continues for a long time if we do not again have recourse to the same liquid (palliative). After exciting somnolence, or rather a deep stupor, by the aid of Opium (primitive effect) it is much more difficult to fall asleep on the succeeding night (secondary effect). Constipation excited by Opium (primitive effect) is followed by diarrhea (secondary effect); and evacuations produced by purgatives (primitive effect) are succeeded by costiveness which lasts several days (secondary effect). It is thus that the vital power, in its reaction, opposes to the primitive effects of strong doses of medicine which operate powerfully on the healthy state of the body, a condition that is directly opposite, whenever it is able to do so."

We must observe from these examples furnished us by the master—and it is always well to cling to his examples as closely as possible—that the reactive energy is always greater than the primitive shock. Were it not for this increase of the expressions of nature in the reaction, a cure might be quite impossible, and it may well be said that woe is man when the vital force does not react against the extraneous noxious influences.

Not so much of value will be observed when strong doses of crude drugs have been made use of. In proportion to the grossness of lack of detail in the primitive effect will there be lack of detail in the reactive effect of the vital force. This lack of detail will often be due to the grossness of the dose administered; a crude dose of drug will be followed by catharsis without specific detail, and when the reaction comes, the constipation will lack the finer sensations which are swallowed up in the intestinal paresis, and nondescript actions and reactions are almost meaningless. This sould point out the lesson to provers, and place a limit on the value of such crude provings. This should teach the advocates of such effects that the individualizing indices are not to be found here.

If we follow out the sentiment of the text, we observe the reactive effect in a given case is generally the opposite of the primitive effect, or as though intended to oppose the primitive shock, whether from a burn, or from freezing, or from a drug, or the fixed disease, as will be observed by carefully re-reading the 65th section. The symptoms or appearance of the reaction are generally found in the pathogensis of the drug causing the primitive shock. The reaction seems to work within the limit of the cause of the primitive shock. The reaction, in other words, is limited to the sphere of the drug causing the primitive effect. In one prover Opium has produced constipation (primitive effect) and in the reaction we observe a diarrhea. In another prover the primitive effect will be a diarrhea, and the reaction will be constipation.—See §65, Organon.

The reaction in healthy people will always be greater than the primitive shock. To state it in another way, the symptoms that appear in one person as primitive effects, appear in another as the reactive influence of the vital force; because the vital force in its efforts to resist the force from without must establish directly opposite actions, and all such reactions are within the line of actions found in the drug or disease cause which the vital force is acting or reacting against. Whatever symptoms or expressions are found in a given reaction will be found in the pathogenetic symptoms of the entity that the given reaction is opposing. There can be no reaction outside of the action of a given entity, whether it be a sick cause or drug.

It must not be supposed that this can furnish a doctrine whereby we can claim or suppose symptoms that have not been actually produced. I am well aware that this doctrine may be criticised before it is accepted, but the study of the provings, thus far, has led me to fully believe in it as a fact.

To understand the action of drugs in the primitive effects, one must not attempt to study it upon the sick, but healthy persons should be chosen, which will give much that is useful by observing what is felt and seen.

Again, to understand reaction one must compare what he sees in healthy persons with what appears in various degrees of sickness in unhealthy people. If we commence the study of the primitive effect through a proving of a drug upon a healthy subject, we will naturally avoid the effect of gross medicines if we would learn much. As has been said, the finer details have been swallowed up in the grossness of effects; but we observe that the few symptoms however seem to repeat themselves with an exactness that is surprising, some appearing on the 1st, 3rd, 5th, 7th and 9th days for many weeks with an exactitude of repetition that is surprising. Especially is this the case if the dose that Hahnemann mentioned, which was the 30th potency, should be the lowest resorted to for proving. In comparison with the gross effects which soon pass off, the effect of potencies upon healthy provers is most wonderful in the variety of the symptoms and in the length of time after

25

the potency was administered. Even many weeks after the proving, we find symptoms coming or occurring in intervals of 7, 14 and 21 days. Particularly did I observe this upon a healthy woman in the proving of Cenchris, who had menstrual symptoms four months after the proving, recurring at each menstrual period with perfect regularity; a symptom that is now a confirmed symptom and valuable. If this could then appear as what we term a reactive effect it would puzzle a philosopher to know why the effect from ten-thousandth potency had not long before disappeared. So that it must be reasonable to conclude that all the symptoms that appear after the taking of the drug that was administered, are the genuine symptoms of the drug, are the primitive and specific effects of that drug, whether occurring in the first day or many months afterwards. Habits and customs have been established by provings that have lasted the provers for years. These, considered as symptoms, have been cured by the same drug under similar conditions, and should be considered a fundamental primitive effect of the drug's use; they are really the sickness of the drug.

If we now undertake to consider the action of the drug when no apparent reaction comes against it to oppose it, we then see still more wonderful effects. If we administer to a patient in the last stages of consumption a drug in suitable form that would have cured this patient when he was yet curable, we now observe wonderful and striking things. We notice that after the administration of this drug that he is made worse, the course of his disease is more rapid, and he may be, by the careless use of such drug, hastened to a premature grave. In this instance we notice the lack of reaction. We notice the continued primitive shock, which united with his disease, instead of curing it, hastens him on towards the grave. We observe then that which we had not observed in healthy reaction, a continued downward course in the primitive action of the drug united with the disease; hence, it may well be said that woe is man when reaction does not come.

We observe this state of things in incurable cases of Bright's disease, consumption, cancer, so that the remedy that was deep enough to cure him, is now poison. We further observe that the remedies that help the severe sufferings in these incurable cases are such as are similar only to the few symptoms in his sufferings. These furnish examples of the primitive action of a drug when not opposed by vital reaction. The primitive expressions become changed by the vital force in healthy reaction, and some have mistaken these for the secondary action of the drug administered; especially this is the case in provings. Then it is that we must consider the primitive, when reaction does not oppose it, that we can know very much of its interior. Observe again the periodicity that comes in symptoms. The periodicity that follows the action of drugs, and what may be studied in a drug may also be studied in disease cause. What is true of the action of a drug is also true of the action of a disease. The most suitable way of studying diseases in their actions is also true of studying drugs in their actions, their conduct. Take for instance an intermittent fever. The paroxysm composed of chill, fever and sweat. The primitive action of that fever cause is attended throughout by the paroxysmal expressions that follow in which the reaction of the vital force has been, either aided or unaided, sufficient to oppose the sick cause.

It might be well to consider the erratic nature of some symptoms belonging to drugs, such as Ignatia having extremes and opposites and alternations of symptoms. Symptoms that change about in a most erratic manner, yet they are all the sick expressions of the one drug. I am aware that I have scarcely touched upon the important part of the truth that is yet to come out of reflecting upon the actions of nature. To be conversant with the signs of drug action is an important road to truth, and the knowledge thus gained must be useful, as a new drug, or the repetition of one chosen will often turn upon what is known about the meaning of actions observed. It is now well known that reaction is going on favorably when mental symptoms are improving and general feelings express a general bodily improvement, even though the symptoms are more painful. The successful healer is one who knows much about the signs of reaction and what is intended by nature. It is well known that chronic symptoms engrafted upon the economy either by drugs or chronic miasms are due wholly to deficient reaction of the vital force.

Incurable results of disease are incurable for two reasons: First, destruction of the tissues of the organism. Second, deficient reaction of the vital force. The latter may be again divided into congenital weakness and acquired debility. But as these divisions of inner complexities belong to other subjects, I will dismiss the subject entered upon in this paper, hoping that sufficient consideration will be given it to expose its weak points, that the strongest light may shine upon the real truth.

THE ADMINISTRATION OF THE REMEDY

It may be supposed by some that there is little to be said about the administration of the homœopathic remedy; by others that there is little to be learned beyond what can be found in the writings of Hahnemann. It should not be expected that Hahnemann could lay down fast lines for the use of the higher and highest potencies when he never used them. What he said about the use of remedies applies largely to the lower and 30th potencies. What he says about these is very useful about the administration of remedies in all potencies, but he gave general rules and nothing more could have been given at that time. An extensive experience with all kinds of potencies and constitutions, varying degrees of sensitivity, will lead a good observer to make no fast lines to be followed by himself or others.

The difference in the activities of a given remedy in the 30th and 10m upon the same constitution is most wonderful, and the difference in the 10m and cm. is still more wonderful in some instances. In some constitutions the 1m is not repeated with advantage and in others stoical, several doses are necessary. The very high potencies seldom require repetition, if clearly indicated, to produce a long curative action in chronic cases, but in severe acute sickness in robust constitutions several doses in quick succession are most useful. In a typhoid with a high fever the best work is done by repeating the remedy until the fever begins to yield, which is at times several days. In a remittent fever the remedy may be repeated until the fever shows signs of falling. While the fever is rising in robust constitutions the remedy may be repeated with advantage, and in some cases it is positively necessary.

It never matters whether the remedy is given in water in spoonful doses or given in a few pellets dry on the tongue—the result is the same. It has been supposed by some that by giving one or two small pellets that a milder effect would be secured, but this is a deception. The action or power of one pellet, if it acts at all, is as great as ten. If a few pellets be dissolved in water, and the water is given by the teaspoonful, each teaspoonful will act as powerfully as the whole of the powder if given at once, and the whole quantity of water if drank at once will have no greater curative or exaggerative power than one teaspoonful.

When medicine is given at intervals the curative power is increased and may be safe if it is discontinued with judgment. When a positive effect has been obtained the medicine should always be discontinued and the greatest mischief may come from continuing to give it. Therefore, it is not always that the technical single dose is the best practice, but the single collective effect is always to be sought.

The correct observer will soon learn whether this is to be secured by a single dose or a series of doses. But after this has been secured there is never an exception to the rule—wait on the remedy. In acute sufferings and in emergencies the above plan is best suited. In chronic diseases for the first prescription the single dose dry on the tongue will be found ever the best. After several doses have acted well, and when given at long intervals, the action is growing feebler and feebler, and the symptoms still call for the same remedy, a series of doses will show a stronger and deeper action, and this is even true if the potency is given much higher. Furthermore, it becomes safe to do this after several doses of a given medicine have been given singly and at long intervals, when it would not have been good practice with the first doses. When the 30th and 200th potencies are used it is much oftener necessary to give the medicine in water than when using higher potencies. These potencies have much milder curative action than the higher and highest potencies, and therefore, they are far more suitable to the very nervous and excitable women and children and to some men.

To suit all degrees of sensitivity in chronic diseases the physician must have at his command his deep acting medicines in the 30th, 200, 1000, 10m, 15m, cm. and mm. potencies. With many chronic patients, if the remedy fits the symptoms or is the similimum, any potency will do all the curing it can in two or three doses at long intervals and a higher potency must be selected. It is better to begin low and go higher and higher. Each change of the potency brings new and deeper curative action. It has been said by some, go very high at once and accomplish it at once, but it is not true that the cure is accomplished. In many chronic diseases the patient must be kept under the remedy a long time, and the remedy must be managed so that the curative power will not be thwarted. This continued action is best secured by the conservative method. In this way the cure is always mild, gentle and permanent. Again, to give the very high potency to the feeble and extremely sensitive, we bring back old complaints and symptoms too violently and too hurriedly, and fail to sustain the curative action long enough to eradicate the underlying miasm.

To avoid the shock or aggravation some give at night, others in the morning, but there is no difference. A deep-acting chronic remedy should seldom be given in the midst of a paroxysm or exacerbation, but at the close. This is an old settled rule that nearly all follow. To give a deep-acting remedy in the midst of great suffering would be to court aggravation and increase the suffering and use up the curative power of the remedy uselessly. The dose would be worn out, and when repeated would often fail to act. It is necessary to nurse the case on to a fortuitous moment and then give the medicine. That moment is after the excitement has past—when there is a calm. If it be a menstrual suffering, after menstruation, if it be chronic sick headache, after the headache, if it be intermittent fever, after the paroxysm, will be found the best time to give the dose of medicine.

The management of incurables differs widely. No two are alike, and it is soon observed that medicines ever so carefully selected aggravate and palliate, and the force of the remedy is soon used up and a new one must be found. It is seldom that the remedy works in more than one potency, and it is not uncommon that the remedy acts but a few hours. The rapid change in symptoms and states compels the patient to be ever near the physician.

The following axiom should always be held in mind: When the symptoms change the remedy must be discontinued, as it ceases to be homœopathic; therefore, whatever action it may exert cannot be curative and may be detrimental.

The single dose in all sensitive people anticipates this change of symptoms and must be the safest for general practice.

The repetition of the dose to intensify the action of the remedy must not be considered as the rule, but the exception.

It is unsafe for the beginner to indulge the desire to repeat too much—it should always be restrained.

The physician who prescribes in water universally will cause suffering in many of his sensitive patients, and it will appear to him that the disease is growing worse and he will change his remedy when he should cease to give medicine.

The higher the potency the greater the aggravation caused by this kind of repetition.

Physicians who practice only in the country among people who are strong and live out-door lives do not see the sharp aggravations that are seen in the city. The country people will stand more abuse from repetition as well as from crude drugs.

THE BASIS OF FUTURE OBSERVATIONS IN THE MATERIA MEDICA OR HOW TO STUDY THE MATERIA MEDICA

Homœopathy is an art and a science of life because it is a study of living objects. The law is revealed by phenomena evolved in living people, not in dead substances. Observations on dead substances are so far removed from living things, and from life itself, that they may properly be considered entirely outside of a science of living beings. They form a purely external science, an abstract science, and should be considered removed and apart from the object to which the Law relates.

In the laboratory has been discovered no remedy for living people, and its investigations have not benefitted the dead. The laboratory conducts study not of life, nor of disease, but of results of disease. That causes are sometimes continued into effects is true, but knowledge of the endings of causes is useless except in relation to knowledge of their beginnings and the course by which they develop. The beginnings of perverted life are not found in pathology nor in the laboratory, not even by use of the microscope.

Symptoms of sickness, are the only dicoverable manifestations of the perverted vital economy. In the symptoms we can see clearly the likeness of every disease and the likeness of the curative remedy for each. Symptoms are the only manifestation by which disease can make itself known to an intelligent physician. It is not the fault of nature's God that man is not wise enough to read these symptoms.

Men who are the victims of self-intelligence think that they can work out of dead matter the cause, the progress, and the curative agents of sickness. This never has been done; in time this idea will be looked upon as the whim of antiquity.

The law of cure known as the Law of Similars is a law of God; it was always so acknowledged by Hahnemann. It has always dealt with manifestations, not with results of vital changes, dead substances; so must it ever be. When man knows the Law and the significance of the phenomena he will perceive the relation of sick-images in sick people and in our pathogeneses.

When he knows the science of Homœopathy he will perceive beginnings of disease in childhood, its progress through life, and its ultimates after death. When these are considered collectively they make one grand whole;

when they are considered separately there is always something lacking. When the ultimates, only, are known, there is a dead science worked out on the dead, useless to the living.

An eminent pathologist once said to me: "We shall know how to cure this patient when we know the pathology." I then asked him: "When shall we know the pathology?" He replied: "When we have made a postmortem.' '

Nothing has been discovered on the dead separated from the living subject to which it was related, that has ever lead to a remedy for sickness. Only dangerous palliatives and makeshifts, that kill as often as they cure, and harm more than they benefit, have ever been discovered. Any that can be mentioned will be found to be of small value in comparison to remedies that conform to real remedial action whereby all living manifestations have been called into use through intelligent application.

When the laboratory can tell us what man loves and what he hates; when it can give us a complete image of his rational mind with all its deviations from the normal; when it can tell which are sensitive to cold, to heat, to dry weather, and to storms; then may we look to this dead science for help outside of symptomatology.

The sooner we learn to see the true classification and individualization by life-signs during sickness, the sooner shall we cure sick people so satisfactorily that we shall not hunt for remedies in results of disease.

Contemplate the millions of dollars squandered in laboratory research without yet yielding knowledge of the cause of bacteria.

Has it ever shed any light upon the soil or the precise condition of our vital fluids, to furnish us knowledge of the lack of resistance and of susceptibility?

Has it told us of the real condition of inherited ten-

dency; what is that weakly condition which ends in tuberculosis, cancer, and wasting disease?

Yet these conditions that tend toward tuberculosis and
cancer are so well known to the wise followers of Hahnemann, by signs and symptoms, that at this day all can
be cured, *yes, cured,* of their inheritances. They can be
tested and cured: tested not by laboratory discovery, but
by methods familiar to the modern followers of the immortal Hahnemann.

These things must be discovered by studying the
things of the will, the understanding, and the physical
signs and symptoms, as they exist in the similarity of
drug-provings. Study of the living must aid us to cure
the idiotic and weak-minded children; laboratories cannot
do it.

A physician is one who knows how to heal the sick.
To be a pathologist and not to have a careful knowledge
of materia medica and of how to use it, is not being a
physician. I have known some good prescribers who did
excellent curing of sick people and had a limited knowledge
of pathology.

The thoroughly-rounded physician is one who adds to
his knowledge of the art of selecting remedies according
to the Law of Similars a knowledge of diagnosis and
pathology. There are times when he must give advice to
patients that are incurable; he must know pathology and
diagnosis. There are kinds of pathology most useful to
the intelligent prescriber, but this knowledge never is
useful in the mind of the man ignorant of the art of
prescribing.

The pathologist considers the disease instead of the
patient; the physician considers the patient, and perceives
the sick patient in the symptoms that represent the per-
sonality of the sick man.

Diseases and results are much the same in all beings,

both man and lower animals, and no individualizing is possible by studying a disease or its pathology. All people produce the same pathology when affected with the same disease. *What is common will never lead the physician to perceive what is peculiar in any individual.*

THE HEALING PRINCIPLE

The vital principle that pervades all simple and complex organisms and substances manifests itself through various media and under varying circumstances. The grain of musk that was exposed for seventeen years in an open atmosphere, constantly revealing itself to all who entered its aura, was not perceptibly reduced in weight or power to impress the olfactories.

The protoplasm reveals its life to vision by the aid of the microscope, in motion, which is an actual observation.

The class of inert substances, of which silica is a prominent member, demonstrates its life force when acted upon by the elements of the animal and vegetable kingdoms, by the change produced in the elements of these kingdoms. This class, therefore, negatively demonstrates that there is life in so-called inert substances.

There is no substance know to man that does not possess life, lower or higher in proportion to the complexity of its organization, growing higher and higher in order and manifestation until the image of the Creator of all things has been reached. Shall it stop with man? No; the higher type is yet to be seen in God, the author of life and its every medium.

We observe that the animal body loses its identity or individuality vital energy, and the elements instantly manifest their own individual vital forces, each to its kind, like busy bees, until the shapeless mass has been transformed to its original dust.

The acting and acted upon, the lively and the inert

bodies and substances are observed throughout nature. To make use of the lesson of life is the demand of the day, through which the healing principle or life can be measured and its nature as a force perverted, an idiosyncrasy is to be corrected, or, if you prefer, cured.

The blending of these forces are the complexities of living and healing. We see the blending of life and death into each other, until the one disappears within the other. If it be life perfected and pure, it is the complete absence of visible death. Midway between life and death we see perfect equilibrium. This condition becomes the necessity of all reproduction or nutrition, through which we observe life living and acting upon its media. The slightest defect in the vital operations creates friction, and the machinery wears out rapidly, becomes heated; death increases and this that was a slight defect, becomes a threatening monster; yet, great only through results, as we know that the very gentle force, properly applied, corrects the original defect, and the grand old machinery soon returns to normal action. The defect may or may not be an idiosyncrasy. Reduced resistance against common things is an idiosyncrasy. In olden times we said, "this patient cannot take Calomel" because she is so susceptible to its action that the smallest dose has been known to salivate and do great injury. People are often susceptible to a substance that will do them great good if the positive and negative of life are duly considered and applied. Cure is often contagion as well as disease. When the vital energy of the disease cause be taken in too great incept, disease is the result, but if the sphere of vital plane of the same cause be elevated to the quality that becomes corrective, the contagion becomes cure. Cure must seek the same *via* as cause; in entering the economy, it must rap at the same portals.

The aura of a given substance causes sickness. This has been observed by long distance inhalations of the Rhus vine. The rose causes sickness in some people. This has been observed in the painter who takes colic from the aura of his brush, even when painting in the open air, or the same colic may come from sleeping in a newly painted room. If so small a quantity can make him sick why would it not be a wise experiment to attempt to reach a quality so subtle that it would make him well enough to resist this aura on other occasions. If the vital wrong can be corrected he is well, and his resistance has returned, which is his protection. If a chemical antidote should be suggested it would surely be reasonable to enquire, what we expect to antidote, as the substance known as the sick-prdoucing cause was too small to be observed by the aid of the microscope, and was an insoluble, and yet it was so powerful that it made the individual sick. Not all are so affected. Quite likely the healthy man is not so affected; therefore the contagion, for such it was, could not be due to nothing but lack of health, or sickness. Then this, which is a recognized idiosyncrasy, is sickness. Was he sick before he took the colic? Was he sick before he was sick? What is sickness?

The curative remedy is sometimes pointed out to the intelligent physician by accident through symptoms.

The animal organism can generally resist the crude substances when the lower attenuations may make him sick, and this is especially true of substances inert and insoluble.

It has been observed that the negative state may be intensified by large incepts of a given poison. A subject is rendered more sensitive to Rhus after once having been poisoned by it.

The causes must be very similar when the effects known by symptoms are so nearly identical, hence it is that persons susceptible to the poison of Rhus are also equally susceptible to the curative or correcting principle.

Rhus apparently cures Rhus poisoning in some cases, but actually cures the patient because he needed Rhus or a similar dynamis as badly before as after he was poisoned. The incept that caused him to become sick was too large to cure and it made him sick. The highly potentiated Rhus cured him of the sickness he had before he was poisoned and the disease that he *has* instantly ceases, as its cause is overcome by the normal vital reaction, he, not having taken enough of the poison to make a well man sick, but only enough to make a sick man sick or worse, recovers his normal state in a few days. Then Rhus has not cured Rhus poisoning, but the patient of his susceptibility to Rhus poisoning.

How different is this state from the state of large dose poisoning, by Morphine or any other crude drug, which must have its own antidote. In one case the patient is poisoned because he was sick, and in the other he is sick because he is poisoned and was not susceptible to the drug that made him sick, and cannot be impressed by that drug only in toxic quantities. This again brings out the positive and negative state of the human system, in which the individual may be as unable to protect himself against cure as cause, as unable to resist cure as cause. Cure and cause are different planes in the same sphere.

What is contagion, as understood, and what is cure, but the irresistible appropriation of some unknowable energy applied by accident or intelligence. We have seen that Rhus cures the patient of his sensitiveness to Rhus as well long after as before he was poisoned by it. This is not Isopathy, as it was not Rhus that was cured, but the patient, and is was simply pointed out to the intelligent physician by the accidental poisoning wherein Rhus was pointed to as one of the medicines that he is sensitive to; it being fully understood that the patient is always highly sensitive to his needed medicine. This, therefore, is but a centering of a complex of symptoms in a homœopathic problem.

The negative state of the body as observed is utilized by the electrologist or magnetic controller, demonstrates many facts. The mesmerist, by his peculiar movements so acts upon the negative subject that the latter is deprived of sensation; his tongue can be punctured and a needle passed through; he can be managed like an automaton, without sensation; but the positive subject cannot so easily surrender himself that he is negative enough to be influenced in the slightest degree. Some can by slight resistance oppose the mesmerist, others are at once controlled and made unconscious. In this state the forces of the body are alone disturbed, the tissues are unchanged. Can disease be more than this primitively? It need not be more. It is not more, while all tissue changes are the *results* of disease. With this thought in mind, it must seem strange that men study morbid anatomy to be able to find means to correct a wrong that is wholly vital. It must seem strange that a learned professor will still hunt with the microscope for the germ that causes the cholera, yellow fever, and zymotic sicknesses; searching among the results of disease to destroy its cause. As well examine a grain of wheat under the microscope to ascertain how tall a stalk it will grow, or to ascertain whether it will grow anything; as the lens has never discovered the vital spark in that grain of wheat, it will not likely become a safe guide to the nature of a vital energy in disease cause or curative force.

The pathological anatomy is the intermediate state, while the external image, made up of sensations, is a perfect likeness of the primitive state; the true disease and these only correspond with each other, and in these only do we see fathomable harmony.

The study of morbid anatomy can never reveal the

remedy to correct the ills of man, no more than the study of the bark of the poison oak will reveal the cause of its life force being such a disease producer or poison. As well to study the root of aconite under the lens to see what it will produce upon the animal force, as to study pathology to ascertain what entity will subdue it and drive it from the human body. The curative principle is not found in that way.

Two negatives make an affirmation.

Take it for granted that there is a minus state that we call susceptibility. If we apply the drug power we shall see, that much of the drug makes sick, a small amount of the drug still makes sick; so small an amount that people ordinarily are not disturbed, yet this sensitive one is made sick; extreme reduction of the quantity still makes sick until a plane is reached similar in quality to that of the dynamis of the sick-making cause, then it is, that the two minus states or conditions are fulfilled and sickness does not follow and the susceptibility has been unconsciously removed. This has been observed in seeking cure by change of atmosphere, and cures have been known to be cures when consumptives have fattened in malarial swamps.

When the curative power of the corrective agent is observed, it may be said that two negatives have met and a positive is the result, or health or cure. Similars have sustained the great law.

The sensitive state has been produced by a peculiar atmosphere and cholera is the result, or small-pox is the result. If it be the latter disease that is prevailing all people not protected become susceptible, and the poison or noxious influence takes life in the negative condition of the medium. If the poison or cause be attenuated to such a plane that the most sensitive person is only slightly disturbed by proving it, the terrible disease can be prevented. It would seem better to protect from small-pox in this way than to vaccinate. Either by vaccination or neutral contagion there is a monster poison ir the economy. Who dare talk of filth and ignore the fact that the natural contagion is more than the charge? If the small-pox virus is so subtle that even when diluted with millions of volumes of atmospheric air is yet a poison, who can say what attenuation may not produce the disease until faithfully tried on sensitive persons. The trial in a season when small-pox does not prevail would not satisfy the enquiry, as the sensitive ones are not manufactured so frequently. The trial then of a single person could not better the matter. The proving of all attenuations of variolinum would be a great gain to our philosophy, as the provings of the morbific products have helped the study of our chronic miasms. Dr. Fincke has made a good beginning toward finding out what the variolinum will do.

The wise ones who stand off and sneer often come in after the truth has been discovered at great sacrifice, and say, "I told you so." These people are often useful, as they create opposition enough to stimulate thorough search after facts. They have a place in the world but they do not know it; and often cover up the regret that they have been born by sneers at decent people.

THE LANGUAGE OF THE REPERTORY

INTRODUCTORY NOTE: To many who have not been thoroughly trained in repertory study, the practical value of such work remains uncomprehended. The following article has been prepared to shed light on some of the difficulties that confront those who have not learned to appreciate the immense value of such an index as is afforded in the modern Repertory, and how familiarity with it unlocks the store-house of our materia medica.

The physician must study the homœopathic principles until he learns what it is in sickness that *guides to the curative remedy.*

He must study the materia medica until he learns what is needed to meet these demands.

He must then study the repertory until he learns how to use it so that he can find what he wants when he needs it.

It must be admitted that many do mechanical work and fail to realize that any other kind is possible. The physician must read over and over the rubrics in the repertory in order to learn what is in it and how symptoms are expressed. Often he will see a rubric or a symptom that he would not have thought of seeking in that place; he should then settle in his own mind where he would have looked for it; then he should make one or several cross-references to guide him in the future to that rubric or symptom.

Many fail to use the repertory because they think of symptoms in pathological language or because they look for expressions in the language of tradition. It must be remembered that symptoms come to us from lay-provers; that sick people are lay people. Both of these express sickness in the language of the layman and the repertory must be the index of the materia medica. Every effort to convert either the materia medica or the repertory into the language of traditional medicine must result in total failure.

Technical language condenses the thought of a given sickness. That is all that is needed to convey all there is knowable from one physician to another until the question of the remedies comes up: What is the remedy? The answer comes by asking another question: What are the symptoms? The symptoms are the speech of the laity and of nature: uneducated nature—simple nature— appealing to an educated physician. The symptoms of a patient have no meaning whatever to an untrained physician—to a physician untrained in the significance of *symptoms of the patient*, of the prover—hence the repertory is meaningless to him. This explains why so many try to use the repertory and fail: they have had no teaching in our so-called homœopathic colleges.

All who know how to use a repertory succeed, and not one has ever discarded it. It appears strange that all do not try to find some one to teach them to use it when there are so many willing to do it; it appears strange that they do not desire to know how to use the repertory; it appears strange that they have not learned to note the precise language of the patient, the language of the materia medica, and the language of the repertory.

Physicians who are ignorant in these methods see no difference when the same symptom appears in three different patients in the same family, though one has this symptom at 10 A. M., another at 1 A. M., and another at 4 P. M.; one is better from heat, another from cold, and the third not affected by either, and I have known them to ask very promptly: "What has that to do with it?"

Three patients suffer from a similar headache; one is better in the open air, one is better from applied cold, and the third, from applied heat; and again comes the question: "What has that to do with it?" Yet these are only the first and simplest differences to be mentioned.

The inexperienced physician in our art trains his mind to lump and condense and concentrate and this leads in the opposite direction to what is required. We have large groups or rubrics but these are next split up into conditions, circumstances and modalities until every least difference in time, place, degree and manner is brought before the mind so that distinction and individualization may appear. "What has that to do with it?"

I will mention the word "weakness" and even our own students may say: "What a common general symptom to mention," but if he is weak—

after eating, must lie down for awhile,

in hot weather,
after stool,
after mental and physical exertion,
after sleep,

who would not wonder if Selenium would not cure such a case? When such a group of circumstances is associated in catarrh of nose, throat and larynx, or carcinoma, and there are

desire for open air,
lack of vital heat,
emaciation in advanced years,
extreme sensitiveness to drafts
—even warm drafts,

there is nothing left for the homœopathist but to give Selenium.

How can the inexperienced physician work this out without a repertory, properly used?

The proper use of the repertory will lead to correct offhand prescribing in simple cases, in from ten to twenty years. The mechanical use of the repertory never leads to artistic prescribing nor to remarkable results.

Certain mental characteristics go hand in hand; some characteristics of mind are necessary to good, artistic repertory-work others are equally prohibitory.

Some minds cannot comprehend that potentization of any given drug is possible in proportion to the homœopathicity of that drug to a given group of symptoms, and that when the drug is not similar, only attenuation is present. When attenuation becomes potentization is a question that the healing-artist alone can comprehend otherwise than theoritically. The physician who can clearly comprehend this can learn to comprehend the value of symptoms and therefore learn, by the aid of a repertory, to compare the symptoms of his patient; otherwise repertory-work is purely mechanical.

Perhaps a clinical case will best illustrate the subject.

Mrs. S., aged 47, a very excitable—almost hysterical—woman, for many years has suffered—

Violent occipital headaches.

> Compelled to take strong medicines, for years.
>
> Occur every few days; never passes a week without one.
>
> Continue three days.
>
> Heat and pressure give most relief.

Bowels constipated; for a week has no desire; then takes cathartics.

> Says: "I have taken everything."
>
> Stool hard and small, resembling sheep-dung.

Craves open air; cool air.

Heat flushes.

Menstruation absent lately.

Urine scanty and strong.

Eyes have sensation that they do not belong to her.

Cold knees and below knees.

Very tired and excitable.

Over-sensitive; extremely sensitive to touch over entire body.

What are the *strange, rare and peculiar symptoms* in this patient?

The remedies that have *stool in round, hard balls resembling sheep dung* that also have *strong craving for open air* are:

Alum., bar-c., carb-an., *carb-s.,* caust., *graph.,* KALI-S., *mag-m., nat-m., nat-s.,* op., *sulph.*

No desire for stool for many days: ALUM., *carb-an.,* CARB-S., caust., GRAPH., kali-s., *mag-m.,* NAT-M., OP., *sulph.,* and many others not related to the case.

Occipital headache: Alum., *carb-an.*, CARB-S., *mag-m.,* nat-m., op., SEP., sulph.

—— *jarring agg.*: Carb-s., *mag-m., nat-m., sulph.*

—— *pressure amel.*: MAG-M., NAT-M., *sulph.*

—— *heat amel.*: *Mag-m.*

March 4th. MAG-M. 10m.

April 9th. MAG-M. 10m.

May 20th. MAG-M. 50m.

There has been no headache since and she has been in good health.

In this case the headache is a common one, but it was what she came to have cured. The peculiar symptom is the one difficult to explain, viz.: *stool in hard balls resembling "sheep dung."* It is certainly uncommon; it is not a diagnostic symptom of any disease. One might wonder what kind of commotion in the intestine could break up a hard stool into lumps so small and tumble these around until they were flat, oval and round and small as sheep's dung; the normal stool and the common stool are quite different. Then it must be "strange, rare and peculiar."

Now as she longs for the open air it will be best to eliminate with the above rubric from remedies that have *craving for open air*; this gives the start.

Then taking the next most important rubric, viz.: *inactivity* or *no desire for a week* what remains can be in the anamnesis above.

So proceed to the end, taking the symptoms in the order of their importance. The result is a cure.

THE MAKING OF A MAN

Truth is a two-edged sword.

Information that may be used for the good of mankind may be used also for selfish ends. In the former, it elevates the user; in the latter, it destroys him. We see the evidence of this in every profession, in every business; in the artist, the doctor, the lawyer, the merchant, and the politician. We have only to study faces to be convinced.

The face of the homœopathic physician who has used the great homœopathic truth for the good of man has a benign expression, while he who has first counted on what it will bring in cash has a crafty face which the children shun. In either case, he smiles if successful; but if he fails, we shall see accentuated the two casts of expression. One reveals patience; and the other deep lines of disappointment and hatred.

It is important to know how it is that truth can become a power to change the faces of men. Truth is so powerful that it will elevate him who uses it for the good of man, and degrade him who uses it against his fellow. It carries with it a penalty for falsifying it, or using it for improper purposes.

When one listens to a great truth, he says to himself that truth *should be known to the world,* or that it can be used to increase wealth.

Truth first enters the memory, and may go no farther and soon may be lost; or it may be admitted into the understanding, and flow through it into the voluntary and then into life. This is the course intended by Divine Providence whenever he gives truth to man. It is that he shall use it for the common good, and not for himself. Whenever man perverts this, he destroys himself; but when he carries out the purpose of the truth, he becomes wise. The highest aim of man is to become wise, and the only way to attain wisdom is to do for the good of others.

Truth first enters the mind by the way of the memory. There it is inspected by the understanding, and it is settled upon whether it is true or false, or detrimental. If it is approved, the understanding admits it to the middle chamber, where it is treasured for use. When Homœopathic truth is thus admitted, the healing artist waits for an opportunity to confirm it. Finally the patient comes, and the truth is called forth; the law and doctrines there treasured are called upon, used, and confirmed to be true. The patient recovers and is grateful to his doctor. The doctor is delighted and smiles. He shows forth upon the face his inmost feelings; a tear comes to his eye and he says, "Blessed be Hahnemann, Blessed be the Lord."

Then it is that truth passes through the understanding into the voluntary—into the affections—and is revealed upon the countenance. Now, truth is made, alive, and can be maintained alive so long as the doctor continues to use it. It now fills his life. He loves it, knows it and remembers it. If he does not love it and use it, he does not grow in wisdom. But by loving it he loves to use it, and thereby learns more of it. The more he loves it, the better he knows it.

If there is one who is wise in the law, it is because he loves it and obeys it. If he is wiser than others, it is because he loves it more than others—but for the sake of the good it will do for man. To love it for the good it will bring to oneself is another form of hatred of men; and hatred of men, or love of self, closes and pinches and contracts and distorts the understanding, and the face becomes crafty. Any violation of the law carries with it its own penalty.

Woe unto him who uses the truth to glorify himself or enrich his pocketbook.

Truth will make man miserable or happy. Man is never happy except when working for others. Man is most miserable when doing most for himself, and the misery is shown on his face. Behold the successful miser. He who has most is most miserable. The wise man is always happy. He has grown wise while loving, and is loved while acquiring knowledge. Peace, happiness and contentment are upon the face of all who live for the good of the human race.

When man appears to know what he does not make use of, his understanding will soon force it out into the memory, and finally the memory holds it no longer. In the understanding is treasured only so much as is loved and used.

The love of truth for the sake of truth, in the voluntary, conjoins with an equivalent of truth in the understanding; and this is the measure of wisdom in any man.

The crafty man memorizes facts, to use for a given occasion in order to acquire remuneration or fame, and should be known as smart in proportion to the success of his undertaking. This is not wisdom. Wisdom cannot be removed from the love of uses.

Love, wisdom and use make one, and inasmuch as they are one in the life of man they make him a man; and wherein he lacks these, he falls short of being a man. These in man are the wherein he exists in the image of God, and when he has thus made truth alive in him he has become "free indeed."

THE PLANE OF DISORDER AND CURE

I have tried many methods for opening the mind to receive explanatory terms, in the effort to study simple substance; to lead the material mind to the realm of immaterial mind. There is a strong tendency to depend on what is gleaned by the senses, but the realm of immaterial or simple substance must be recognized by the reason. Material substances, in the form of ordinary food, are best suited to nourish the cells of the body, to repair the waste of material cells, resulting from their normal activities. To educate the mind (inclined to receive only that which can be received through the avenues of the senses, only those reports at the sight, hearing, smell, taste and touch), so as to cause it to think interiorly, requires considerable care and study.

It is necessary to transfer the mind from the concrete to the figurative to perceive something of the character of immaterial substance. Material substance is fed and treated from the plane of nutrition, but the immaterial substances are affected from the plane of disorder and cure. Some think there is as much curative substance in crude drugs as in potencies. Holloway, in his address at Kansas City last year, took his ground from Hahnemann's position, that curative powers in drugs cannot change the affections and intellect without working in the realm of potencies.

Let us consider the light of day, the light of the Sun. We, living on the earth's globe, rotate with it. When the side on which we live is toward the Sun we enjoy its light, but when that side is turned away from the Sun we are in darkness. People are not in the habit of thinking of the light as anything, but if it were not something it could not disappear. The Sun, from which this light emanates, is approximately ninety million miles from us, yet we receive its light. A man who weighs 140 pounds on the Earth would weigh two tons at the Sun's margin owing to the attraction of the Sun, which is twenty-eight times as much as on the Earth. As soon as material substance comes to the Sun it is hurled into the Sun; the nearer it approaches the sun, the stronger is the velocity and attraction.

Light, however, is something proceeding from the Sun, radiating in every direction. When it reaches the Earth it is attenuated through ninety million miles, the distance between Sun and Earth. How much it is attenuated we can scarcely conceive, yet we can see things from, in, and because of light, but cannot see light itself. It is so attenuated that we cannot see it, but there is

enough of it that we can see to read by it. The light of
the Sun must be diametrically opposed to material substance. Material substance is drawn into the Sun, light is
thrown out from the Sun. It, then, must operate by opposite laws to those that affect material substance. The
Sun ceased to be material substance when transformed
into light and hurled outward to the planets. If light is
thus attenuated through ninety million miles, it is so
great an attenuation that we can scarcely think of any
greater, yet it was a simple substance at the beginning.

Nutritive substances are material; curative substances are immaterial, simple substance. There is always
a tendency to influx where simple substance is active.
When there is a disturbance in the inner planes of man's
economy there is an influx, from the atmosphere, of some
deleterious simple substance. If there were a curative
immaterial substance, it would be drawn in by influx and
act as an antidote. If remedies are given on the plane of
disturbance they will cure.

Man is affected in the internals and in every cell
Every cell has all the planes. Every cell is what man is as
a whole. This elevates the thought to the curative principles. Hahnemann says it is strange that medicine in the
old times could not go in the opposite way from that which
it took and perceive these things.

Crude drugs produce the opposite effects from the
attenuated dose. Crude whiskey, when taken into the system, produces a drunken condition; an attenuated dose
makes a man who appears drunk, feel better. The pri
mary action of a drug represents the effect of the crude
drug. The effect of the attenuated dose is similar to what
would be experienced long after taking the crude form. In
attenuated form, primary and secondary effects, opposite
effects, are found. The attraction of matter and repulsion
of light account for these effects. It may be that one of a
material cast of mind may perceive that these things are

true and thus the mind can be elevated to think higher than the fingers and toes.

A class of men, at present, think they discover the cause of disorder in bacteria, hence they search for pathological bacteria to be grandparents, and establish a family. Here is a material idea which indicates the trend of the Old School and all the theories they manufacture, and the trend of Homœopathic doctors who are not Homœopaths, believing in the bacterial etiology. If bacteria cause disease, we have many things to think about. Let us reverse the problem, and bring out things to think about in a different way. When out in the frontier country, I found the earth covered with a bed of lava from fifty to seventy-five feet in depth. The outer surface was decomposed from the influence of light, rain and heat (oxidized), forming a soil in which trees, grass and shrubs grew in abundance. Fire swept over the land and cleared it completely, destroying everything. The next season there was a vast growth of fireweed (*Erechthites*). Immediately I said, looking at it: Did this fireweed cause the fire that spread over the woods? What a wonderful thought, brilliant idea. I was then anxious for a body of men to tell it to. No one ever sowed the seed over that vast area where thousands of acres are spread over by the fireweed. Then I said: No, the fireweed did not cause the fire. The fireweed came from the fact that the land, burnt from the fire gave a soil, prepared by the heat, rain and air, in which these things worked a spontaneous development to cause the fireweed. What, spontaneous development? Why that idea was given up long ago. Yes, by whom? Given up long ago by SCIENCE.

Another time I was hunting in a place where the lumberers had their camps. They had cut off the woods, used the lumber, and moved off, leaving the shanties and stables and pens where their pigs were kept to rot away. Where the pigs were kept there was a copious growth of pigweed,

(*Cycloloma Piatyphyllum*), where the cattle were kept smartweed (*Polygonum Punctatum*) grew in abundance, where man had deposited his fecal waste was a copious growth of nettle (*Urticaceae*). We do not say that the pig-weed was the cause of the pigs, that the smartweed made the cattle grow, etc. I had elevated my mind above that, and came to the conclusion that these forms of growth were the result and not the cause of the men and the cattle and the pigs.

In my own garden, on the north side of the house, in the shadow, where the ground is copiously watered, the moss has crowded out the grass. So the preparation of the soil preceded the development of any growth. Changes in the blood, when health is disturbed, make a preparation of soil in the blood for the spontaneous development in the body of various forms to correspond to every change in bodily disorders. To assume that these spontaneous growths cause the sickness is absurd.

Fluids that contain bacteria and evolve them will act as agents of infection. You can kill the bacteria with alcohol, and inject the fluid, remaining, into the body and cause a condition in the blood similar to that in the body from which the fluid was taken. The cause of the disorder is on the plane of simple substance. When it floats forth into the ultimates it evolves spontaneously into bacteria. This is direct evolution from cause to effect. You cannot become normal in soul, affections, and uses, so long as you reason from effect to cause. This trend of thought is essential to our school, to check our expenditure of millions in laboratory analysis. Blood analysis is of no use to help me to help a patient. Everyone who is seen to go deeply into bacterial study loses all love for it because it has no use. Causes are continued into effects. Germs are caused from the fluids. These fluids are infectious but the germs as living beings are not infectious. Sepsis comes first,

then the germs appear. There is spontaneous development of sepsis in the blood. If the germs are left long
enough they will kill off the poison. This is illustrated in
the case of a cadaver. The scalpel that pricks the hand in
the course of a post-mortem examination is more poisonous than the scalpel that pricks the hand after using it on
the cadaver that has lain for six weeks and is mortified
and green.

THE SECOND PRESCRIPTION

EDITORIAL NOTE: What perplexing problems we often meet in
practice! How we crave, at times, the advice of a master mind!
We are so often the victims of prejudice, over-confidence or ignorance, and our patients suffer in consequence of this. Could we but
understand the intricate laws governing the inner man, disease,
and remedies, how much more wisely might we adjust ourselves to
the far-reaching problems which endanger the life of a father, a
mother, a noble son or an affectionate daughter. We would not
then, as is so often done, impede or pervert the action of a carefully selected remedy by our impatience to get results, or by our
impetuosity in hastening certain conditions which will not be
hastened, or by our ignorance in so quickly changing remedies
before one of them has had time for definite action. To help us
in this noble work we reproduce below a masterly paper by Dr.
J. T. Kent, read before the International Hahnemannian Association
at Niagara Falls in 1888.—G. E. D.

What is more beautiful to look upon than the bud
during its hourly changes to the rose in its bloom. This
evolution has so often come to my mind when patiently
awaiting the return of symptoms after the first prescription has exhausted its curative power. The return
symptom-image unfolds the knowledge by which we know
whether the first prescription was the specific or the
palliative, i. e., we may know whether the remedy was
deep enough to cure all the deranged vital wrong or
simply a superficially acting remedy, capable of only a
temporary effect. The many things learned by the action
of the first remedy determine the kind of demand made
upon the physician for the second prescription.

Many problems come up to be solved that must be
solved, or failure may follow.

How long shall I watch and wait? Is a question
frequently asked but seldom answered.

Is the remedy still acting? Is the vital reaction still affected by the impulse of the remedy?

If the symptoms are returning, how long shall they be watched before it is necessary to act or give medicine.?

Is the disease acute or chronic?

Why is the second prescription so much more difficult than the first?

Why is it that so many patients are benefited when first going to the physician and thereafter derive no benefit?

I presume that most good prescribers will say: "We have often acted too soon, but never waited too long." Many physicians fail because of not waiting, and yet the waiting must be governed by knowledge. Knowledge must be had, but where can it be obtained? To know that this waiting is right is quite different from waiting without a fixed purpose. This knowledge cannot be found where its existence is denied; it is not found with unbelievers and agnostics.

When the first prescription has been made and the remedy has been similar enough to change the existing image, we have but to wait for results. The manner of change taking place in the totality of symptoms signifies everything, yet the manner of the return of the image, provided it has disappeared, signifies more.

First.   If aggravation of symptoms follow;

Second.   If amelioration of symptoms follow;

1.   Aggravation of existing symptoms may come on with general improvement of the patient, which means well; but—

If aggravation of the symptoms is attended with decline of the patient the cure is doubtful, and the case must be handled with extreme care, as it is seldom that such patients recover perfectly.

2. If amelioration follow the prescription, to what does the amelioration apply?

It may apply to the general state or but to the few symptoms. If the patient does not feel the elasticity of life returning, the improved symptoms are the facts upon which to doubt recovery.

The knowledge that the disease is incurable often is obtained only in this way. In such cases every remedy may palliate his sufferings, but cure does not come. The symptoms that are the expressions of the debility are there, and hence the totality of the symptoms is not removed.

After the curative impulse has entirely subsided, the symptoms will appear one by one, falling into place to arrange an image of the disease before the intelligent physician for the purpose of cure.

If the first prescription has been continuously given, there has been but little if any chance of a pure returning image of the disease, therefore this image must be very unreliable.

When the remedy has been fully exhausted, then, and only then, can we trust the symptoms constituting the picture.

If the first prescription was the similimum, the symptoms will return—and when they return—*asking for the same remedy.*

Too often the remedy has been only similar enough to the superficial symptoms to change the totality and the image comes back altered, therefore resembling another remedy, which must always be regarded as a misfortune, by which the case is sometimes spoiled, and the hand of the master may fail to correct the wrong done.

Whenever the symptoms return the same image, calling for the same remedy, then it is that we have demonstrated, that—for a time, if the disease be chronic—we can but recommend the range of dynamics to cure this

27

case. This rule is almost free from exceptions if the remedy is an antipsoric.

What must the physician do who has not the knowledge of dynamic medicines? He must sometimes see sick images come back without change of symptoms, though I believe it is seldom.

The symptoms may call for Phosphorus as strongly as when he began, and Phosphorus 6x has served and no longer cures. What can he do but change his remedy?

Can it be possible that man can be so ignorant of how to cure as to give a drug that is not indicated because the one that is indicated does not cure?

These ignorant mortals condemn the system of Homœopathy and feel that they have performed their duty to the sick, forgetting that ignorance was the culprit.

I have observed in cases where a low potency had been administered in frequently repeated doses, that some time must elapse before a perfect action will follow the higher potency; but where the dose had not been repeated after its action was first observed, the new and higher potency will act promptly.

When the symptoms come back—after prudent waiting—unchanged, the selection was correct, and if the same potency fail to act a higher one will generally do so quite promptly, as did the lower one first. When the picture comes back unaltered except by the absence of some one or more symptoms, the remedy should never be changed until a still higher potency has been fully tested, as no harm can come to the case from giving a single dose of a medicine that has exhausted its curative powers. It is even negligence not to do such a thing.

PROPER TIME TO CHANGE

When the demonstration is clear that the present remedy has done all it is capable of doing—and this demonstration can not be made until much higher potencies than usually made have been tried—then the time is present for the next prescription.

To change to the next remedy becomes a ponderous problem, and what shall it be?

The last appearing symptom shall be the guide to the next remedy. This is so whenever the image has been permitted to settle by watching and waiting for the shaping of the returning symptom-picture. Long have I waited after exhausting the power of a remedy, while observing a few of the old symptoms returning; finally a new symptom appears. This latest symptom will appear in the anamnesis as best related to some medicine having it as a characterisitic which most likely have all the rest of the symptoms.

It is not supposed that this later appearing symptom is an old symptom on its way to final departure, for *so long as old symptoms re-appear and disappear it is granted that no medicine is to be thought of.*

It is an error to think of a medicine when a symptom-image is changing. The physician must wait for permanency or firmness in the relations of the image before making a prescription.

Some say, "I must give the patient medicine or he will go and see someone else." I have only to say that it were better had all sick folks gone somewhere else, for these doctors seldom cure but often complicate the sickness.

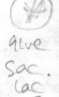

give
Sac.
Lac

The acute expressions of a chronic disease have a different management from the acute disease, *e. g.,* a child suffers from bronchitis in every change of weather. It may grow worse if treated with the remedy for the acute symptoms.

The miasm that predisposes the child to recurrent attacks must be considered.

One recently under my care had received Antimonium tart., Calcarea, Sulphur, Lycopodium, etc., in such indiscriminate confusion that the child was not cured. The waiting on Sac.-lac. through several attacks permitted the drug-effects to pass off, and the true image of the sickness was permitted to express itself through several of the exacerbations taken as a whole.

When western ague is complicated with a miasm, a single paroxysm does not fully express the totality, but several must be grouped and the true image will be discovered. If the acute disease be complicated with a miasm the indicated remedy will wipe it out *"cito, tuto et jucunde."*

AVOID HASTE

All things oppose haste in prescribing. In very grave diseases haste is a common error, more frequently with the second prescription than the first. Many doctors suppose that a diphtheria demands a medicine immediately because "something must be done." This is an error; many a life has been saved by waiting and waiting.

For example:

A little girl was suffering from a severe attack of diphtheria and the mother had treated it four days with Mercurius 3x, and Kali bich. 3x, in alternation. She was poor, and therefore I did not refuse to take the case which was then in a very bad state: nose, mouth and larynx full of exudate.

After a long study the child received Lycopodium cm.. one dose, dry, which cleared out the exudate from nose and fauces, but did not touch the larynx.

I dare not tell you how long I watched that child before I saw an indication for the second remedy which it would have needed had the Lycopodium been given when the child first took sick. I waited until the poor child was threatening dissolution when I saw a little tough yellow mucus in the mouth. Kali bich., cm., one dose, cleared the larynx in one day and there was no further medication necessary.

The first prescription is made with the entire image of the sickness formed. (People usually send for the doctor after there can be no doubt of the sickness to be treated.)

The doctor watches the improvement of the patient and the corresponding disappearance of the symptoms under the first prescription, and when the case comes to a standstill he is uneasy, and with increasing fidgetiness he awaits the coming indication for the next dose of medicine.

This fidgetiness which comes from a lack of knowledge unfits the physician as an observer and judge of symptoms; hence we see the doctor usually failing to cure his own children. He cannot wait and reason clearly over the returning symptoms.

While watching the prescriptions of beginners, I have observed very often the proper results of the first prescription. The patient has improved for a time, then ceased to respond to any remedy.

Close investigation generally reveals that this patient improved after the first dose of medicine, that the symptoms changed slightly without new symptoms, and the new "photo" seemed to call for some other remedy, when, of course, the remedy was changed and trouble began. Constant changing of remedies followed until all the antipsorics in the CHRONIC DISEASES had been given on flitting symptom-images, and the patient is yet sick. This is the common experience of young Hahnemannians trying to find the right way. Some of experience make lesser blunders and some make few, but how many have made none? All of these blunders I have made, as I had no teacher, until I blundered upon the works of the great Master.

WAIT AND OBSERVE

The first prescription may not have been well chosen medicine, and then it becomes necessary to make a second effort.

As time brings about the re-examination of the patient, new facts are brought out in relation to the image of the sickness, indicating that the first medicine had not been suitable; perhaps several weeks have passed and the re-examination finds no change in the symptoms.

Shall I compare all the facts in the case to reassure myself of the correctness of the first prescription, or shall I wait longer?

Yes, to the former, of course, and if the remedy is still the most similar to all the symptoms, wait, and watch, and study the patient for a new light on his feelings to which he has become so accustomed he has not observed.

Commonly the new study of the case will reveal the reason why the first prescription has not cured: it was not appropriate.

If it still appears to be the most similar remedy the question arises: "How long shall I wait?"

At this point it should be duly appreciated that the length of time is not so important as being on the safe side, and "wait" is the only safe thing to do. It may have been many days, but that matters not, wait longer.

The finest curative action I ever observed was begun sixty days after the administration of the single dose.

The curative action may begin as slate as a long-acting drug can produce symptoms on a healthy body. This guide has never been thought of by our writers, but it is well to be considered. Why not?

It is the practice for some to go lower if a high potency has failed.

This method has but few recorded successes but should not be ignored.

The question next to be considered is the giving of a dose of medicine in water and divided doses. This has at times seemed to have favor over the single dry dose. This is open for discussion, requiring testimony of the many, not of few, to give weight. The best reports are made from both methods, and both are in harmony with correct practice.

IMPROPER ACTION

The next important step to be considered is when the first prescription has acted improperly, or without curative results. Then it becomes necessary to consider a second prescription. The first prescription sometimes changes the symptoms that are harmless and painless into symptoms that are dangerous and painful.

If a rheumatism of the knee goes to the heart under a remedy prescribed for the one symptom, the remedy has done harm. It is an unfortunate prescription and must be antidoted. In incurable diseases when a remedy has set up destructive symptoms, an antidote must be considered.

If the remedy changes the general symptom-image, and the general state of the patient is growing worse, the question then comes up, was the prescription only similar to a part of the image, or is the disease incurable? *Knowledge of disease* may settle this question. If the disease is incurable, the action of the remedy was not expected to do more than to change the sufferings into peaceful symptoms, and the second prescription is to be considered only when new sufferings demand a remedy.

But suppose such a change of suffering comes after the first prescription and the disease is undoubtedly curable, then the conclusion must be that the first prescription was not the true specific, and that the true image has not been seen.

Wait until the old image has fully returned is all there is to do.

It is hazardous practice to follow up rapidly all the changing symptoms in any sickness, with remedies that simply for the moment seem similar to the symptoms present. The observing physician will *know by the symptoms and their directions, whether the patient is growing better or worse,* even though he appear to the contrary to himself and his friends.

The complaints of patient or friends constitute no ground for a second prescription.

The greatest sufferings may intervene in the change of symptoms during progress of permanent recovery, and if such symptoms are disturbed by a new prescription or palliated by inappropriate medicine, the patient may never be cured.

The object of the first prescription is to arrange the vital current or motion in a direction favorable to equilibrium, and when this is attained it must not be disturbed by a new interference. Ignorance in this sphere has cost millions of lives.

When will the medical world be willing to learn these principles so well that they can cure speedily, gently and permanently?

There can be no fixed time for making the second prescription; it may be many months.

The second prescription must be one that has a friendly relation to the last one or the preceding. No intelligent prescription can be made without knowing the last remedy. Concordances in Bœnninghausen must not be ignored. The new remedy should sustain a complementary to the former.

REMEDIES SUITABLE TO FOLLOW

In managing a chronic sickness the remedy that conforms to an acute experience of the illness is worth knowing, as very often its chronic may be just the one that conforms to its symptoms.

Calcarea is the natural chronic of Belladonna and Rhus;

Natrum mur. sustains the same relation to Apis and Ignatia;

Silicea to Pulsatilla;

Sulphur to Aconite.

When Pulsatilla has been of great service in a given case and finally cures no more, while the symptoms now point to Silicea, the latter will be given with confidence as its complementary relation has long been established.

On the other hand Causticum and Phosphorus do not like to work after each other, nor will Apis do well after Rhus.

How physicians can make the second prescription without regard to the experience of nearly a century, is more than man can know.

These things are not written to instruct men of experience in the right way, but for the young men who have asked so often for the above notes of our present practice.

I am told almost daily that this kind of practice is splitting hairs, but I am convinced of the *necessity of obeying every injunction.*

CAREFUL RECORDS

You should have no confidence in the experience of men who do not write out faithfully all the symptoms of the patient treated, and note carefully the remedy, and how given. Especially is this necessary in patients likely to need a second prescription.

The physician who has in his case-book the notes of every illness of his patients has wonderful hold of any community. He has the old symptoms and the remedies noted that cured, and he can make indirect inquiry after after all the old symptoms long ago removed.

The pleasure is not small found in consulting such a note-book.

Experience soon leads the close prescriber to note all the peculiar symptoms and to omit the nondescript wanderings indulged in by sick people; however. it is important to be correct in judgment.

Many physicians make a correct first prescription and the patient does well and cheers up for a while, but finally the test is made for the second and then all is lost. Homœopathy is nothing if not true and, if true, the greatest accuracy of detail and method should be followed. It is fortunate that the physicians who repeat while the remedy is acting are such poor prescribers or their death-list would be enormous.

THE SIMILIMUM

I had supposed that this question had been settled, but it seems I am not informed, as many are saying the only thing necessary is to find the name of an agent capable of causing similar symptoms on the healthy and the similimum is that agent, I cannot accept that as the teaching of the master.

These perverters of truth claim that the self-same agent will cure in any dose or any potency. My statement is that similimum, the curative power or force, is not essentially the curative drug. The similimum may be found in Aconite 200th where Aconite 3x has failed. Then Aconite is the curative agent but not the similimum, but Aconite 200 is the similimum. When Aconite tincure cures, and cures permanently, I believe it does so because it is the similimum. I have recently seen Arsenicum 200 fail in a case so clearly indicating Arsen, that a tyro could not fail to see it, and the same 200 is known to be genuine and had for years served well; the 10m cured promptly. The remedy was Arsenicum, but the similimum was Arsenicum 10m. I have seen this same Ars. 10m cure when the 3x, 6x, 30, 60, and 200 had failed.

Then the stimulation must be the curative power and not the name of any given drug. I may conclude that Ars. is the remedy and the case is not cured. I must next choose a suitable potency and as suitably refrain from its repetition. The smallest part of the conclusion has been wrought when the name of the curative agent has been decided. I admit it is seldom necessary to be so exclusive in finding the curative power, but that it does sometimes occur I am more than convinced. A friendly doctor said to me a few days ago in my office that he was curing a case of psoriasis with Ars. 3x. He stated that the patient had been taking it off and on for a year, and that when he stopped the medicine the disease seemed to come back. Nothing can be learned about such a case, as there was no clear statement of the facts in the case. But it is much more satisfactory to use a very high attenuation of any drug believed to represent the curative powers in a single dose. It is the safest and surest way to avoid a mistake. If the remedy acts, it is so permanent and almost sure to be similimum. If it does not act, there is no harm done and a lower potency may be selected. If a lower potency is selected and repeated, as often has to be, the over action spoils the case and sometimes precludes the possibility of a cure. If the remedy is homœopathic to a given totality, a single dose very high may cure the whole case; if, however, it seems necessary to repeat, and the disease only disappears while the remedy is being repeated the selection is a bad one and had better be changed.

This knowledge we gain while using a high potency if a given case leads us slowly but surely in the way of success.

It is a grand mistake to fly to a low power because a

high has failed to act, yet it may be tried as a manner of convincing man of his own weakness.

The similimum is the curative power that every true healer is in search of, and I take it for granted that every physician in his heart is searching for truth. Then it must appear to all unprejudiced minds that the name of a drug is no more the curative power than the name of a disease is the disease to be cured. As any given disease has an individuality in causes of varied intensity so will its cure be in antagonism of varied intensity. One drop of Aconite root may cure the Aconite mental picture in one person and fail signally in many, and the 200 cure the case in a few hours. I would not say may, unless I had seen the work.

I had once under my care a patient whose symptoms were like those of Sulphur. As I had not advanced in knowledge beyond the 6x, I gave that remedy in the potency named with what seemed to me astonishing relief. Finally, Sulph. 6x failed to give the continued relief, although the agent (for it was not a remedy) was continuously repeated. I compared Sulph. with the patient, and Sulph. seemed still indicated, but it would not cure, I must change.

I changed and changed, and finally the patient changed, I spoiled my case, and felt like "cussing" somebody for it. Nobody to blame but myself. Some three years later this patient finding nobody that could do any better than I had done, bad as it was, came back to me, and by the way I had changed I had opened my eyes, this patient had taken my crude drugs, but I then knew how to develop a case and cure it. He took Nux 2m for a few weeks with improvement, but the same old burning on top of head and soles, the same II a. m. hungry stomach; the same itching, and the same "not very well myself" all there. These symptoms had never met similimum.

The famous Sulph. 55m one single dose and S. L. made astounding changes that lasted for nearly two months, when the returning symptoms were the signal for another dose. Three doses cured the case permanently. Sulph. 55m was the similimum. Sulph. 6x was therefore not the similimum. Sulph. was his remedy but the attenuation was next to be chosen. Why is this not true of any agent in the materia medica? There is nothing new in these facts, but it seems so strange that there can be found a man with brains too small to comprehend it or too dishonest to own it or too skeptical to believe it.

The microcephalic panderers to the loud-mouthed ignoramuses are seeming to rule the world by their mighty majority, but pure Homœopathy has continued to grow and will continue to grow, and the educated, thinking people of the world will support it just as rapidly as they are made acquainted with it. No man shall tie me down to the limits of a microscope or to his own narrow sphere of observation or accepted truth. The man that remains in the lower strata of potential similimums and demands that everybody worship with him is too narrow to be called a healer or a benefactor of man.

The similimum may be found in the lowest attenuations, but is positively found for all curable diseases in the high and highest genuine potencies.

THE STUDY OF OUR MATERIA MEDICA

The artist studies his model until he feels the lines and shadows, and in his mind sees the image on canvas or carved in stone. He builds a model and carves in granite the similar. The student of our *Materia Medica* must study a proving until he feels the image of the totality of sick feelings of all the provers as if he had proved this remedy and felt all the morbid feelings of the provers.

The doctor that prescribes for symptoms as they look

on paper fails to feel the weight of responsibility of the true healer. The physician that first places all the morbid feelings of his patient on paper and then ponders over that complexity of symptoms until he feels and sees what that patient suffers, and next searches the *Materia Medica* till he finds the same image, will be able to cure the sick as Hahnemann did. This gives him the sphere of sicknesses either produced by disease or by drugs. This sphere is an important feature of the study of cure and sick-making causes. Through this study we discover the sphere of action of Aconite as it differs from Sulph., of Belladonna as it differs from Calcarea, of the natural successors, complements and inimicals. We may study pathology until the dawn of the twentieth century, and it may not reveal what we need in the art of healing the sick, but the careful study of each picture of sensations may reveal to the student and artist the sphere of medicinal powers and curative possibilities.

Some may study much longer than others to reach this mastery of a drug image, but study will bring out the picture in time. There are drugs that are largely proved, yet so badly proved that the true image has never been brought out. This is generally the case when man has meddled with the statements of the simple-minded lay provers. The language of nature cannot be interfered with if the proving is expected to be a guide to the cure of our fellow-man. Modern provings are commonly a farce and will not lead to the elevation that Hahnemann's remedies sustain. The old masters knew how to do it, they were governed by the principles of the Master, they were governed by the philosophy, and their provings will stand and forever be safe guides to the cure of all animals and man.

The wrangle between the material and the immaterial philosophers may end in some good; both sides have truth, but to some extent perverted. Both sides evade the facts that oppose their own methods of reasoning, and their own conclusions. Some will not accept a cure as a fact, because it was made with an infinitesmal medicine. Some will not accept a proving because it has been made with infinitesimal doses. The actions of such men do not change the facts that exist, but they do retard the study of *our Materia Medica*. A proving that was made under my own eye, under the proper rules for proving, demonstrated most clearly that real symptoms were produced by the 10 millionth potency of Lachesis. I had heretofore not believed it possible to procure symptoms from this potency. The prover did not know what the dose was that she took. She brought out one symptom as perfectly new, and it might be doubted as a genuine Lachesis symptom, but the fact that I had discovered the symptom several years before clinically, and confirmed it and verified it. Such a symptom the prover did bring out; and such a symptom known to belong to the drug, and that in the very high numbers, removed all doubt in my mind of the possibility of procuring symptoms in such high numbers.

This prover was not in perfect health, I am willing to say in answer to the proper question. She was a very nervous person, extremely sensitive, and a subject of many nervous symptoms. This must of course greatly impair the value of the proving in the eyes of many. A singular fact that I want fully stated here, is, the symptoms of the prover were entirely new and ran their course as an acute miasm should have done, completely subduing all the symptoms peculiar to the prover (with exceptions mentioned), and when the proving or drug symptoms departed, all her old symptoms came back. This shows that she was not proving a similar, that it was not a Homœopathic aggravation, but that it was a genuine proving. The proving of Lachesis was so clear that Dr. B. Fincke and Dr. P. P. Wells have made remarks on it to the effect that there can be no doubt about the genuineness of the proving. That the proving suspended the old symptoms of the prover is the proper thing, and what is constantly observed when scarlet fever or measles or small pox run their course; and as all know the symptoms come back after the acute disease has run its course. It may be gleaned that a proving may suppress a given sickness. That is just what happened in this most wonderful proving, and is just what happens in some of our best provings. If this be true, it must refute the idea that no value can attach to provings on persons not perfectly healthy. No one denies that healthy men and women are the proper provers, neither is it true that provings on sick persons may not have a high value.

Another grand lesson is found in the proving, viz.; that highly dynamized medicines are capable of suppressing the symptoms of natural diseases, and implanting themselves instead. Another warning to the beginner, that he may not be too hasty in giving medicine to sensitive, nervous patients.

In presenting this proving, as it comes from the pen of the prover, it is my purpose only to say for it, it must stand or fall on its own worth as a proving made to throw light on the great pathogenesis of Lachesis.

LACHESIS

Mrs. H. W. A.—Proving of Lachesis 10m. Beginning February 14, 1887. A very nervous little woman who has never been very sick, but always very sensitive to surrounding atmosphere, so that she proves every thing she breathes.

February 14th—Took a few pellets dry on tongue, 1:30 p. m. Head felt better in a little while. Soon felt a severe, heavy, ache in both thighs as though they would come off or break. Slight amelioration by morning. Felt warm blood circulating in legs and feet; from knees down, are usually cold. Felt happy and jolly, in spite of severe aching. Could not stand as usual during shopping. Upper arms began to ache, 3 p. m., left worst. Pain in legs diminished, as pain in arms increased; could not carry a small parcel. Left arm *aggravated* by hanging. Left arm *ameliorated* by resting in coat. Aching moved upward to the shoulder, as though arm would drop out. Aching extending under scapula. Subsided into an *uneasy* ache after 5 p. m. Weight diminished. Was told I look *pale*. During evening had to rest the *left* leg on chair, and take off the shoe. Elevation relieved the leg, but *left* arm began to ache. Aching pain again went under scapula and *posterior left lung*. Could not lie on right side because of drawing sensation around the heart. Lying on left side *agg.* pain in arm, shoulder, lung and heart. Wondered if I would have heart disease, as my mother died of atrophy of the heart. Restless and suffocated all night.

February 16th—Could not study or give due attention. Heart ached and would stop breath as though it would palpitate, but it did not. Went to sleep that night listening to the beating in head and ears synchronous with heart beat.

February 17th—Aching of entire left side from crest of illium to first rib. Aching under both scapulae, *left* the worst. Upper arm so heavy could hardly raise it. Sensation in arm as if it were pulled. Intense aching between heart and scapulæ, and was afraid to stir or breathe, and would raise and lower the shoulder to get relief. Slight palpitation and pain in apex.

February 18th—Pain in apex followed by palpitation. Afraid some one would see and speak of the anxiety. Could hardly hold anything, would slip out of my hands. Feared the increasing palpitation which aroused me frequently in the night. Dreamed of riding in a strong wind which took my breath. Dreamed of riding on horseback. Going swiftly through the air gave me a sinking

28

feeling in the stomach and left thorax. Waked holding my breath. Desire to unfasten dress from sternum to waist line. Could not study in evening, hated everything, books, paper, pencil, lectures; and medicine. Felt like squirming; has often come on since I began taking the drug. Afraid to go to sleep after retiring; put hand on heart to watch its beating. Could rest comfortably upon *left* side, with hand upon heart; so slept.

February 19th—During shopping, at noon, felt weak and sinking, from heart to stomach. Palpitation during lecture, 2 p. m. Kept moving about in chair. Sore under left scapula. Pressure of chair back caused palpitation, followed by cough. Could breathe better in open air, so took a long walk. Heart seemed to stop beating, then made extra exertion. Attacks of palpitation until 11 p. m. causing hacking cough each time.

February 20th—Slept well all night. *Dreams,*—toward morning dreamed I was almost dead with heart disease, but did not wish my friends to know of it. Was in a crowd; was suffocated and feet so cold, like walking on ice. Wished to get in the air, but trying to get through the crowd caused palpitation. Thought my body had become mottled like a snake skin; thought it would be soon on my face, so that I could not go in company any more. Did not know why this was, but it was a punishment which I would understand in another world. Desired time to die to come quickly, for my heart ached so that I could not be happy; neither make my friends happy. Slight palpitation on rising. Increased so that I could not walk after 11 a. m. Tried heating by grate, no relief. Palpitation every few minutes so that I coughed, could not talk or laugh, must have dress unbuttoned. Aching all through left thorax, a dragging sensation. Frequent pain in second intercostal, seemed to pull inwards and down. (A creamy leucorrhoea on rising in morning, after sitting. Pain boring inwards in right occiput; old symptoms. Leucorrhœa, light green. Red sand in urine, adheres to sides of vessel, menses closed with pus-like discharge.

February 20th—*Sixth Day.*— Burning in right ear and last upper molar. Tooth sore; felt as though it set in an ulcer. Must dry and warm the feet every hour or so. Palpitation in stomach after eating.

February 21st—*Seventh Day*—Violent palpitation while dressing; voice trembled so I could not talk. Great weakness of lower extremities. Then of upper arms. Was asked if I had mental anxiety because the face showed so much anguish. Was unusually happy *unless talking*, which caused palpitation. 10 a. m.; Violent throbbing of arteries supplying abdominal viscera, left side, extending into the rectum. Quick rapid beating, causing change of position. Nerve of the left leg seems to be twitching, throbbing. Wake with coldness, which causes me to crawl down in bed to warm and sleep. 5 a. m.; Sleep, dreams of pure white calf and cow. Waked in slight perspiration. Coldness continues until 11 a. m. and the cough comes on. (An old symptom now worse, K.) Must warm the feet. Stool irregular for a week, requires great effort, though small. Anus protrudes like cushion before pieces are passed. Try several times to appease the unfinished sensation. Must push tissues back, smarting long time after stool. Cough pains in left side abdomen and from perineum upwards. Copious leucorrhœa at stool or during any exertion. Back-ache relieved by passing hot creamy slightly stringy discharge—faint acrid odor. This flow often relieves knot-like feeling of left ovary; old symptoms. No appetite for breakfast or lunch because of throbbing in heart and left side. Eat well at 6 p. m. Burning in stomach. Cold water nauseates. Can feel cold water all through the abdomen. Hands burn. Veins in hands so distended must hold them up to get relief. Cold morning. First day that have felt like study this winter.

This dose did not produce left sided sore throat. Ulcerated odor from stomach. 4:30 a. m.; for week have awakened cold and sensation of squirming. Coldness over heart, stomach, back. Flesh is cold. Amel. by moving about. Awake at 6 a. m. in slight perspiration. Sweat again p. m. Odor slightly of garlic. Frequently must arise at 5 a. m. to relieve backache by urinating. Old symptoms more prominent since taking the dose. Scarcely noticed before, (Kent).

February 28th—*Fourteenth Day*—Frequent quivering aching. Extensor proprius pollicis lame, nearly let me fall when standing on tip-toe. Aching in hypogastrium and inguinal region. Pain in uterus, going upward, while leaning forward. Burning in different spots of the body. Can spell correctly but not form letters rapidly, mix words. Feel quite happy. Smell of turpentine caused distress in lumbar region, extending downward and forward into ovarian and hypogastric region, like dysmenorrhoea.

March 1st—Cold feet, a. m. Felt lame and sweat while heating them offensive (subjective). Left upper arm cold, as if ice were upon it. Very sleepy, heavy eyelids. Waked early, with terrible distress in bowels and stomach. Followed by much flatus. Diarrhoea at 7 a. m.; watery, leaving burning and tenesmus in rectum for several hours. Left arm cold. Hands very hot and swollen. Burning in stomach after breakfast. Throbbing in left thorax and abdomen. Leucorrhoea better, catarrh worse. Pain in right fibula.

March 3rd—*Twentieth Day*—Slept better waked unrefreshed. Dreamed of birds and animals. Dreamed I was dying of dropsy from kidney disease. That water was collecting about the heart. Headache. Pain in back of head. Golden flashes above the eyes on closing them. Discouraged. That those despised who knew me best and had lost confidence in me. Felt that none understood my motive, which is good. Have lost the power to exert any influence. Am so tired that I fail in all undertakings. The physical and spiritual will not harmonize. Longing to break the tie that binds the spiritual to the physical. The influence of evil is uppermost. Morbid tendency to decide that wrong is right. Realize this only after it is committed, then feel crushed. Cannot rise above it. When alone the mortification of such mistakes nearly drives me wild. Cry for help and receive mockery. Lost all consolation so long derived from the unnumbered words of my mother. These griefs *agg.* by mental efforts to rise above them causing me to despise myself. Remorse, followed by tears. No strength of will to do desperate deeds. In moments of self-forgetfulness duties are performed with surprising ease and success. Self-consciousness that cannot be overcome. Grief at committing actions which at the time seem proper, but afterward seem improper. Grief crowds all else out of mind.

March 4th—*Twenty-first Day*—Chilly a. m. and p. m. Went to bed to get warm. Hot spot on vertex and over eyes. Cant think, forehead too tight. Heat from vertex into throat and back of neck.

March 5th—Awoke 2 a. m. troubled dream, crowding thoughts. Tried to study, but old impressions crowded the subject out. After lengthened effort broke into tears and dropped asleep. Awoke at 4 a. m., cold, aching back, relieved by micturition. Slept, waked later tired and discouraged. Distress in lower abdomen from running to take street car at 10 a. m. Nearly fainted over the simple operation of reducing a hernia (reducible). First time in four years. Slept p. m. Waking, arms felt like limbs of trees, numb. Stomach, over which arms are crossed, greatly distressed. Distress going downward to the uterus. Arms folded across stomach causes distress. Taste of blood, because of bloody mucus from posterior nares. Offensive perspiration. Several nights when going to sleep, have felt the bed was floating, as it seemed in childhood.

March 21st—Deep yellow, mucous stool sinking into the bottom of vessel; watery, with floating white particles upon the top, like rice. 3 p. m. Great bearing down in the rectum, as though it would protrude. Stool at 8 p. m. So hungry and thirsty, ate soft part of raw oysters, which seemed to satisfy. Relief from the throbbing of heart, which has endured for a week.

March 22nd—Slept well; *dreams natural. Dreamed* that on preparing for lectures, could not hurry. There was such soreness and gone feeling in the stomach. Back of head ached. No motion of bowels. First evacuation of urine, thick, deep orange color; unsatisfied feeling, causing burning and smarting of parts. Cold from knees down, ankle aches. But little of the burning and smarting, sensation (scalded) of mouth and stomach, present yesterday. A. M.; bloody mucus from left lung. Weak in attempting to walk. Yesterday, while standing for the first time at foot of bed, felt very tall and bed looked small. Felt three feet taller than usual. Toast, raw oysters and "cambric tea" seem to suit. Crave sour things, which for two years have *agg.* my bowels, so also salt. Blisters in mouth, on lips, under nose, disappearing. As eager as a thirsty child for a glass of water. Small moulded stool covered with mucus; feel better.

March 26th—Mournful, dreamy state of mind, as though something very sad were transpiring, took Lach., 9m.

March 29th—Cold, sweaty feet when not near a grate, a. m. Walked a long distance in p. m. 4 p. m.; pain in or over right kidney caused by desire to urinate. Followed by distressing sickened feeling in stomach. Pain went from stomach to left heel, then up the leg, ending in dull ache. Numbness in great and second toes, *left,* as though something pressed from the end. Same symptom occurs in bed. Wake in night with urgent desire to urinate, pain in *right* kidney. Feet warm and feel swollen.

Inclination to sweat after returning to the bed, especially when surfaces come in contact. Tossing until day-break, then slept. Most comfortable lying upon the stomach. Tired when called to get up. Fall asleep on the pillow, but if waked will slip the head off and roll on the stomach. Burning sensation from vertex to last dorsal vertebra. Perspiration just before sleep turn on back to make it warm. Perspiration musty and old, as at one time during the ague; when I would wake in night with profuse sweat, making me sick at stomach.

March 30th—Left toes numb. While packing, cramping in hypogastrium. Occasional pains from left of cervical vertebra to right, to left elbow. Heat in forehead. Eyes sensitive to heat. Left heel feels as though ice were pressing upon it. Uneasiness and fullness in kidneys before urinating. Urine profuse and colorless. Bowels feel insecure as from impending diarrhoea. Weight in rectum from long standing. Frequent pains in back opposite lower end of sternum. Itching over whole body after sitting a long time. An eruption size of small pea sometimes festered always sore and itching. Feel if I could break constriction in the forehead, could reason clearer and think more deeply.

April 6th—Itching in roof of mouth and base of tongue; must rub it. At times burning and pricking on the edge of tongue, agg. by smell of tobacco or turpentine. All gone feeling in stomach amel, by eating. Slow urination, especially after waiting. Sweat middle of night, or after first sleep. Throat feels full. Mouth feels sore. Agg. of the burning in mouth and stomach by salt. Dyspnoea agg. by slightest exertion. Constriction of the throat, as if something tight were about it. Coughing at night caused by itching in left side of throat, extending to ear. Amel, by warmth of hand. Hands puffy and often very warm. Sweat followed by chill (caused by dampness of clothes) ; then heat, then sleep. Fourth toe joint sore upon under side. Moved to first toe and thought it would be a bunion. So sleepy at 8 p. m. am obliged to retire. Right foot and leg feels large, warm and heavy. Left foot and leg feels small, numb and cold. Quivering in both ears when lying down at night, at times relieved by change of position. Aching back of both ears. Aching a little above the apex of heart. (Soreness about the edge of mammary gland before menstruation, Old Symptom.) Throbbing in left side. Slight pain in left ovarian region, sometimes both sides, and then in hypogastrium. During past two weeks swelling induration and smarting of the ducts of sublingual glands. Relieved. Feeling of prolapsed rectum, only relieved by lying on the stomach. Top of head sore and hot. Throat burns and feels raw. Lungs dry and tight. No expectoration after long coughing. Burning smarting with itching.

April 7th—Constipation; feces hard, bleeding from rectum. Feels like cut after stool. Bearing down in rectum, long time after evacuation. Gray spots drop in front of left eye while reading. Caused blur and nervousness. Agg. by looking to the left. *Amel.* by continuing to read. Mouth sore; herpes, lower lip, right side.

April 8th—Numbness extending from lumbar region to lower extremities after long walk. Menses p. m. Bloating in epigastrium. Sensation of an opening in abdomen from umbilicus down; *i. e.,* upon either side of bladder. Bladder distended, cold, before menses. Also aching in left arm, thoracic and abdominal cavities. Crawling sensation for several nights, in anus after retiring. Severe aching in left leg, first four hours of catamenia.

April 9th—Waked from sound sleep by severe colic, followed by loose stool, dark almost green. During stool cold and prostrated. *Amel,* by stool. Weak before menses, had gushing, hot milky-white leucorrhoea. (At cessation of menses, continuous itching above the coccyx; worse at night. Has been customary for several months, Old Symptom.)

April 10th—Twitching in first finger (left) extending through tendons to wrist. Back of neck so weak that must have a high back chair. Catarrh in head better. Two attacks of coughing; 4 p. m. Repeated 2d day. Can't cough deep enough. Smarting and itching either side of trachea into ears. Cannot recall unfamiliar easy subjects. So sleepy by 7 p. m. am obliged to retire but am wakeful for some time after lying down. Before and during menses, sweat at least exertion. From thighs upward warm, sweaty and suffocating. From above the knees downward, cold necessitates a warm iron. Cramping in left great toe before the menses. Worse in bed at night. Worse in turning from back to right side. Crawling sensation under seat of cold sore. In various places when tired. Same sensation would appear as a spot before eyes, during the blind headaches of my childhood, 16-20 years.

April 12th—Extreme pleasure causes trembling and twitching for hours, more than would severe fright or sudden surprise. That and mental exertion caused wakefulness until midnight. Waked very early. Annoyed by sudden loss of subject of sentence, in attempts to speak. Effort to hold an idea until it can be expressed. Expression or the real effort, drives subject matter quite out of mind. Aching in occiput, extending to cervical vertebrae. Same pain extending down the arm when walking or upon receiving a jar.

April 18th—Constant desire to lie down, can think better. An hour's study and strength gives way. Pain in occiput, neck and eyes feel cold, head hot. *Ameliorated* by warming feet. *Ameliorated* by lying down, finally. *Ameliorated* by open air. Such an anxious feeling to be strong and think quickly. Became quickly exhausted. Long for physical strength. Sleep until 4:30 a. m. Awaked refreshed, but work of the day before engrosses me to that extent, that when I rise, am already tired. Desire to lie down again after breakfast. Tired feeling from forehead downward and backward through cervical region. Many times obliged to give up writing and throw myself on the bed.

THE STUDY OF PROVINGS

It is nearly useless to cram students with the language of provings. If they cannot be made to see the clinical image to be met, they fail to make good prescribers. The student needs to know something of what we do, and what can be done with provings. Dry study of provings without application to clinical images, will not do for the neophyte.

Rarely do we find a student with sufficient acumen to formulate these images for himself; so, after puzzling over them for a time, he falls to grumbling over the imperfections of the Materia Medica, sometimes even, making fruitless efforts to correct the imperfections. Imperfections do exist, and some of them are fully recognized by good men, but how they are to be corrected is not so well known, even by the best men of today. Dr. Hughes has demonstrated that he thought he knew how to correct those imperfections, but he has failed to demonstrate satisfactorily to the profession, that he knew even one remedy.

There is no short road to a fair knowledge of therapeutics.

The physician who masters the use of the repertory, usually makes the most rapid prescriber.

The symptoms that are in the way, are the ones we do not understand. Suppose each egotist were to throw out all symptoms he does not understand, what portion of the Materia Medica should we have left? Hahnemann made most wonderful use of the Materia Medica that he left us; we ought to do as well as he, with the many added provings, but if we tear down, we should be quite positive that the building would not result in improvement. The best symptoms of the Materia Medica have come, and must come, from the provings of potentized drugs. Throw away all such symptoms and we shall be compelled to practice medicine upon the thrown away Materia Medica, for the portion left and accepted, will not sustain the law for universal application. This is demonstrated by the fact that those crying for crude provings, constantly confess their inability to cure the sick. The very cry for a revised Materia Medica is an ample confession. The use of quinine, whiskey, and compounds, testify loudly in the same direction. The grumblers never recognize the possibility of the difficulty being a personal one, nor think of their confession as the guilty pleading of their own lack of knowledge of the Materia Medica and how to use it. A confession of the inability to use the Materia Medica as it stands, is not a qualification necessary to the erudition of a compiler of a new Materia Medica. They have confessed, we have not accused. The confessions extend so far, there is little left for them to learn pertaining to cures. The most startling confession recently made, the assertion that the 30th and 200th potencies do not make symptoms (!) but has a negative result; either the doctor did not select sensitive persons, or he refused to recognize symptoms.

Not all provers bring out symptoms from potencies, but the sensitive ones furnish symptoms of inestimable value. If the physician makes a careful study of his willing provers, he will be able to select for them, such remedies as they can get symptoms from, i. e., by studying the natural traits of their life, he can see their weaknesses and make use of them. A lady expressed a wish to prove drug, she was carefully observed, and thought to be sensitive to Phosphorus. She proved the drug in a high potency, confirming many old symptoms of Phosphorus about which she knew nothing, neither did she know the name of the drug she was proving.

These facts stand, nor do they become less than facts when other doctors fail to obtain symptoms the same way.

It is grievous to demonstrate one's inability to find a remedy fitting to subjects, for the purpose of proving, after making numerous trials. It means something. It means failure. Not of the law, not of the potentized drug, not of the patient or prover, but of the physician. He knew not how to select provers or remedies for provers, therefore he is become an agnostic. The chemist says to a friendly physician: "I hear you have become a Homœopath?"

Physician: "Yes, that is true."

Chemist: "Well, you do not mean to say you believe in the 30th potency, do you."

Physician: "I understand you are a chemist, that you make a living by your knowledge of chemistry, and that your science is based upon the hypothesis of molecules and atoms, etc."

Chemist: "Yes, I am a chemist by profession."

Physician: "Well, now my friend, have you ever seen a molecule or atom?"

Chemist: "Let's go; we'll have a bottle of wine."

The chemist knows the molecule is not very well determined, that it is entirely hypothetical, but he does not care so that he produces the results that previous experiments enable him to expect. The results are not changed, even though the molecule be argued out and not believed in. Facts stand in spite of unbelief.

THE SYMPTOMS AND ASPECTS OF SUCH CASES AS PRESENT AN UNFAVORABLE VIEW AND CAUSE AN UNFAVORABLE PROGNOSIS

The difference between a symptom complex and a symptom image is partly a question of knowing from training and partly from experience. To one who knows the totality as written out it may mean a clear symptom image and a sure index to a remedy the patient needs, which generally goes with a prediction of speedy recovery. To one who lacks training and experience the totality as written out is a complex of symptoms that means chaos. As one gains knowledge by training, reading, and experience, the symptom complex is less common until he is capable almost at a glance of saying of some cases ever so carefully taken that the whole case has the stamp of complexity. Yet some of these after much study will reveal the image in the totality, and it can be seen what is the remedy, but it must be known of any case that so long as it is chaos, just so long a favorable prognosis is to be withheld.

In this great question there is ample room for artistic perception and judgment to manifest themselves, but there are scientific rules to be followed which constitute the foundation of art and experience. The beginner who has been properly taught may soon be able to judge of the relative magnitude of a given record of symptoms and know to which class it belongs.

There is more to be learned about diagnosis and prognosis by studying the complex of symptoms than by any form of physical examination, but both and all methods of investigation should be used, as they confirm each other, and often where one is defective the other is strong and helpful.

To know symptoms in cause, beginning, purport, direction, and ending is only that acquaintance with sickness so often urged by Hahnemann. To distinguish the symptoms that are natural or common to fixed morbid states should be the earliest acquirement of the physician in order that he may learn to discover what is queer and unaccountable.

To distinguish an incongruous symptom complex can

scarcely be expected until one is able to say what is required in any symptom totality to constitute it harmonious.

Experienced homœopathic observers know very well that the burning, stinging, enlarged glands, infiltration, hardness of the part, weakness, loss of flesh, in a scirrhus of a mamma will not lead to a remedy that will act curatively; also that oedema of extremities, weakness, albumen in urine and heart symptoms, dyspnoea and anxiety furnish no basis for a remedy for the patient. All know that remedies given on such symptoms are only expected to comfort, and will not restrain the progress of disease nor very much prolong life.

All know that the above manifestations are the representatives of the sickness that ultimated upon the patient, but do not signify or show forth the signs and symptoms of the patient. The particulars of the disease are there, which are the common symptoms, but the generals and particulars of the patient are left out. Now it matters not whether these generals and particulars are masked, suppressed by previous drugging or never existed, except in the ancestry of the patient. They must be discovered in any case or a favorable prognosis cannot be declared. It simply sums up by distinguishing from well settled evidence what is order from what is disorder.

It is not to be doubted that sickness may appear in order or disorder. Many or most sicknesses will appear in an orderly form if permitted to do so. The acute sicknesses all have order so that we are able to declare their course and termination. Many chronic sicknesses present a form of order which is well known to observers. The order so far as knowable is a guide to distinguish that which represents the disease from that which represents the patient. The hysterical patient presents an incongruous symptom complex that always deceives the neophyte. It seems natural to gather all those queer, incongruous

uctuations, imaginations and sensations and prescribe
or them. Who has not done just this thing? Who has
ot had his lingering cases over which he has toiled for
months, while the patient improved in no manner, and
he friends wondered if the doctor was ever to be of any
se? When one has learned the nature of the hysteria
e sees that he has been trying to fit the remedy to the
ysteria and not to the patient. The writer has been
sked to prescribe for such cases many times when the
ymptomatology was beautifully presented, where the
ysteria was there in all of its richest neurological exag-
eration, but not an idea could be drawn from it to por-
ay the state of the patient. Such a case remains incur-
ble until the symptoms that stand for the patient are
lso known. These generally are found, if they are discov-
red to be changes of desires and aversions, loves and
ates. These are most difficult to secure, as every hysteri-
l patient conceals her real loves and hates, and relates
uch as are not true of her; hence it requires the skill
nd power of an experienced strong mind, which cannot be
eceived, to question her when she has lost her guard.
his case is incurable until the case can be taken in a
anner to present what is true of the patient. It is always
ue that what is predicted of the disease is easy to secure,
ut what is predicted of the patient comes out under dif-
culties by cross-examination or by accident and prolonged
bservation.

Let it not be supposed that the symptoms that are
redicted of the disease are to be ignored or considered
alueless in selecting the remedy, but they are to be con-
dered subsequently to the symptoms that are predicted
f the patient; and it has often occurred that a remedy
as made brilliant cures when it suited the patient, even
hough it was not known to possess a strong likeness of
he disease; but let the likeness be first to the patient and

last to the disease. The patient is first and the disease is last. It is like initiation, direction and termination.

In the prospective phthisical patient we see a patient with few symptoms of the patient himself, but weakness, loss of flesh, anaemia, coldness, tired from all exertion, bad reaction, easily disturbed by eating, drinking, exposure, loss of sleep and weather changes. These states are common to so many remedies that it will at once be seen that the patient is not represented and no promise can be made, though there is no sign of tubercles. A favorable prognosis must be withheld until a series of carefully selected remedies has been used and the symptoms that represent the patient begin to appear, such as mental symptoms and other generals too well known to need description. There is enough to be told about this subject to convince any one who thinks with his head that a knowledge of diagnosis and prognosis is not limited to the traditional doctor, as is claimed. Indeed the most of these quasi-learned class investigate with their heels, like the mule, instead of with their heads; i. e., they go about things to kick them into pieces and not to know them. They do not love truth for the sake of truth.

There are three conclusions to be put into axioms:

First. When there are tissue changes with no symptoms to represent the state of disorder in the economy.

Second. When there is a complex confusion of particulars and no generals.

Third. It does not follow that the patient must die because the symptoms are such as to persuade the physician to withhold a favorable prognosis. It may only mean a lingering sickness.

THE TREND OF THOUGHT NECESSARY FOR THE COMPREHENSION AND RETENTION OF HOMŒOPATHY

It is important to avoid thought destructive to the fundamental principles of Homœopathy. I desire to have

my friends shun some things leading away from Hahnemann's thoughts. True Homœopathy is the object of this
association; to maintain the thought and trend of Hahnemann's reasoning. As long as I have practiced there has
been no inducement to depart from his doctrines. He
used the 30th potency and said certain classes of cases were
incurable,—those that had been drugged and disorders
thereby suppressed. However, the experience of past
years, added to thirty years of personal experience in prescribing and study, has revealed that these cases can be
cured by use of higher potencies, without departing from
the trend of Hahnemann's instructions. The tendency to
depart from Hahnemann's methods is the largest danger of
pupils today.

For illustration, suppose a case appears with hip-joint
disease or tending toward it. Following the plan of
Boenninghausen of studying the case to find a remedy by
consideration, 1st, of the part effected; 2nd, the symptoms
of the part; 3rd, the modalities of those symptoms; and
4th, the concomitants; where will it lead? This patient
with hip joint trouble thinks of that as the affection to
be eradicated, and the doctor thinks from that in search
for a remedy. You will perceive that this is the opposite
of considering the patient. That is not following Hahnemann who says that the sole duty of the physician is to
heal the patient, and taught how to do this by sketching
the image of the patient in the totality of characteristic
symptoms. He never recommended concomitants of a part
affected. Concomitants cannot come into consideration
except as in connection with an objective condition. Study
the patient and everything of the patient. If you do not
grasp this you do not receive Hahnemann's idea of training the patient. I would urge you to shun concomitants
as it leads away from the idea emphasized by Hahnemann.

The hip-joint patient has pain in the knee, perhaps
some trouble in the uterus, or headache which is said to be

29

due to constipation. To what is the constipation due? Perhaps they had not thought of that. Which are the concomitants? By thus centralizing on a part of the body you fail to grasp Hahnemann's thought which is essential to the existence of Homœopathy. With the thoughts centered on a thing in one part of the body, then on the concomitants and then the modalities, as recommended in the preface of Boenninghausen, you are led far away from the trend of Hahnemann, and Homœopathy is destroyed by such methods. If that method were successful, I would not oppose it; but it is not in line with Hahnemann's methods,—it does not lead to the charcteristic symptoms of the case. What you want is to be led easily, simply, to that which characterizes the patient.

If you do not work with this aim you stray from the idea of going from center to circumference and go to the other idea. It must be from center to circumference always, from first to last, from things prior to things ultimate. I have thought along this line for twenty-five years, and must make it most forcible in maintaining the idea of Homœopathy.

1. The center of man is his loves. When the loves go wrong he is sick in his will, the very center. This we find in dealing with those who threaten to destroy their own life or the life of another. A faithful, noble wife has no fault to find with her husband in her natural life, but finds herself with an aversion to him, does not want him to touch her. This is a symptom of the innermost of man, it is not on a par with the skin and the toe-nails. According to the other plan, this is only a concomitant. Love of things is not always all in the brain. Cravings for things for acids, for sweets, etc., are expressions of the patient's loves, but must be expressed through the stomach. In the loves which are affected and are different from the normal, you have a description of his sick self. Tempera-

ments which are natural demand no consideration. Hering introduced temperaments into the Materia Medica, but temperaments are not in the provings. Morbid changes of the mind are the basis of the prescription. Proceeding toward the circumference, work on those remedies related to the disordered affections first. Any remedy not in this group cannot cure.

2. The second point of consideration in the study of the patient is the intellectual functions, the reasoning faculties. As many remedies suited to disturbances of the affections are found also to have intellectual disturbances, you proceed next to consult those related to the intellectual disturbances and may thus eliminate a few more remedies. Among symptoms related to the affections, also those related to the intellect, some are common, less important than those more rare. Consult the most important, those most strange, first.

3. Memory disturbances come next in order in the mind but in study are less important. The lists of remedies are so long that you will seldom eliminate many remedies from those of the preceding lists. Memory disturbances are the most common of mind symptoms.

4. Next to the mental symptoms in importance are the physical generals. The physical generals cannot be cured with remedies that do not have the mental conditions. The physical generals are those things which can be predicted of the bodily condition in its entirety. First of these to be considered is the patient's relation to heat and cold. He may be very warm, desiring cool things, cool air, cool applications, cool food and light clothing; or he may want heat, cannot be too warm. He may be so cold that there is lack of vital heat. Now what has this to do with the hip-joint, the kidneys, the liver, the stomach or the uterus? Nothing, yet these things relate to the man as a unit. They are general in their application to his entire bodily

condition. His desire for motion or rest is the next important physical general. Perhaps he cannot keep quiet, never comfortable unless he is walking. At the same time his shoulder may be more painful on motion of that part; working the arm from the shoulder, and all that relates to that part, may be worse from motion. The patient is better when walking, but the shoulder is worse from motion. It would be foolish to start with the part to try to see the patient himself. Many remedies have the modalities of the part differing from those of the patient. Take first the things first; the patient is first before his parts. Again you may have the patient himself worse from motions, and all his aches and pains worse from motion. How he is affected by the air is another physical general. He may be better or worse in the open air. If the patient is a woman, her menstruation must be considered. This is not particular,—menstruation is a function of the body, and she will say that she is worse or better during menstruation, or worse just before or just after menstruation. The patient as a unit may be worse or better after eating; himself all over may be better or worse after the rectal evacuation, better after stool; these are important generals of the body. Two things run through the conditions, and must be distinguished, the bodily conditions which are aggravated from various modalities, and the particular aggravations from them.

Among the conditions relating to the bodily condition are weakness, pallor, and, frequently, the color of discharges when the color is due to a condition which represents the loves. As the blood is, so is the love. The color of the discharge expresses the condition of the blood when there is a deterioriation which renders them greenish. The greenish color to discharges from the vagina, as in cancer, represents the condition of the blood. A laudable condition of the discharge is common. When a symptom is common to all or to many remedies it is not important. Hahnemann's emphasis is upon the symptoms strange, rare, and peculiar. These are most important. The common symptoms in each group are left until the last in the symptoms of the affections, of the intellect, of the memory and of the physical generals. These are all generals. We go first to the generals and then to the particulars, proceeding from center to circumference. You may have a long list of symptoms that would baffle a strong mentality in a man, without an idea of order. In a case without symptoms of the affections, no intellectual symptoms, no physical generals, with only a long list of particulars, what can you do? When a patient is properly examined and all is reduced to writing, then, as Hahnemann says, the greater part of the work is accomplished.

When a case is properly taken, with all these symptoms brought out, it is easy to work it out to a small list of remedies. It is not a short cut,—there is no such thing as a short cut. It is the proper way, working from center to circumference of the man himself.

When you come to the physical generals perhaps only one in the list of mental symptoms is worse from heat. Then what need you care about the particulars? You have the man himself, and the particulars will take care of themselves. As the affections are, so is the man, extending from center to circumference. When you know his affections you know what trend is taken.

5. Then we come to the particulars,—the thing for which the patient comes to be treated. Referring again to the hip-joint case, perhaps none of these remedies now are found in the hip-joint list, which was the point from which you would start by the other plan. Most cases of hip-joint disorder cured by me in the past twenty-five years were cured by remedies not in the hip-joint list. This list contains those remedies that have been observed

to cure hip-joint cases, but this remedy with which I cure a patient who has hip-joint trouble may not cure another hip-joint case; hence it is not in the list, nor is it included as a clinical symptom.

A man with a rectal ulcer was advised to be operated on to relieve the copious hemorrhages from the rectum. He was urged to consult me before having an operation. I found a persistent mental symptom was the need of intense restraint to prevent himself from destroying his own life. Natrum Sul. had this symptom, but has no rectal ulcer recorded. A few other symptoms present, together with this strong mental symptom, led to the use of Nat. Sul. and he had no more hemorrhages.

When you come to investigate the particulars, if you have a half-dozen remedies left over, proceed on through all the particulars. In this hip-joint case, you may have also liver affection, and all circumstances belonging to these symptoms must be considered, though they are classed as concomitants by the other method. Starting with these particulars, which is the concomitant? Working out the case on that plan, you may work out to an entirely different list of remedies for the different particulars, but they are in the same patient. By beginning the investigation in relation to the patient, you may find none of the particulars in the remedy selected, but the remedy cures the patient, and the particulars disappear.

A doctor brought a patient to me for consultation one cold Winter day, saying he had tried for a long time and failed to benefit him. The most troublesome symptom was a dry, hacking cough for which he had prescribed Arsenicum. He said the young man had been steadily emaciating, and he thought I might help him. I looked at the young man and noticed he had no overcoat on though it was very cold weather. Asking him why he wore no overcoat, I found that he was never chilly, but wanted the cold air, felt better in the open air, wanted to walk and work rapidly, had been emaciating for some time, and had this dry, hacking cough. I asked the doctor why he did not give him Lycopodium as that fitted the patient and the patient was clearly of the opposite type to Arsenicum. Lycopodium stopped his cough and he increased in weight and was cured.

I started out to follow the Bœnninghausen plan but it did not cure the patients. You can give different remedies in succession without holding to any one, and after years, the patient is no better, they are not curing the patient. Very sensitive patients should not be given too high a potency. For oversensitives it is best to begin not higher than 1m. This can be repeated two, or sometimes three times, and then a higher potency used. Each potency can be used two or three times with benefit. Sometimes he will need to begin again at the lowest potency and go through the series. Thus you will perhaps cure the patient without change of remedy.

Failure of best success with the Bœnninghausen plan led me to study Hahnemann's teachings more closely. This dawned on me twenty-five years ago and I have been practicing it all these years. Starting with the patient, as above outlined, we find in each group many remedies to be eliminated because they are not related to the patient. This is especially true in the particulars. Remedies will seldom be found in the lists of all the particulars; you must omit some, but be certain to omit the particulars and not the generals. The least important are to be omitted. Start with the most important, proceed to the less and less important, on to the least important. If you do not follow this plan, you work in a helter-skelter way and are led to confusion.

A patient comes with something to be cured. That is usually not the thing to begin with, for you must get at the thing that is at the bottom. Each one must use his own method of eliciting the symptoms. There is a tendency among those working in modern scientific falsities to have remedies for pathological tissue changes to cover the results of disorder. Although it may not be known to fit the pathology, if it is the patient, the remedy will cure the patient. By becoming expert in this method you can do wonderful things. You must recognize that the loves and thoughts extend through the body; they are not only in the brain. Man thinks with the fingers, the eyes and the skin. The volitional system extends throughout the body. You will find the patient himself has a lack of vital heat yet the suffering part is aggravated by heat; the patient is cold but the part is aggravated by heat. The things of his affections are represented in his physical loves, and he says he does not like this or that. These things are close to the patient, close to his vital loves; they express the patient.

By the Bœnninghausen method, there is no opportunity to distinguish between the patient and the particulars. This method has retarded the development of Homœopathy. It has obscured Hahnemann's Homœopathy, based on the idea of the patient first and the focusing the observation on things strange, rare and peculiar. These do not relate to the particulars (the part affected). You will cure inflammation of any part when guided by the symptoms of the patient, whether the remedy thus selected has produced that sort of inflammation or not.

There prevails a tendency to say that one is sick because the liver or the stomach or the uterus is disordered. One patient will visit a gynecologist, to be told that all her troubles are due to the disorder of the uterus, and a course of local treatment will make this in order and then she will be well. The local treatment does not improve the patient, and she consults a spinal specialist who tells her

the troubles are due to the spine, and treatment to cure
that will restore her to health. Then the eyes are examined. Yes, says the oculist, all the troubles are due to
errors of refraction; a change of glasses will improve her
condition. Next the heart specialist is consulted, with the
assurance that correction of the heart trouble will make
her well.

None of them had directed any attention to the
patient, but the condition of the patient was said to be due
to her organs. The man himself is prior to his organs,
more interior than his organs. The condition of the organs
is the result of disorder more interiorly. It is necessary
to proceed from first to last, from things beginning to
things ending, to grasp the idea of Homœopathy. I have
seen results of treatment in my cases that few have seen,
and this is the reason. Long experience results in expert
facility in perceiving symptoms and surmising what has
preceded them, in leading the patient to reveal what is
there without asking leading questions. You can turn the
patient aside and lead him to reveal the very center of the
case. You become expert in the use of the repertory, increasing from year to year, as long as you live. It is a
lifework, a beautiful work, worth living to perform.

In the woman the menstrual symptoms, of all particulars, are nearest to the generals; they are close to the
life of the woman. Sexual symptoms, especially desires
and aversions, are analogous to loves and aversions. Discrimination of the value of particulars is important. It
is a question for meditation to determine how closely the
symptoms of a part pertain to the generals. Symptoms
occuring in many parts are more general than those of
only one part as illustrated by discharges of similar character from several parts. The condition of the blood is
analogous to the loves. Few remedies have recorded the
condition of the blood, that it will not coagulate, but it is

a high grade symptom. It is common for blood to clot, and rare for it not to clot.

There have been many criticisms for this use of the term generals, but it is the best word that meets the needs. The idea is that of systematic dominating from center to circumference. It is Hahnemann's system ultimated to a more scientific basis. The discoverer and founder comprehended without much thought and study. There are many difficulties to be explained. For their explanation it is necessary to study Homœopathy, and then study man. Holding these things in the memory, we meditate upon it all, then decide that it is good, and employ it in use. The result delights you, and you love it. Thus it extends more interiorly and cannot be forgotten. You love Homœopathy, as you apply it, and, as the love is, so is the life. It is in you and part of you if you love it; you are a vessel of the truth. It grows and expands a million fold, extending out from the interior. We proceed from center to circumference, perceive how men are sick harmoniously from center to extremities. If this philosophy is not in the life, and only in the memory, it is not a part of you—it is only with you. If something comes up to delight you more, it can be laid off. Nothing can come to delight you more than Homœopathy if it is in you and part of you.

There was once a poor man crippled and sick, an artist, whom several of us thought should have an opportunity. I gave him some medicine, and told him if he was better when that was used he need not return. We united, several of us, and paid out much money to keep this man at Paris for several years. Long afterward he returned with a gift that he had made, chiseled from marble, a beautiful piece of work. I said to him that his work differed from mine,—it was very beautiful but returned no response, while the poor crippled dishevelled man whom I was able to restore, returned in gratitude and warmth of vigorous life. His cold marble, crude and rough in the beginning, was only a cold, unresponsive object after all his work was expended upon it.

THE TREND OF THOUGHT NECESSARY TO THE APPLICATION OF THE HOMŒOPATHIC MATERIA MEDICA,

or

A RATIONAL USE OF CURATIVE AGENTS

It is not of the material stone, earth, ore quartz and mineral salts; nor is it the colors of plants, leaves, buds and flowers; nor of stems and stalks; nor of the chemical and physical properties of animal substances used, and the natural eye to behold, *that one should think.*

It is not the density of the platinum, or the whiteness of the aluminum, or the yellowness of gold, or the toxic nature of arsenic that one must turn his thoughts.

Think of the nutritive wheat, corn and barley used for foods, and then of the deadly aconite, belladonna and fox-glove; and while thinking of one group as nutritive, and one of the other as poisonous, we make no progress. But when we observe that they all grow and thrive in the same atmosphere and in the same soil and by reflection remember that one builds up and the other destroys man, *i. e.,* one builds up the physical body and the other disorders and destroys the vital force of man, can we but conclude that there is some primitive substance, too subtle to see with the external eye, that becomes the medium of power? This is the field of action and causes.

These substances of the three kingdoms must be examined, *i. e.,* they must be looked into by the internal eye, and the quality of each must be ascertained.

This does not mean that the internal surfaces of crystal forms must be examined with lenses. Neither the interior of man, nor living plants, nor the so-called dead, earth elements have ever approximated the visual realm of external man. But the vital test brings a response from the lowest and most inanimate elements as speedily as from the most poisonous plant or most venomous serpent virus, when *circumstances* have turned disordered life into the delicate degrees of susceptibility necessary to the homœopathic conjunction and affinity. To behold the interior of nature with the interior eye, the understanding must have long training and the purpose must be for the use of man; when an apparent *sacrifice* is a work of love one may see, when men and women devote life and property to science simply to benefit the human race. This may be disputed, but only by the unenlightened, who know not the dreadful sacrifices made by the provers of septic poisons, serpent viruses, specific substances and poisonous drugs.

The abstract vital force is, to the untrained understanding, unthinkable, and as all internal examinations are upon this plane, then it must follow that a preparatory training *must* precede the actual examination of the internal qualities of the three kingdoms.

It is not generally known that the three kingdoms exist, as to their interior, in the image of man. Neither is it generally understood what it is to exist in the image of man. It is not even known what man is, nor what the plant kingdom is, and much less what the mineral kingdom is. If all these statements related to geology, botany and anatomy, they could be presumptuous, as these sciences are highly cultivated, but they treat of the kingdoms only as to their exterior or material relation. The internal qualities have been left for the homœopathist, and such an exploration is within the province of homœopathics.

To discover that man, as to his will and understanding, is capable of extremes, requires only that one shall examine our statesmen, our professional men, our scientists, and then the lowest types in civilized countries and cities. To examine original tribes would not reveal the growth possible to the human race, nor the degradation reached by fallen man. The human race at its highest plane of development is only man. No matter what attainments, what expansion, we see but the possibilities, the capabilities and nobility of man. He is but man and as such is but the image of his Creator. Rise as he may, he does so only within himself, and at his highest he is but himself, and even that is borrowed. So much as he has fallen below this highest point of the human race, and of any man, has he failed to reach his own individual possibilities, or fallen into degradation, so much is he but an image of himself, of man. When he is but the image of himself he profanes himself, and likewise man, and how much more so must he profane God. Look at the animal faces in the degraded streets of our great cities. We see but the degraded forms of man. Disobedience, sin and sorrow have brought depravity, and the souls within revel in hatred and crime as much as they will in the land beyond. *This* is not the *real* man whom we see. It is but an image of what each one might be, but *it is* the real of such beings. A misspent life can here be contrasted with the life of usefulness, and the life of hatred with the life of orderly love.

In one *all* to hate, and in the other *all* to love.

In the one despised, in the other beloved.

The one, then, is man with his love for the degrees of uses; the other but an image with his hatred of uses.

In man is heaven; in his image is hell.

The fullness of man is but his capacity for growth as a receptacle for love, wisdom and use.

The image of man is hatred, ignorance, and to be cared for by local protectors and penitentiaries.

Independence contrasted with dependence.

Freedom contrasted with bondage.

Inconceivable gradations exist between these ex-

no disease
that doesn't
have ·
coverage
in nature

tremes. These varying shades of changes in man come by
inheritance, vocation, opportunity, disease and drugs.

There are no changes possible in man that cannot be
produced, caused and aggravated by drugs. Man's diseases
have their likenesses in the substances that make up the
three kingdoms. Man himself is a microcosm of the elements of the earth. The earthy elements strive to rise,
and do rise through the vegetable kingdom into man, and
they strive to equal man; but, as they are not permitted
to do so, they appear to degrade man they they may ap-
proximate him. Every element and creature below man in
the created universe seeks to degrade man, which, however, is only an appearance, by exercising such an influence, as will elevate itself at man's expense, as if
through jealousy.

We see this emerald quality on all sides. Man's every
inferior seeks to belittle him, and in every gradation down
through to the lump of aluminous clay we see the tendency
to lift up itself by depressing the interior of man in order
to make him a brute. So we see that man, with his depressing load, may rise within and become a glory or sink
and become a brute. Even his external form in time resembles the face of an animal, but not until long after his
internals have assumed the disposition of that brute which
he in face most resembles. He grows Godlike in proportion
to his struggle against his inherent evils, i. e., his loves
mould his face and figure into the image of his real life.

The study of man as to his nature, as to his life, as
to his affections, underlies the true study of Homœopathics. Whether we study him in the cradle of innocence,
in the hieroglyphics of Egyptian sandstone, in the cunie-
forms of Assyrian clay, in the sculptor's marble, on
ancient and modern canvas, in Grecian architecture, in the
vocations and trades of modern and recent progress, in
the electrical telegraph, in the ships at sea or the mighty
system of railroads that span the landed universe, we are

but viewing the growth, action and qualities of this one, sole object of our attention, viz., man. When we have reached the highest that is of man, and know him in all that he is and can be, then may we begin to study all the gradations down to the lowest image.

Man may be a physician to his equals and inferiors but he cannot know his superiors in a manner to fully grasp the expanse of that great and glowing vital furnace that melts the metal to fill the moulds of human exigencies. Then the physician must rise to the pinnacle of man's growth; perceive his changes, even to the lowest degradation. The physician must rise above bigotry, prejudice and intolerance that he may see that in man which will furnish the basis of comparison.

A rational doctrine of therapeutics begins with the study of the changes wrought in man. We may never ascertain causes, but we may observe changes. A physician highly trained in the art of observation becomes classical in arranging what he observes. It will be hardly disputed that the changes in man's nature, without an ideal natural man, would not be thinkable. Whether we observe the changes wrought in man through his own will, through disease, or through drug provings upon the registration page, we have but one record to translate, viz., that of changes wherein man has in all cases been the figure operated upon. The record of changes in the abstract is nothing. But when we see in that record the speech of nature, we then see the image or effigy of a human being.

Hahnemann emphasized the symptoms of the mind, hence we see how clearly the master comprehended the importance of the direction of symptoms; the more interior first, the mind, the exterior last, the physical or bodily symptoms.

SUMMARIZE.

Man.

Disease in general.

Disease in particular.

Remedies in general.

Remedies in particular.

The only possible way to conform to the above trend of thought and thereby establish a system of therapeutics, is by proving drugs as Hahnemann taught. We may now see clearly what is to be understood by proving drugs, and we may define it as that conjunction of the given drug force with the vital force of man, whereby a given drug has wrought its impression upon man in a manner to make changes in his vital order, so that his sensations, mental operations and functions of organs are disturbed. When a large enough number of provers have registered sensations, mental changes and disturbed functions so that it may be said of a drug that it has affected changes *in every organ* and *part of man* and *his mental faculties*, then may it be said that it has been proved; not that all of its symptoms must be brought out, but it has been proved sufficiently for us. In other words, its image has been established. It is then known what there is in man that through its conjunction has been brought out. When this particular perfect image of man has been observed fully by a rational physician, the nature of the sickness that this drug is capable of curing may be fully perceived. The danger of using drugs whose properties are known only as related to a single organ must now appear, as drug is curative, or is a remedy, only because it is capable of producing symptoms on the entire man similar to such symptoms as the man is capable of having. The remedy finds its place in man and develops its own nature; but if it has not in it that which can rise up and so impress man, it could not be capable of developing these symptoms. Man's image is therefore in all elements of plant and earth, and when that susceptibility exists in man then the proving may be wrought; but if that corresponding image is not in man at the time, then man is proof against the drug, except in increasing and larger doses. Such provings exclusively are not desired, as they only impress a single organ with gross symptoms which are so unlike natural disease that a rational physician sees not therein the image of man, and stumbles into the grosser observation of artificial sickness, and is led to the ultimates, viz., pathological anatomy, rather than a rational study of the Materia Medica. Many of our provings are wonderfully defective for the above reason. Hahnemann's remedies will stand forever, as they are well-rounded provings from many degrees of strength in drugs and susceptibility.

The examination of an epidemic is in all nothing but the consideration of a similar number of provers. The steps from the whole group to individuals are in all cases the same. The case is as follows: When a given epidemic, or endemic, comes upon the land, as many cases, most carefully written out, as can be gathered, are to be arranged in the Hahnemannian scheme, all symptoms under regional headings, so that prevailing disease *may be viewed collectively*, as a *unit*, or, *as the image of a man*, or as though one man had suffered from all the symptoms observed. The same course applied to a large group of provers will bring the totality of the symptoms before the view as though one man had felt and recorded all the symptoms obtained, and the image of man may be then seen in the totality of the symptoms of the scheme. The particular or individual study in the epidemic cannot be properly made until the symptoms are studied collectively, and in this kind of study is the same as after a proving has been arranged in schematic form in order to ascertain what other remedies and diseases are like it—diseases as to their symptom image, and not morbid anatomy—the same as to remedies as to their symptom image. In this there can be no theory nor theorizing. The record of symptoms is to be considered either in natural disease or in the proving of a drug to ascertain so far as possible all

30

the remedies that are, in general, similar throughout, in their fullness, to this one now under study. Books have been so arranged. *Bell* on *Diarrhoea* is but an anemnesis of all there is of that prevailing disease, and so must every single case, either in mind or on paper, be presented. Here we see the series to work out our cases by. Every epidemic and every man sick must be so wrought out; first the general and the particular; remember that the particulars are always within the generals. Great mistakes may come *from going too deeply into particulars before the generals are settled.* An army of soldiers without the line of officers could not be but a mob; such a mob of confusion is our materia medica to the man who has not the command.

Hahnemann was not able to manage psora until he had completed his long and arduous labors which ended in the anemnesis of psora. After he had gathered from a large number of psoric patients all the symptoms in order to bring before his mind the image of psoric man, he was able to perceive that its likeness was in sulphur, *et al.* Boenninghausen arranged the anemnesis of sycosis which has been perfected by recent observers. The anemnesis of syphilis must be arranged in this same way by every physician before he can treat it successfully. By this means we may settle in a measure the miasmatic groups. The vast labor that Hahnemann put upon psora, before he discovered that this was the only way, shows how difficult it is to bring before the mind the full image of a prevailing disease. It is many times more difficult to solve the problem and find the similar remedy in isolated diseases and uncommon acute diseases. Boenninghausen's *Repertory of Chronic Diseases* (never translated), is arranged on this plan with symptoms and remedies graded. An experienced eye glances over the repertory and arranges in his mind the anemnesis by singling out the remedies that are suitable to the general image of the disease that he has fully mastered. The expert prescriber has fixed in his mind the image of the sick man before he takes up a book or thinks of a remedy. He masters the sickness before he asks himself what is its likeness.

We must avoid the confusion of mind that often comes from thinking in the old way, not knowing what to call disease, and what to consider as only results of disease. When advocating the above principle, I was once asked how to go about an anemnesis for epilepsy, for Bright's disease, diabetes and other so-called diseases that have been arranged by old nosology. It must be first understood that these so-called diseases are not disease as the homœopathist thinks, but the results of diseases known as miasms. Psora, syphilis and sycosis are the chronic miasms to be arranged in schematic form, and the arrangement in such form includes all the symptoms of each of the three. Thus we have a foundation to build upon, and all curable cases, if properly studied, will be cured before they become structural. An attempt to arrange a schema for disease results could only fail, as the group worked at is but fragmentary.

A practical illustration comes to us at once when we think of Hahnemann's prevision, inasmuch as he was able to say that Cholera resembles *Cuprum, Camphora* and *Veratrum.* This he saw in the general view. When La Grippe comes the natural course to pursue by him who follows Hahnemann will be to write out carefully, as in one schema, the symptoms of twenty cases, more or less, the more the better, and then, after careful consideration *by the aid of repertories,* make a full anemnesis of all remedies, and the ones showing a strong relation throughout will be the group that will be found to draw from in curing the epidemic. Only occasionally will the physician need to step outside of this group. But no man can predict which one of this group will be required for any single case. But, in time of such hurry, when a large number of

sick people must be visited in a day, the physician knowing the constitution of his patrons, much time may be
gained in selecting for each sick person, from this group,
the remedy he needs. In a large proportion of the cases,
the remedy will be found in this group. One will suffer
with strange symptoms corresponding to the characteristics of one of the remedies in this group, and another
will show forth the demand in like manner for another.
As there are no two sick people alike, thus no two persons
will give forth an identical display of peculiar symptoms.
Though several persons may need the same remedy, each
one of the several persons must call for the remedy by
virtue of the symptoms peculiar to himself. When all of
these features are properly understood, it will be clear
to the mind how it is that every prover contributes his
portion to the grand image that makes the disease likeness into the image of man.

Now, as like causes produce like effects, and as the
causes of natural sicknesses have never been discovered,
we can only reason from the effects of natural causes as
we reason from artificial causes.

The teaching of Hahnemann, in the Sixteenth Section of the *Organon*, is to the effect that the vital principle cannot be assailed by other than dynamic agencies,
or spirit-like agencies. This must be accepted as true. To
prove that it is not true would require us to prove that
scarlet fever, measles, small-pox, and in fact all acute in-
fections and contagious diseases do assail the economy by
other than spirit-like means.

With all the instruments of the *scientific* school of
medicine, with every effort and ambition, no progress has
been made by them to establish their material hypothesis.
Therefore Hahnemann's statement must stand as true.

The more dynamic, the greater resemblance to the life
force and *vice versa*. The septic virus is dynamic because
it has been vitalized or dynamized in nature's laboratory.

It is a product of life operating upon matter, and the most dynamical toxics are animal ferments and ptomaines; no matter how concentrated they exist in a highly dynamic form.

The fluids and substances, ferments, ptomaines, etc., are the viruses, are the dynamic causes of fixed diseases; they are the causes of bacteria in all forms. It is not argued that the miscrosopical bacterium may not convey the fluid dynamic substances upon its body as perfectly to the detriment and hardship of men as a fly, a dog, or an elephant may. Fluids containing bacteria of well-known disease producing character may be diluted until the bacteria is no longer found, and that fluid is just as active in its power to reproduce its own kind of sickness as when it was surcharged with microscopical animalculæ. Of course there is a difference—the susceptibility must be present in diluted virus, while any person may become ill from the concentrated ferment applied to any abrasion or injected hypodermically.

This condition once understood, the Materia Medica prover is prepared to consider the difference between the proving of drugs in full strength and in potentized form. But as there are no bacteria in drugs, and as they are as potent sick-makers as ferments, when properly selected, it will be seen at once that it is not due to the bacteria in the concentrated virus, but to the virus itself. It is the life force of aconite, of silica, of virus of septic fluid, and not bacteria that makes man sick.

The susceptible prover catches the disease that flows into him when he proves Cuprum the same as the person who catches cholera when he becomes infected by the dynamis of cholera. He cannot protect himself—or the vital force cannot resist the deranging influence of cholera any better than it can resist Cuprum—If he is susceptible. If he is not susceptible to cholera, he cannot take cholera; if he is not susceptible to Cuprum, he cannot prove Cup-

rum. But, by increasing the quantity or by changing the
quality into quantity, of either, he may, without susceptibility, become sick, but it is not then in the same manner
or course as that of natural contagion. Natural contagion
and infection are only possible through the susceptibility
of man to the noxious cause.

The doctrine seems to be essential to the perfect understanding of the image of man in drugs and diseases.
When man has lost his equilibrium, so that he is not
protected against deleterious influences, he is but an image
of man, as man, in the order of his existence, cannot be
assailed by any of the spirit substances that pervade the
atmosphere in which he lives. Even if influenced by concentrated artificial sick-making causes, he does not suffer
from the fully developed image of the disease, as when
susceptible, unless he is kept under the influence a long
time, as is the case in alcholic, opium, arsenic and hash-
eesh subjects. When momentarily affected he soon reacts
and becomes himself.

Reflect upon the mental state of the man who has
used alcoholic stimulants in great excess for many years.
His manhood is gone, he is a constitutional liar, and will
deceive in any manner in order to obtain whiskey. It may
truly be said he is but an image of his former self, and
much more an image of what he might have been. This
is no exception. Indeed, every drug is capable of rising in
its own peculiar way and making such changes in man as
will identify itself in the image of man. There is no disease that has not its correspondence in the three kingdoms.

It is the physician's duty to know that every proved
drug contains the image of man, and the likeness of the
disease and diseases it can cure. To be able to see a drug
in its totality, to see its symptoms collectively as it assumes the human form—not the body, but the character of

the man, or his image—must be the end in view in order to use the Materia Medica for the healing of the nations.

TO ALL HOMŒOPATHS

"If you give quinine, go on with it; if you give an opiate, go on with it; do not go back into Homœopathy. The man who does these things is a homœopathic failure. Some men are incapable of grasping the homœopathic doctrines, and fall back into mongrelism which is a cross between Homœopathy and allopathy. I would prefer an allopath to one who professes to be a homœopath but does not know enough Homœopathy to practice it. . . . If a doctor has not the grit to withstand the cries of the family, the criticisms of the friends, the threatening of his pocketbook and of his bread and butter, he will not practice Homœopathy very long. An honest man does not fear these things. There is but one thing for him to consider: "What is the right thing to do in this case?" . . .

The attitude of the public must never furnish the physician with indications as to what he shall do. . . . But the doctor who will flinch and tremble at every threatening is one who will violate his conscience; is one that can be bought; can be hired to do anything; . . . becomes a coward and a sneak; is ready to do almost anything that is vicious and cowardly, and will abandon his colors in time of emergency. . . . The doctor who violates the law also violates his conscience, and his death is worse than the death of the patient."

THE VIEW FOR SUCCESSFUL PRESCRIBING

The success of prescribing depends upon the view taken of the totality of the symptoms. The view of any given totality affords the indifferent or the marked success of any given prescription.

The grasp of the symptoms, in part or as a whole, is firm or lax in accordance with the view taken of the parts and the whole collection of symptoms. What else can be understood by the image of any case expressed in symptoms?

To be able to view the totality of symptoms so that the most similar remedy will appear to the mind is the aim of all healing artists. As the view varies, so varies the success.

The examination of the patient is always made in accordance with the view of the totality the physician is in the habit of taking. Some can never learn to examine a patient so that the symptoms, when written out, will have the form required for a review. Any successful prescriber would know by the reading the totality what is lacking to make up an image. But let us now suppose that the case has been properly taken, and that it is a full, well rounded case, with all the various symptoms that belong to perfect case-taking.

One will view such a case from its pathology, or from its probable pathology.

Another will view it from the temperature, color of hair and eyes, or what star he was born under.

Another will view it from the keynotes he can find in it.

Another takes the usually set phrases of the patient with the opinions and wordings of tradition, or the opinions of some previous physician.

In such a manner, a distorted view of the whole case is formed.

Again, it is observed that the totality contains an alternating image, or one set of symptoms one time and a different set another time. The prescriber's view may be formed from one group today, and from another after the change has come, which leads to change of remedy with every shift; but at the end of the year the patient has grown steadily worse. Yet he has cured (?) each group of symptoms to his and his patient's satisfaction. Such work is a failure from the imperfect view had of the whole case. He fails to view the patient from the totality of the symptoms: from all the symptoms.

Removing symptoms may not restore health to the

*patient. Curing the patient will remove the symptoms
and restore his health* (ORGANON § 8).

We have assumed that the symptoms have been well
taken, and therefore the view of the case is possible, which
must be, of the symptoms which represent the patient as
a whole; the symptoms that represent all the organs and
parts; all the symptoms and conditions and circumstances
of the organs and parts; all the pathology of the organs
and parts; age, sex, habits and business.

Suppose the symptoms to be viewed come directly
from the patient, what can be seen, heard from the patient
and companions,—all are presented without interruption.
One reader will ignore all but the pathology; another will
notice only the keynotes; another will notice only the diagnostic symptoms. In each instance, something is ignored
or neglected; or, at least, the view of the case is absent.

Hahnemann's teaching has never been improved upon.
We must be guided by the symptoms that are strange,
rare, and peculiar. How shall we do this?

By first fixing in mind what symptoms are *common*,
then it will be easy to discover what symptoms are *uncommon*, or, in other words, strange, rare, and peculiar.

Common symptoms are such as are pathognomonic of
diseases and of pathology, and such as are common to
many remedies and are found in large rubrics in our repertories; e. g., constipation; nausea; irritability; delirium·
weeping; weakness; trembling; chill; fever; sweat.

When such symptoms have taken their places in any
given case, it will be seen at once that what remains must
be uncommon, therefore peculiar and, as such, are always
predicated of the patient as a whole, and of his parts in
particular.

However, some of these common symptoms may become peculiar where their circumstances are peculiar; e. g.,
trembling at any time or at all times all over the body and
the limbs is a strong and most troublesome symptom, but

it is not peculiar nor uncommon. But trembling *before a storm*, or *during stool*, or *before menses*, or *during urination*, is rare and strange.

Weakness is also common if constant, but it comes only *before menses*, or *before stool*, or *during a storm*, it is at once quite uncommon, and changes the view of the case.

Chilliness, if constant, is common to many people, and is a strong common general as it is predicted of the whole patient, but if it comes only *before* or *during menses*, *before* or *during stool*, or *while urinating*, or only *when in bed in the night*, or only *while eating*,—then it is strange and peculiar, or uncommon.

All of these are common to no disease known to medicine, hence they become striking and help to form *a view* of any given totality.

It must now be seen that the physician who has in mind only the pathology as a basis for his prescription has only what is most common, and therefore has no view of the totality, and therefore violates the first principles of prescribing. He prescribes for results, for endings, and not for things first, not for causes.

It must be known that the symptoms that exist in childhood, and such as were present before any pathology existed, are the corresponding symptoms of causes, as all causes are continuous into effects. They are not causes, but they represent causes, and often are all that can be known of causes, and they furnish a view of the case from causes to endings; from causes to ultimates: to pathology. It is important to discover early these symptoms in any chronic sickness. The symptoms through childhood down to the present describe the progress of the sickness. These give an experienced physician a good view of the case, with its probable endings or pathology.

It is well to have all such results in view, but these ultimate symptoms are of the least value, and without the

fullest representation in symptoms they are of no value as
showing forth the view of the case by which to find the
remedy.   But a physician must have a good and full
knowledge of all these, as well as of anatomy and physiology, or he will not have the basis for good judgment, and
hence will form a distorted view of the totality.

The symptoms that represent the patient as a whole
are of great, and often of the greatest value, especially
such as are expressed in the patient's own speech.

The mental symptoms, composed of his reasoning
powers, loves and hates, and memory.

And then his general bodily symptoms and their circumstances, such as worse from cold, from warmth of
every kind, from weather, wet and dry, from motion or
rest, time of day, etc.   These are of highest importance
when they apply to the whole body.

Two sets of aggravations and ameliorations must come
into view, viz: those that apply to the whole being and
those that apply to his parts.   These are often the opposite
in parts or organs from what they are in general bodily
states of the patient, and must be looked up in the repertory in sections that relate to the part mentioned.

A woman consulted me for a violent rheumatic pain in
the shoulder. She came into my office with her arm bound
to her side to prevent moving the arm, as the motion of
the arm increased the pain in the shoulder, yet the patient
walked the floor constantly to ameliorate the pain in that
painful shoulder. The pain in the shoulder was worse before a storm. DULCAMARA cured at once. This shows how
a part may have an opposite modality from the whole body.

Nothing has harmed our cause more than books that
generalize modalities, viz: by making a certain aggravation or amelioration fit all parts as well as the general
bodily states. Cold air may aggravate the patient but
ameliorate the headache. Stooping seldom aggravates
headache, backache, cough and vertigo in the same degree,

yet Bœnninghausen compels you to look in one place for all of them, and they are marked with the same gradings.

The patient is often better by motion, but his parts, if inflamed, are worse from motion.

Lying aggravates backache, headache, and respiration in different degrees, and the patient in still another manner. If each symptom is not inspected, and considered with a view to its own circumstance, the result will be widely different. Parts are better by heat when the patient is better from cold, and vice versa. The headache is better from cold, and the body is better by heat.

If we do not consider these circumstances, we do injustice to the patient and his parts. Therefore the circumstances that relate to the general bodily states and the circumstances that relate to the parts and organs must be vastly changed.

Ever so perfect an understanding of the pathology and pathological symptoms in a given case gives no view of the case for homœopathic prescribing. The common symptoms, without the peculiar symptoms, may give a good understanding of a given case except for prescribing. Common symptoms alone will lead to failure of the prescription. We might as well attempt to prescribe for nervous dyspepsia, gastritis, jaundice, gall-stone colic, enteritis, constipation, or a bilious temperament. The beginner often fails because he has secured only the common symptoms.

The symptoms of the organs and parts taken by themselves give an imperfect or one-sided view of the case. They fail to give the symptoms of the patient in such a form as to present a perfect view. There is something lacking. Many cases coming for advice express the particulars, and fail to give the symptoms that characterize the patient. This must be one of the most frequent causes of failure with the young physician.

This can be illustrated by the study of discharges.

Discharges are common to inflamed mucous membranes of ear, nose, throat, trachea, vagina, etc., and as such each is only a particular, but the part or the inflammation does not cause it to be green, bloody or viscid. Therefore this must be due to some change in the whole economy which makes it general, and increases the value of the symptom from common to peculiar, and therefore changes the view of the case. Laudable discharges are natural and common. Therefore, let me repeat that if the part is inflamed there will be discharge, but that does not cause the *color*.

So it is with blood when it is fluid and fails to clot; it is peculiar.

The symptoms that characterize the whole mental and bodily states sometimes present such a *view* that the remedy may be seen at once; again, all the foregoing classes of symptoms are necessary to furnish a *view* of the past and present. When such a complete view presents itself, the prescription becomes easy.

If prescribing is to be made easy, it is to be done by securing such a perfect view of the *whole case* as would be expressed by saying that "The sole basis of the homœopathic prescription is the totality of morbid signs and symptoms," as Hahnemann taught so many years ago. It will be seen, therefore, that carelessness in taking the symptoms, as well as in *viewing* the symptoms after they are noted, must lead to indifferent results. Remember that it is not the totality of the symptoms taken by a careless or ignorant physician that constitutes the basis of a homœopathic prescription, but the totality of all the symptoms the patient has.

With menses too late or suppressed or scanty, the patient weeping, with aversion to fats, nausea, vomiting, weight after eating, the young man will say Pulsatilla at once; but wait a moment. The patient is very chilly, likes the house, never needs the open window, is worse from motion, wants to keep very quiet; now you change your mind

and give her Cyclamen. Or, if she is better in motion and
in open air, and craves it, and is too warm, then Pulsatilla.

The physician cannot be careless, and cure as Hahneman did.

WHAT IS HOMŒOPATHY?

This is a very broad one, and hence its answer cannot
be limited or contracted. To say that Homœopathy is based
upon the law of *similars* is but the bounding of a cone
by describing its base and leaving its apex undiscovered
and projecting into space; to say the least, the answer is
unsatisfactory. When similars are mentioned, the novice
immediately wonders what similars are referred to, and
how are given similars related to each other. It is simple
to affirm that similars nullify each other, and it is easy
to demonstrate the fact, but other questions arise of
greater importance and much harder to answer—how are
these similars recognized, and how are they utilized to
cure disease?

After hearing the statement that similars nullify each
other, and having accepted the law expressed by the
formula *similia similibus curantur,* what Homœopathy
really is, is yet to be learned. The knowledge comes after
due conversance with disease and drugs. One must acquire knowledge of disease in all its relations to the human
body. One cannot afford to neglect any resource whereby
he can gain information relative to disease. Causes,
morbid anatomy, duration, and course of every disease in
particular must be thoroughly studied. The habits of each
and every fixed disease must be observed to acquire a
knowledge of its true nature. One must be able to predict
from the present what will likely take place in the immediate future. He must also know the sick-making substances and the sicknesses they produce, their course and
duration, beginning and termination. From these the
homœopatist arranges his similars. These are his *media*

through which he develops a knowledge of the art of curing homœopathically. Without a careful and thoughtful study of the two, he can never answer the question which has been selected as the subject for this paper.

If he neglects a part he is ever crippled and in darkness as to the whole or totality. If he neglects to study disease in any of its many sides, he gropes in darkness during his lazy, half-useful life. If he reads morbid anatomy, and attempts to apply remedies by such knowledge, he must live and die with a life filled with numerous failures. The man who reads his symptomatology, as found in drug pathogenses, may do fine work, but he has neglected the half that he should have learned. The human body, the house of both health and sickness, must be searched until familiarity breeds contempt.

Homœopathy is the science of healing based upon the law of similars as a law of selection. To select under this *law,* one must be acquainted wih parts and counterparts, positives and negatives—*similars*—that his *conclusions* may be made by *exclusion,* that he may demonstrate to himself as well that remedies are not indicated, as that the one similar only can conform to the disease in hand; appropriate, because it of all the known medicines is most like unto the disease to be cured. It is well known that many want to be called homœopathic physicians: some desire the appellation who in practice have not this information mentioned above. They are not even acquainted with sick pictures. They only recognize disease in parts, not seeing the whole. These men alternate, or practice, by using a part of the picture of one drug and a part of the picture of another drug to cover the two portions of a supposed disease which they see only in a fragmentary state; not being acquainted with disease in totality, they cannot shape a picture in a single drug to fit any but the fragmentary disease. Only a few days ago one of these men said to me: "I have just prescribed Arsenicum and

Sulphur on the pathology of the case." Being anxious to learn the pathology that furnishes such an infallible guide to these remedies, I made a pressing inquiry, but that which I learned was so vague I am unable to comprehend it.

The study of true pathology should be encouraged, and is essential to the science of Homœopathy, and no homœopathician has ever discouraged it. Pathology is any discourse upon disease; it is broad and all-embracing. The study of disease as manifested through subjective and objective symptoms a study of lesions or results of diseases as made known by physical inspection, etc., etc., down to morbid anatomy, all should be known by the homœopathician, with a full appreciation of the true value of all. The disease in its course, history, and every known manifestation should be considered that the individuality may appear in one grand picture.

Not until this picture, this totality, this individuality, is clear in mind, is grasped completely, can the physician deal with it intelligently; he will then see, in some pathogenesis, a picture with a similar totality and individuality standing out with the same bold relief. Now if he is acquainted with both, and acquainted with the grand law of selection expressed in *similia similibus curantur,* he will administer the medicine possessing in its pathogenesis this likeness to the experienced homœopathician. These are the primary and essential tenets of Homœpathy. The rest of the science is made up of degrees that perfect as they advance, and are qualitative in character and quantitative in appearance. Under these degrees we learn to play upon the strings of a vital harp with a tactus eruditus.

The next advancement deals with dynamization. Many are satisfied with the primary tenets of Homœopathy and want no more. They do not wish further instruction. They do not wish to be made conversant with the fact that all non-surgical diseases are dynamic in character (cause), and must be cured, even are cured *only*, by dynamic effects. They lose confidence in the potency of *Aurum* when it becomes too attentuated to guarantee visible gold, and yet they know that visible gold cannot be appropriated by a living stomach. Dynamic power begins to evolve very low in the scale of potentization, and may be evolved from the crude substance of some drugs. Experience, not philosophy, can satisfy the hungry mind as to the truth of this grandest achievement of the immortal Hahnemann.

When fully convinced that the dynamic power cures, another advancement awaits the student. He is then presented to the mysteries of dealing with automatic forces of living body when influenced by disease. He observes the effect of a dose of potentized medicine selected by the law of similars. It is indeed a small part of his observation to see the patient recover with no medicine but that contained in the dynamized drug. For greater things remain to be seen and studied. The aggravations and ameliorations found in peculiar diseased states are not so simple. The disease that may arise from a single dose of Sulphur in the last stage of phthisis is most astonishing; and the beginner cannot convince himself that the potentized drug was the cause of it. When I say to my class, you must not give Sulph. to the patient in the last stage of consumption, they all look at me in surprise. It is often observed that Phosphorus does great harm to low forms of organic disease. I have several times known a chronic invalid to go on with little suffering for a long time, and with a hope to stay the progress of her disease, administered a single dose of a very high potency of an antipsoric medicine, only to distress her, put her to bed, and from which time her downward course was rapid, while I am convinced that had I avoided antipsorics she would have lived and suffered much longer. If a carefully selected antipsoric aggravates a low form of disease sharply, and

31

the aggravation is protracted and no amelioration of the general condition follow, no more antipsorics should be thought of for that patient; the hope of cure must be abandoned, and short-acting medicines resorted to to palliate. In gout, cancer, phthisis, and organic diseases of this kind generally, the rule holds good. Any physician who has followed the use of high potencies for a considerable time must feel it. Then who can say there is no power developed? Only he who has not found this method of treating the sick. The physician that sees not these aggravations only demonstrates that he has made few or no homœopathic prescriptions. The closer the homœopathic relation between the remedy and disease, providing the disease is of low origin and well advanced, providing the disease incurable, the sharper and more distressing will be the aggravation.

Once a fleshy, robust-looking lady, came into my office for professional aid; she looked so well that I suspected only a slight illness. Finally, a close study of her symptoms revealed the history of rheumatism, endocarditis, suffocation, amenorrhoea of eight months' duration, and great bodily suffering, indeed, I was surprised that she manifested so little of her suffering. I compared her symptoms closely, and found that no remedy but Pulsatilla could correspond to her symptoms. This remedy was administered dry, one small dose, and Sac. Lac. She went home and felt very badly. Pelvic symptoms became marked, and she sent for me. She believed her flow would resume, and I hoped from her report that I had made a homœopathic prescription. But she struggled on and no flow appeared; her pelvic symptoms were such as should accompany her menstrual *nisus*, but greatly intensified. I dare not repeat; success depended upon permitting the remedy to have its own way. She was made comfortable as possible, and I waited on the remedy during this struggle for one or two weeks. The endocarditis then began to show itself with all its terrors, dark blood began to well up from the lungs, which grew worse from day to day, pulmonary oedema became marked, and blood-spitting increased from day to day. I felt that I must interfere and make an effort to save her life. The only result of the remedies selected was simply palliative. She passed quietly.

I have treated several cases of gouty rheumatism in which I could plainly see that every dose of medicine advanced the original malady. Many times I have been forced to feel that the dose of dynamized drug added new force to the old disease, and it progressed even more rapidly. I never saw such striking results from low attenuations. Not long ago I was called to the bedside of a patient in the last stage of phthisis. She had a diarrhoea, and passed large quantities of colorless urine; other symptoms accorded, and she took a dose of Acetic acid, which controlled the diarrhoea and polyurea, but immediately her chest symptoms came on with greater force than I was able to control, and she sank rapidly, I am sure she would have lived much longer had I permitted the less harmful conditions to go on. These things look strangely to the inexperienced physician, but they are facts; and, above all, show the great power of our potentized remedies. The truly appropriate remedy commonly develops the evidence of extreme sensitiveness in all kinds of sickness, and the extreme danger of repeating remedies is here illustrated.

If there is anything I dread it is an incurable disease. My experience in this line has been greater than I could ask. While these things have shown the danger of repeating medicines, they have also taught me another thing; viz. I am generally able to predict the gravity of the disease: I have seen troublesome aggravations, a pleasant increase of the existing symptoms or even new symptoms appearing as presumptive evidence of a good selection. In the western country our diseases are so mixed with that

unknown quantity, or something that we call malaria, it
is necessary to repeat medicines oftener in acute disease
than in most countries. Malaria disease and states are so
cumulative in character that the effect of a single dose is
soon exhausted and another becomes necessary. Therefore
I find myself repeating frequently in many acute cases. I
begin by repeating once in two hours in a fever that is
continued, but as soon as I see signs of a remission I stop
all medicine and wait on Sac. Lac. When a fever is going
up I repeat, and the instant it has ceased rising, I cease
medicine, in agues I generally administer one or two doses
in the apyrexia and wait results. I seldom administer
medicine until the paroxym has been completed. When
the first dose is followed by a perceptible aggravation, a
second dose should never be administered until the amelioration, which follows the aggravation, has ceased. When
a medicine aggravated it will generally influence the
patient much longer than when no such aggravation has
been observed. An amelioration that begins forthwith also
demands that all medicine be stopped, but such amelioration is seldom so striking as when the amelioration has
been preceded by a slight aggravation. Immediate *amelioration* often indicates the *absence* of deep-seated disease.
Especially in this case with the use of long-acting medicines. These go so deeply into the life that they shake the
very foundation of the automatic existence. When these
powers are so clearly demonstrated, can any man desire
Morphine to quiet a patient in any kind of agony? Can
any man feel the need of greater force to combat disease?
Yes, there are men who do not know this force; it cannot
be evolved at will by anybody who wills to evolve it. This
force is never observed, except by him who has learned
the philosophy taught in the *Organon* of Samuel Hahnemann; and it is after, *not before*, looking upon the wonderful effect of a remedy conforming to the law of similars
that one can appreciate the power he has with which to

combat the ills of life, and with which to defend frail man against the assaults of his natural enemy.

Then to the question, What is Homœopathy? I must answer, *no man knows,* God only knows, the length and breadth of the intricate, unfathomable mystery, the knowable part of this science, if I may use the word, consists in observing the sick-making phenomena of drugs and the phenomena of sickness, gathering and grouping the similars, selecting with the likeness in view and waiting for results

While we are observing the folly of others we must learn to avoid extremes in our own midst. We must not despise the original thirtieths of the master because we have found the Cm in so many cases useful. While reveling in the higher degrees of the true healing art, the younger and weaker must be fostered while tremblingly climbing the pathway up the hillside so familiar to most of us. While the way is beset with thorns, it is nevertheless the way of truth, and no part of it is to be despised. With the young and old our faith must be pinned to the law of similars, the single remedy, the smallest dose, the dynamic *power*, and last, but not least, the *proved drug.* These coupled with our organic philosophy, we shall continue in doing good and living to do good.

"WHAT SHALL WE DO WHEN THE LAW FAILS."

There is a large number of earnest believers in the *law of cure,* who desire to limit or restrict its application, not realizing that this limited acceptance makes it to themselves no law, but a rule of management of a few cases. With them it is not a law that has any relation to their failures, but some other kind of medical practice must be called into use to fit the uncured cases which are, as a rule, the majority. These expect to cure all cases of disease with medicines in crude state, and failing to do so, condemn the law as only applicable to "certain cases."

They say that certain diseases must be treated with strong medicines; that a congestive chill must have large doses of quinine. They deny the dynamic activities of medicines and ask foolish questions and manifest wonderful ignorance of medical philosophy. They do not admit what they cannot demonstrate, and their demonstrations have been very meager, therefore their useful medical knowledge is admitted to be very small. They are not willing to learn the part that does not permit itself to be accounted for through the action of visible particles of matter.

The dynamis and identity are unexplained, and yet we see them. Call them by what name you please, they are present. I am asked what I mean by the dynamis and identity. By a slight digression I will explain myself in a few words. The power, each identity possesses to produce its kind is unquestionably a most singular force and may be latent or active. The power to grow from and out of the acorn the mighty oak, is no less a force in the dry acorn than when surrounded by congenial environment, heat and moisture or the earthly implantation. What this force is has not been revealed to man. It may be a vital force or a formative force. The acorn has never been known to grow a sycamore; nor has the button-ball ever grown an oak. What is this identity that is not transferable?

This dynamis is found again in animal life producing its kind. In crystalography this formative force is apparent. In symptomatology we again see it, each drug producing its own and no other identity or individuality. But it must be remembered that the peculiar environments must under each and every circumstances be suitable to the identity or the evolution will not occur. The vital energy may be a complex force composed of heat and electricity, but as such our subject is not endangered, and at present there is no clear demonstration. It has been stated that the vital dynamis cannot exist apart from electrical vibrations. Even this is hard to demonstrate in view of the fact that the vital spark in its latency exists in the acorn without electrical activities. From these it is clear that life is not motion, although motion is one of the evidences of life, as it is of heat, of electricity and of light. It was recently said in one of our public meetings that without motion there is no force. The statement needs no further refutation. Again it has been stated that the amaeboid vibrations are the only evidences of life in protoplasmic cells, but the analogy will readily lead one to conclude that the motion is not *the* dynamis. The vibratory activities in protoplasm increase with types up to the highest cell life, but the vital dynamis, or formative energy becomes no more typical or perfect that in the lowest order of such activity. Then to develop the activities of each and every sickmaking substance is the aim of the Homœopathist. He must study the most favorable relations for the evolution of the manifestations of each identity, or he has not performed his whole duty as a physician. Hahnemann was acquainted with these necessities and potentized, or attenuated medicinal substances to place them in a favorable relation to sick making causes to conform to the law of similars. They who are willing to learn of the master himself find the law universal in its application to the demands of the sickroom, because they do not attempt to limit the environments of a drug in its curative evolutions. They are willing to use a drug from the lowest to the highest attenuation, only to find the most suitable relation to sickmaking cause and alteration of health as expressed in symptoms. As to myself I have no longer a doubt, in fact I am more than convinced that I could not universally apply the law curatively with the exclusive use of lower potencies.

Then it should be expected that the law would fail in the hands of men who do not admit the essentials to

its universal application.   Crude drugs cure disease
promptly under certain conditions, and the lower potencies
when carefully selected are generally potent enough to
cure most diseases, but shall we permit prejudice to deprive the world of increased usefulness. The dynamis and
its identity are unexplained, yet they are facts. No method
of reasoning can forecast such things and no method of
reasoning can do away with these facts. Can it be said
that the law has failed when, in a given case, the dose administered is yet too large to cure? The failure of the law
to help us out comes at all times from its non use. We
think we are the law, we try to use the law, but we don't
use the law. Homœopathy is an applied science, and is no
part of man's imagination or belief. It cures disease when
the law is applied, and not when misapplied. When man
fails it is man's failure, and the law stands unimpeached.

Again the law seems to fail where the selection has been
perfect, and the potency suitable by meddling with the action of the remedy. This fault is a common one and depends
upon ignorance of the philosophy of Homœopathy. I have
many times heard the law condemned for not curing an
incurable sickness. The physician who expects to cure the
sick must know of disease what is curable, and he must
know how to observe and how to interpret what he sees.
I remember a chronic rheumatism of all the joints in the
body to have so changed in six months that the ankles
and toes only were painful. The general state had greatly improved, and the patient was nearly well, but she said,
"I cannot walk and I must be cured;" so she went to a
neighbor who bathed and rubbed vigorously, and the
ankles and toes became better immediately, but the whole
trouble came back, and I was never again able to relieve
her. There are many things that a physician must know
to prescribe homœopathically outside of what drugs may
do. He may know the appropriate remedy and then not
know how to use. The patient may say he is better, or he

is worse, and the statement is of little value. If it relates to his general state he is competent, but if in the direction of his symptoms he is incompetent. Pain going from place to place must be observed for a purpose. A deep seated trouble changing under the action of a remedy, coming to the surface, though the suffering be increased ten fold the remedy must not be disturbed or the cure may never be realized. Though the patient say "I am so much worse, just see how I suffer," he must have Sac. lac. The physician who does not know these things can never follow the law closely enough to make it universally successful.

The treatment of chronic complaints demands an investigation entirely different from self-limited diseases. A man may disorder his stomach by gluttony and establish morbid phenomena, which may continue as long as the cause is continuous, but will cease when the cause is removed. Should such diseases be called chronic? I think not. These are an intermediate class that need for remedial measures instructions for the patient and very little medication. These diseases tend to recovery, which is unlike the disease properly called chronic. Any disease having no tendency to recovery may properly be called chronic. This must not be interpreted to mean a symptom. A symptom may have a tendency to disappear, and soon be followed by another equally as dangerous. The ulcer may close and a diarrhoea appear as intractable as the ulcer. This shows that the proper disease has no tendency to recover.

The question will then arise, as to what is understood by chronic disease and how it is defined. It must be understood first of all that all diseases when leaving the body —when cured or self cured do so under unvarying rules or laws. The vital manoeuvres are not one way today and another way next week. Nature operates under fixed principles. Now it must be known first of all that diseases recover from above downward from within out and in the reverse order of their coming. When the phenomena of disease do not follow this circumscribed limit of directions the disease is growing worse or at least progressing. When any given disease has existed a considerable time and its changes present phases in the reverse of the above formula though the supposed causes have been removed, it is of necessity a chronic disease, and will only change or reverse its order of direction by suitable homœopathic agencies. A knowledge of these principles *only* inform the physician *when*, and *when not*, to interfere in the treatment of the disease. It is so common for a patient to return after a correct prescription saying, "I am much worse today." The physician must now look into the case. If the new symptoms are such as were noticed in the early progress of the disease the cure is certain if properly conducted. If the new manifestation is felt on deep organs that have not heretofore been touched or given rise to symptoms, the disease may be known to be deep seated and most likely incurable. Sharp aggravations after a prescription the direction being from within out is a sign of speedy recovery. Following a prescription for chronic rheumatism, if heart symptoms intervene the patient never will recover. If the acute symptoms following a careful prescription are prolonged, the recovery will be slow.

The vital reaction to the remedy may be estimated by the intensity of the aggravation that follows the remedy. In acquired disease, such as are the result of indiscretion in diet and debauch, are seldom followed by any reaction as they do not belong to any specific chronic miasm of a progressive character.

I have hinted at a few things that a physician should know, and there are thousands of the kind. But it must be known at this time that the *law* will fail to be of serv-

ice to him who knows not how to apply it. It helps him in
proportion as he becomes acquainted with it.

Some days ago a physician who had graduated a few
years ago and settled down in a malarial district, remarked
that he could not cure the chills without quinine in large
doses. I began to question him, to see if there was a good
reason for the statement. He never had listened to a lecture on medical philosophy, and seemed to have no con-
ception of its meaning. He was well educated in everything but Homœopathy. He had a fair knowledge of the
Materia Medica but he knew nothing of how to apply the
law of cure. I am perfectly willing to say what I know
to be the truth; that the professed Homœopathists of this
or any day claiming to need large doses of drugs to cure
the sick are like this young man, ignorant of the philosophy of Homœopathy and remain so during life. The colleges have neglected this philosophy hence the *law* fails to
help the physician who should have the most confidence in
it. Confidence comes from acquaintance that is ample and
of long standing.

Another doctor says, "I must do the best I can," when
the law fails. "I must break that chill or he will go to
some one else, and he would then get quinine; I might as
well give it to him as for some one else to." You have
then concluded to do your patient harm, because if you do
not somebody else will. If I see a pocket-book on the
street, I can as well say that I may as well steal that, if
I do not somebody else will. The patient may have a skin
disease and want to recover. You know that it can be
made to disappear by outward applications. Now will you
consent to do that man harm because if you do not you
will lose a fee, or he will go to the next doctor? Will you
not warn him of the danger? Is he not better with that
disease on the outside than within the body? But you say
I have tried homœopathic medicines and the law has failed.
Then because of your ignorance of the law, you propose

to be hired to drive that skin eruption back into the body
You might as well be hired to give the patient a dose o
poison. "Then what shall I do?" When you do not know
what to do, why do you do anything? The great mistak
rests in the ambition to do something. No man shoul
consent to do a wrong as a substitute for an unknow
right way. These things are hard to see. I have man
times convinced myself of my own ignorance after a lon
and hard struggle, but had I been called ignorant of thes
self-same things, I am satisfied I could have argued th
point satisfactorily to myself. This is a man's stumblin
block, and is in the way of progress.

Many of our best followers of the law are not so we
acquainted with remedies as they would like to be, bu
they cure their cases, and the redeeming feature wit
them is that they know how to *avoid doing wrong*. "B
sure that you are right, then go ahead" will do in thi
place.

To avoid frequent failure under the law it is necessar
to know something not taught in allopathic colleges.

"When we have to do with an art whose end is th
saving of human life, any neglect to make ourselves thor
oughly masters of it, becomes a crime." (Hahnemann.)

WHAT THE PEOPLE SHOULD KNOW

All who know and desire the benefits of the homœo
pathic system of medicine, or art of healing, should ac
quaint themselves with the customs of the strict practi
tioners in order to avoid the deception of pretenders wh
are willing to imitate for diminutive fees, having no con
sideration for the patient nor the art of healing.

There are physicians who call themselves homœopaths
but are so only in name, as they do not follow the method
worked out by Hahnemann. They give two medicines i
one glass or alternate in two glasses, or in some cases give
medicine in three or four glasses. They do not conform

to Hahnemann's rules in taking the case and writing and
preserving full records of the cases. The people who are
acquainted with these facts cannot protect themselves
against such impositions. The false and the true pervade
all experiences and conditions of life, and the unenlightened
and simple suffer by the deceptions of the false. The time
has come when the followers of Hahnemann should furnish
information to the people in order that they may recognize
the genuine if they desire the benefits of the homœopathic
art of healing.

It should be known, first of all, that true homœopathicians write out the symptoms of each and every patient,
and preserve records for the benefit of such patient and the
art of healing. A moment's thought must convince any
person that human memory is too uncertain to be trusted
with the long record of symptoms, even in a small practice;
then how much more does the busy practitioner owe it to
his patients to keep accurate records of their sicknesses?
No physician is competent to make a second prescription if
the symptoms upon which the first prescription was made
have not been recorded with fullness and accuracy. Often
in such a case the neglectful physician has forgotten the
remedy given, even the one that has caused great improvement, but as there is no record of the case as to remedy
or symptoms, and many of the latter have passed away,
there is nothing to do but guess at a remedy, which generally spoils the case or so confuses it that the case seldom
ends in a cure, and the sufferer always wonders why the
doctor, who helped her so much at first, lost control of the
case. Many cases that should end in perfect cure result in
failure from the above negligence. Under such circumstances, when the physician has made a bad guess, he goes
on spoiling his case by guessing and changing remedies to
the disgust of the patient and injury to the art of healing.
Such failure leads to the experimentation and temporizing
which lead to disgrace. The people should be able to know

whether a physician is what he calls himself, or is of another sect. The temptation is very strong to be "all things to all men."

The people should not expect to obtain homœopathic results from a physician whose methods are not in accordance with the homœopathic art of healing.

If a person wants mongrelism, regularism, polypharmacy, etc., by knowing the methods of the homœopathist, he will be able to discriminate and select the kind of his preference, and it is reasonable to suppose that if he does not want a homœopathist he will be glad to know how to shun him. Nothing is more humiliating to a Hahnemannian than to be called to the bedside and find that the people do not want him; but actually want one who gives medicine in two glasses because some old family doctor did so. Therefore, this information is as useful to him who would avoid a homœopathist as to him who desires one.

Homœopathic patrons going abroad and those far removed from their own physician, often ask for the address of a good Hahnemannian. Such address cannot always be given, yet there are many reserved, quiet Hahnemannian physicians scattered over the world, but they are sometimes hard to find. As far as possible, traveling homœopathic patients should carry the address of Hahnemannians. In the absence of this a test may serve the purpose. Go to the most likely man who professes to practice after the manner of Hahnemann and tell him you want to consult him; but unless he writes out all the symptoms of the case as directed by Hahnemann, and continues to keep a record for future use, you cannot trust your case with him, as you have learned to have no confidence in the memory of the man. If he refuses to do this because of lack of time or ignorance, he should not be trusted, and it is best to bid him "good day" at once. If he be what he professes to be, he will be delighted to find a patient that knows so much of his system of practice, and the patient and physician will become fast friends.

There is another matter that the people should know about; that the homœopathic physician cannot prescribe on the name of a disease; also, that names are often the cover of human ignorance; also, that two sicknesses of the same name are seldom given the same remedy. If a physician could prescribe on a name there would be no necessity to write out the many pages of symptoms that some long cases present.

The name of the disease does not reveal the symptoms in any case of sicknesses; the symptoms are the sole basis of the prescription; therefore it will appear that the name is not necessarily known, but the symptoms must be known to the physician in order that he may make a successful prescription. It will now appear that if a physician has not time to devote to the patient in order to secure the symptoms, he is likely to be just as useless to the patient as though he were ignorant, as he will, in either case, fail to procure the symptoms which are the only basis of a homœopathic prescription. A little thought will enable a patient to ascertain whether this work is being done with care and intelligence or with ignorance, inexperience and laziness. It matters not from what excuse, if the physician fails to ascertain all the general and particular information in a case, he should not be trusted, as this labor, well performed, renders the rest of the work easy and a cure possible.

The people should also know that when such a record is on paper it is in such form that the patient may become the object of great study. In no other form can a likeness of his sickness be presented to the understanding of the true physician. Any physician who sneers at this plan shows how little he values human life and how much he falls short of a Hahnemannian.

The people should also know that the true physician

may now compare such a record of facts with the symptoms of the Materia Medica until he has discovered that remedy most similar of all remedies to the written record. And when the patient has become intelligent, he will say to his physician: *"Take your time, Doctor. I can wait until you find what you think is the most similar of all remedies, as I do not want to take any medicine you are in doubt about."* This statement makes a grateful doctor, as he now knows that he is trusted and known, and has a patient intelligent and considerate. Under such circumstances the doctor can do his best and such patients obtain the best and uniform results.

People who are not thus instructed become troublesome to the physician, and even suspicious, when they need to inspire him with full confidence, and sometimes they even change physicians and do the one wrong thing that is against the best interest of the patient. It is possible and desirable for the people to be so instructed that they may select the safest physician and know when he is working intelligently. People who are instructed do not intrude upon the physician's sacred moments, but, on the contrary, aid him with trust and gratitude.

Only the ignorant suggest this and that in addition to what is being done, and the more ignorant the doctor the greater is the number of things resorted to to make himself and others think he is doing something. The intelligent physician does what law and principles demand and nothing more; but the ignorant one knows no law and serves only his wavering experience, and appears to be doing *so much* for the patient, in spite of which the patient dies.

The physician must often long for a patient so well instructed as to say: *"Doctor, if you are in doubt about what to give me, don't give me anything."* Such words could only come from one who knows that there is a law governing all our vital activities, and that law must be invoked or disorder must increase to the destruction of all order in the human economy.

If it were not true that the human race is ignorant of the highest principles of science, mongrelistic medication could not find support upon the earth. It is true that if the people would study Hahnemann's Organon and thereby secure the safest medication for themselves and their families when sick, crude compounds and uncertain medication would not be the rule as it is at the present day. In all trades a man must be somewhat skillful in order to gain entrance to an intelligent patronage; but in the profession of medicine, personal tact excuses such lack of training and ignorance of all science of healing.

People who know what homœopathy really is, should seek to introduce the principles among the most intelligent people by reading, and not by urging upon them a favorite physician.

32

PART III.

CLINICAL CASES

PAIN IN ABDOMEN OR SUSPECTED TUMOR

Case II.—Murex Pur: Mrs. K., aged 40, a midwife. She complained of the abdomen; she believed she had a tumor. Severe knife-cutting pain in the region of uterus running up to left mamma; pains, undefined, running up and through pelvis, worse lying down, aching up and through the pelvis, worse lying down, aching in the sacrum, dragging down in the uterine region as if the uterus would escape. Empty, "all-gone" feeling in the stomach. Greenish-yellow leucorrhoea, with itching in labia and mons veneris; intense sexual desire. The os uteri was said to be ulcerated and eroded, and it was sensitive to touch. The contact of the finger with cervix brought on the sharp pain that she described as running to the left mamma. The uterus was enlarged and indurated. She had been the mother of several children; had had several abortions, and was accustomed to hard work. She had been treated locally by a specialist of acknowledged ability, and she had taken many remedies of his selection as well as from her own medicine case, all very low. Her catamenia quite normal.

To take up the important and guiding features of this case we must compare several remedies, but principally Murex and Sepia.

The cutting pain in the uterus has been found under *Curare*. *Murex* and *Sepia,* but Murex is the only one producing a cutting pain in the uterus going to the left mamma.

The "all-gone" empty feeling in the stomach is characteristic of Murex., Phos. and Sepia.

Throbbing in the uterus, belongs only to Murex. The dragging down is common to both Murex and Sepia, but the sexual teasing only to Murex. Both have a yellowish green leucorrhoea. Pain in sacrum is common to Murex, Sepia and many others. "Enlargement of bowels" is found in *Allen* under Murex, not mentioned in Minton's *Uterine Therapeutics*. The pains in Murex go upward and through, worse while lying down. In Sepia the patient is better lying down, and the pains go around.

Murex 200, one dose was given. She was much worse for several days. Then improvement went on for two weeks. The remedy was again repeated. One year later she complained of a return of her symptoms. One dose was followed by relief, since which time she has made no complaint, but praises the individualizing method.

ABDOMINAL TUMOR.

M. A. W., aet. 30, asks treatment for abdominal tumor, which is large enough to give her the appearance of being about eight months pregnant. She is a house maid, and her friends will not go out with her fearing that people will think they are associating with an un-married pregnant woman. She had consulted two surgeons who refused to operate because of the rigidity and exten-sive adhesions, and also because of the sickly aspect of the girl. The face was indeed waxy and sickly looking. These surgeons told her she would die from the tumor.

The tumor was first noticed five years ago. It became prominent on the right side of the uterus and extended up to the pelvis; was said to be movable until two years ago. The uterus is now immovable and the tumor which hangs over the right side of the pelvis is very hard, as large as a child's head, and cannot be made to move in any direction.

June 1st, 1888.—Pain in the pelvis now and then. Swelling in the pit of the stomach not due to the tumor. Swelling of the feet, indenting on pressure. Constant con-gestive headaches which she could give no description of, only "it aches all over." Eats but little, and what she eats causes nausea. Constipation; no desire for stool;

takes physic, hence no modalities of value. Goes two or three weeks without a stool. Always feels a constriction about the waist, which most likely is due to pressure of tumor, hence it is not a valuable symptom. Sensation of great fullness after eating, and she mentions above that she eats but little. Menses fairly regular "with cramps." She has not drank water for eight years, as it makes her sick. Feet burn so that she must take off her slippers to cool them. Starts in sleep, and when awake starts at the slightest noise. Restless sleep. Pain in left side of abdomen. Teeth decayed when young. They are dark and bad looking. Wants hot things; cannot take cold things into the stomach. Pain in the stomach after cold things. Pain and nausea after water, cold or warm. Pain in left groin. She had this pain before the tumor was felt. *Lyc.* cm; one dose, and *Sac-Lac.* morning and night, dry on the tongue.

July 23rd.—The remedy increased the symptoms so much that she was alarmed and would not return for many weeks, but now is so much better in a general way that she returns to report and ask for more medicine. Upon close questioning it was found that for a week or more her symptoms were on the increase. Her stomach symptoms at first grew worse, then improved and now are worse again. *Lyc.* mm. She got one dose and s. l.

Aug. 2d—Reports that all the symptoms are better, and she is feeling greatly improved.

Aug. 31st.—Pain in pit of stomach. Pain in forehead, vertex and temples. Bowels no better. If she drinks water she feels so full and gets cramps. Sleepless; starts suddenly. *S. L.* No change in tumor.

Sept. 15th.—Feet do not swell now. She vomits and has a pain in stomach after eating or drinking. *Lyc.* mm.

Oct. 28th.—Symptoms all passed away, except that she has a pain in right side, in the tumor.

Nov. 27th.—No symptoms. Calls at intervals but gets only s. l.

Jan. 23d, 1889.—Symptoms returning, especially the stomach symptoms. *Lyc.* mm

June 3d.—She has been improving steadily and was free from symptoms. Bowels move every three or four days. Stool normal. Feels more swollen than for some time. Uncomfortable. Bad feelings return. Pain in right groin. Feet swollen. Headache in forehead and eyes. Pain in lumbar region. Lyc. mm. Feet burn.

August 15th.—Symptoms have been gone since here last, but now all are coming back. *Lyc.* 2mm.

December 31st.—She has reported several times, but there were no symptoms. Bowels regular. She can eat and drink anything. She looks well. She says the last powders have made her well.

The tumor is what most readers will ask about, but has not been mentioned, as the tumor was not treated. The patient was cured and the tumor at last report was small; the uterus was movable and with it the small tumor also moved. She did not mind the tumor as she was so well and shapely.

ABROTANUM: WITH CLINICAL CASES

Irritable, weak-minded, worse from mental exertion. The head topples over because the neck is emaciated; the face is wrinkled and has a sickly look; the temples are marked by distended veins. The face looks old, the infant looks like a little old person. (Also, Bar-c., Iodine, Natr-m., Op., Sulph.) (If from syphilis, Aur-mur.) The whole body is emaciated and wrinkled; the emaciation spreads from the lower limbs upward (which is the reverse of Lyc. and Natr-m.) Enlarged glands, especially in the emaciated abdomen. Diseases change from place to place (metastasis). Mumps go to the mammae or to the testes.

Rheumatism leaves the joints and endocarditis appears with profuse sweat; cannot lie down for the dyspnoea; sinking as if dying, pulse feeble. Rheumatism comes on when a diarrhœa has ceased too suddenly. Piles which get worse as the rheumatism abates. Bleeding from the piles in amenorrhoea. (Graph.) Hydrocele in boys. Distended abdomen. (Ars., Bar-c., Calc., Iodine, Lyc., Puls., Sulph.) Piercing pains in the heart. Piercing in the ovaries, mostly the left. Wakes in a fright and trembles, is covered with cold sweat. The extremities are numb and tingle as if thawing, after having been frozen. High fever after the rheumatism has gone to the heart. The wasting child has hectic fever with a ravenous appetite. Lives well yet emaciates. (Also Iodine, Natr-m.) Abrotanum attacks the white fibrous tissues, the joints, pleura, peritoneum, etc. Gouty nodosities in the wrist and fingers. Rheumatism goes to the heart, compare with Cactus, Dig., Kalm., Lach., Naja., Spig. Spong. The grand features of this remedy are metastasis; marasmus spreading upward.

Case 1. Mrs. P. suffered from gouty deposits about the finger joints, which were very painful during cold, stormy weather. The joints and nodes were sore and hot at such times. The nodes ceased to be painful and sudden hoarseness came; ulcers in the larynx followed; great dryness in the nose and painful dry throat; sticking in the cardiac region. She lost flesh but the appetite kept good. Calc-phos. had been prescribed by her former attendant. After duly considering the case, Abrot. 45m. was given. She suffered for many days after this dose with a most copious discharge from her nose and bronchial tubes; expectoration was copious, thick, yellow. Hoarseness ceased at once. In a month she ceased coughing; the finger joints became painful and swollen considerably. In three months she had no pain and the nodes were scarcely perceptible. She is now perfectly well and has been so one year.

She had only one dose of the remedy, as the case was doing well enough, i. e., as the symptoms were taking the right course to recovery in the proper way. She suffered much pain on the road to recovery but I know of only one way to cure these cases, and that is to let the remedy alone when the symptoms are taking the proper course.

RHEUMATISM OF LEFT ANKLE AND KNEE

Case 2. Mrs. T. had suffered from chronic rheumatism of the left ankle and knee for several years. She rubbed the limb with a strong liniment and the rheumatism was speedily cured. But it was not long before she needed a physician. I saw her friends surrounding her bed, she was covered with a profuse, cold sweat, sitting propped up on pillows. Her friends said she was dying, and I thought so too. She had a small, quick pulse; there was pain at the heart and auscultation over heart, revealed the usual story, which is too well known to all, as there are many such cases. She was six months pregnant. Gave her Abrot., and she slowly recovered. The little one now bears my Christian name in honor of the great cure. She has recovered, perfectly free from rheumatism, and the lad is now several years old.

These two cases show what Abrotanum can do when properly indicated. It is a powerful remedy and must not be repeated. It acts many weeks, in waves or cycles; it is too seldom used.

ABSCESS ON FACE.

Case II.—A middle-aged gentleman had an abscess on the side of the face just in front of the ear. Suppuration was advanced and the fluctuation was marked. Silicea had done some good as it had controlled the pain. The cavity was aspirated by a surgeon several times but it continued to refill. After three weeks there was no abatement of the difficulty. The integument took on a new feature, becoming *bluish, mottled with great burning and sharp cutting pains.* The hardness was extending and the opening gave out a bloody thin excoriating fluid of foul smell. He was chilly and nauseated and had symptoms of pyaemia. After one dose of Tarantula cubensis 12x an immediate change for the better took place, no more pus formed and he was well in ten days. The discolored localization became a bright red and then faded to the natural color. The nausea and general pyaemic symptoms were greatly relieved within twelve hours. No more medicine.

ACONITE OR SULPHUR?—(PNEUMONIA)

Take a case of pneumonia that has advanced to the stage of exudation and let that patient get a little cold sufficient to arouse him to a state of mental anxiety. With a superficial examination you will find Aconite indicated, but just as sure as you give it you will fail. Give Sulphur at once and you will cure your patient. Never mind the fact that Aconite has the superficial show. I say in ninety-nine cases out of one hundred give Sulphur. When I first commenced prescribing I gave Aconite and I never had anything but failure, and have been disappointed many times by giving it.

ADENOIDS CURED WITH TUBERCULINUM

I recently met an old friend who said that he and his sister had lately become interested in a dear little child whose parents had died of tuberculosis. These friends were trying to help the child along through school, but the school-doctor said it was useless effort: that the child's head was all stopped up with adenoids. This child was also stupid; it was sickly, having night-sweats and many symptoms suggestive of TUBERCULINUM. My friend offered to pay for my attention but I said I would be as generous as he and that it would give me great pleasure to help the child; and I did.

I sent Tuberculinum.

After a short time the child was breathing through the nose and was gaining in school. In the course of about four months they thought the child was so much better that they showed her to the doctor to see if he still considered that adenoids were present. He said they surely were there, very marked, but that now he did not see them at all; that he also had heard of those things getting well of themselves.

I have cured probably 100 cases of adenoids with Tuberculinum alone, so that the children breathe through the nose, and close the mouth.

Only four weeks ago, a child with adenoids was brought to me; I couldn't find much of anything else, except a history.

She was irritable;

Extremely stupid;

Unable to breath enough to keep going, day or night, except through the mouth; and the doctor said there was nothing to do with that child but to remove those adenoids by operation.

To-day I received a letter, after only four weeks, telling that the child is now breathing through her nose. Why, that is almost as quickly as you can do it with a knife or a red-hot iron!

Yes, probably a hundred cases cured with Tuberculinum alone; that has some significance.

Another case I had took eighteen months for cure, but the father was a dyed-in-the-wool homœopath and did not give up. He reported that the specialist had said: "It must be operated; you are criminal if you don't do it at once." But the father said: "My doctor don't do such business."

Well, sometimes the child was better, breathing through the nose for awhile; then it would take a little cold and the nose would close again.

In eighteen months the child was entirely well and is the picture of health:

There are several children in the family, and this one, who was such a poor, sickly, good-for-nothing baby that required eighteen months to cure with Tuberculinum, is the healthiest.

Many of these cases could be reported; it would be only about the same story over and over again. I advise you to study the symptoms.

Question: So often we have children brought to us with adenoids, on whom the operation has already been performed. What are we to do?

Dr. Kent: There you will not succeed so often as you would if they let the patient alone. This is your problem.

TUBERCULAR GLANDS

Dr. Kent: Speaking to another point: I have had a great deal of experience with tubercular glands on both sides of the neck. Each had about four or five fistulous openings.

She had had such glands for some time:

The neck was whittled out, and very thin, the fistulous opening persisting.

She had a tuberculosis family history; and:

Other tubercular symptoms, with these glands.

I started her on a series of Tuberculinum bovinum. I used the bovinum in that case because it comes from the glands of the cow's neck. She was kept under a series of potencies, probably to the ten-thousandth. Then those glands all subsided and healed, and the neck there was perfectly smooth.

She afterwards became pregnant and brought forth a healthy, perfectly normal child.

Before she finished nursing the child those tubercular glands rose again.

I then had her stop the nursing, placing her again under treatment.

At the end of about six or eight months she appeared perfectly well and, so far as I have heard, she has not had any return nor any sign from those tubercular glands of the neck.

Another case was operated three times by our excellent Dr. Pratt, here in Chicago; the enlargement repeatedly returned, and he operated three times. When they reappeared for the fourth time, advised by one of her friends she came to me. Her symptoms were clear for Tuberculinum bovinum. There were but two remaining glands, which became inflamed and nodular hard masses and she was suffering from the swelling of the tissues. Tuberculinum bovinum took down all that swelling.

She came to me some time in the winter and I treated her until summer; she appeared to be perfectly well, a picture of health, and gaining in flesh.

Then her mother thought her well enough to spend a week in Canada where she could have a nice home and a big time. So she went up there. I advised and urged her most earnestly to remain where I could keep watch of her, so that when her symptoms should begin to return I might give the indicated remedy; but, No, No, she must go.

So soon as she arrived there in the cold weather and storms, she took cold; the cold went to her lungs and she died of tuberculosis. I am satisfied from the way she had progressed that, if she had been where I could watch her and keep her free from colds, she would have regained her health.

So I have seen any number of patients, with such glands of the neck, entirely restored to health by the aid of Tuberculinum bov.

Dr. Kent speaking to another point: After removing the adenoids the child goes right on with whatever tendency happens to exist in that child.

Every individual born at the present time, with all the fierce tendencies of our living—bad governing, bad rearing, bad clothing and bad feeding, that we have at present in the entire human race—is capable, just as soon as you thwart one mischievous bent, of developing something else! No one can foresee what that will be.

Suppress an eruption: some will then have brain trouble; others, lung trouble, and others will develop abdominal troubles. Whatever is their weakest point will then be manifest.

If this child had been permitted to go right on with the adenoids, the disease-directions would have been continuously towards the adenoids; to increase and intensify the catarrh. But somebody operated: cut out the entire activity there, probably cleared it all up.

If he had left a part of the condition, there would have been, for this particular kind of disease, the things directing his attention there.

When that was carved out, so beautifully removed, then the next weakening that the child had would manifest: in this case, as hayfever; so that has developed.

The probability is that the same remedy would be indicated now as was indicated before from center to circumference.

We can never tell what will happen, or what the direction will be, when you remove adenoids.

If the tonsils are not removed, it may be to the tonsils;

Ear-troubles may develop;

It may be lung-trouble:

Almost anything may appear; but it is generally internal: very seldom is it an eruption.

If eruptions are removed, one can never tell what center will then be attacked.

What I wish to say is, that any part of the body may be affected, according to what is the weakened place.

When I make a test with Tuberculinum, the response for which I first look is:

The mother says the boy feels so much better;

He eats better;

He is feeling better, in a few weeks after he takes it.

If any such response is obtained, it is possible, if the symptoms are pretty certain, that I may test with another dose but generally I am pretty well satisfied that Tuberculinum is the basis of it.

If you have the symptoms of Tuberculinum, of course you will stand by it; but in many instances, with those puny things with large glands, stopped-up noses, breathing through the mouth, and semi-idiotic or degenerate, we have nothing but the physical condition on which to depend: no symptoms. Hunt here, hunt there, hunt somewhere else; you have nothing on which to depend: everything is suppression.

I test such cases at once with TUBERCULINUM; or:

If there is pain with Psorinum; and these tests are legitimate experiments with me.

First, one dose of one of these remedies, according to the symptoms: as the symptoms develop, I try another dose.

The second dose may fail.

If a remedy is specifically indicated by the symptoms, I use this specifically homœopathic remedy and then:

Continue with a series of potencies.

By developing the remedies and working up the vital

strength, the child will begin to give symptoms; the patient will begin to have symptoms, here and there. It is a brilliant sight, to observe the anti-psoric remedy standing out, right clearly; then I follow that out.

After getting indications, I commence to sound first the responses to my test for TUBERCULINUM, to see if possibly there is a tubercular test in this constitution, a tubercular tendency with *that which is indescribable, that thing we have never been able to put into language*; I am guided by that instinct of which I am conscious, but cannot put into words: you will have to imagine it.

Tubercular History Love and Mental Ability Revived

Now another strange case I may tell you: A woman had been sick four years, declining steadily, when she came to consult me.

She had lost all her loves: had not the ability to exercise that function at all. She was ashamed of it: did not like her husband; did not love her children: and she said: "What shall I do! Don't tell of it. I don't want anybody to know that I do not love my husband; he is a good man. And my children; I have lost all my love for my children."

She had no resolution whatever; was entirely irresolute: Was irritable; had no desire to do anything: it was all lost.

Undertaking any mental exertion brought much pain in the occiput; she put her finger directly on the spot: she felt hot right at that spot.

Hers was a marked tubercular history. From her recital I recognized that there was a difficulty—it was clear to me that there was some obstruction—in the passage between the third and the fourth ventricles; it appeared to me that the cerebro-spinal fluid would not flow out of the brain to accomodate her mental exertion, and then she would have congestion.

I could strongly suspect that there were tubercular deposits in the brain; I was convinced of this by her strongly tubercular history. But I did not come to a conclusion until after studying her for more than six months, giving her such remedies as I could.

She would pick up slightly; and then within a week would drop right back again; I would select another remedy, and after another slight improvement she would again drop back.

Finally, I thought: Here is a tubercular history and here are the tubercular symptoms; I am going to test her.

Putting her under a test with TUBERCULINUM bovinum 10m, she responded to it.

She said, "Doctor, I am a new woman." All of her loves came back; her mental ability revived.

She had 10m twice at long intervals and had 50m twice, also at long intervals.

She responded and felt better after the first dose; within three or four weeks her symptoms returned and I gave her a second one. She is now on the third or fourth dose; now, after about three or four doses she is a new woman, perfectly natural in everything.

ANÆMIA

Little Helen, seven years old, presented the appearance of a very sick child when seen.

Jan. 16. Blood on the pillow, on fingers and in mouth. (Sulph.) Has passed thread-worms. (Sulph.) Very hungry by spells. Headache frontal. Vertigo in the morning. Abdominal pains. Faintness. Thirst more than hunger. (Sulph.) Aversion to milk. Craves meat and sweets. Has never thrived but has been running down in general health during past year.

Aversion to milk: *Calc., calc. p., carb. v., cina,* LAC.

33

D. NAT. C. *nat. s.*, nat. p. *phos. sep.*, *sil.*, stan., *sulph.* Craves meat: Sulph., Sulph. 10m.

Feb. 13. Generally improved; symptoms all lessened. Return of some symptoms in mild form occasioned repetition of the remedy—first in 10m, then 50m potency—on Feb. 28, April 1 and May 1; the last time all symptoms reported absent except aversion to milk. She was robust and rosy as a child should be.

This patient presented scarcely anything but common symptoms, yet the prescriber was able to find the characteristics of the patient suffering lack of nutrition, in the abnormal appetite. The most peculiar symptoms of other parts were found to be in harmony with the peculiarities expressed through the stomach and the remedy met the requirements of a successful prescription.

A SERIOUS CASE

C. R. W. aged three years. Parents and grandparents living and healthy. Patient has been fed on modified milk which was invariably sterilized. Teeth appeared slowly but without much trouble. Previous illnesses: Capillary bronchitis soon after birth, for three days; has had it several times since; easily "takes cold," lungs most affected. Whooping cough began when ten months old, very severe for two or three months. Occasional croupy cough since: two or three coughs at a time, mostly at night. Circumcised four months ago. Adenoids removed from pharynx, after which color, sleep, etc., were improved. Depression about the size and shape of the bowl of a table-spoon at ensiform cartilage.

Fell on the carpet several months ago, partially dislocated the hip-joint. After a few days of quiet appeared quite well. At times since that has pain in the knee of the affected side. Strength good last summer. Had rectal injections a few times. Of good appearance and fairly developed.

March 5, 1903. Coryza five or six weeks ago; nose obstructed; restless in sleep; tired and sleepy frequently; grinding teeth in sleep; was better and worse again. Sick following a sleigh ride ten days ago: temp. 101 or 102 degrees; pulse 130 or more. Urine scanty (three to five oz. in twenty-four hours), smoky, high-colored, sp. gr. 1028, albumin plentiful; no appetite; sluggish bowels, feces pasty, white. Was treated with a purge, kept in bed, and given milk-diet. Attempts to give him lithia water failed. Nasal discharge continued only one day. Third day, hot fomentations to kidneys gave some relief. Fourth day, vomiting the milk; unable to retain it in any way it was modified; milk-toast vomited in two hours. Cooked rice, milk, and oatmeal were retained. Fifth day, urine slightly increased in quantity, color improved, sp. gr. 1028, less albumin—granular and hyaline casts, epithelial casts red and white, no blood-corpuscles in casts. Until this time sleep poor; fever and rapid pulse continued. Glands on both sides of neck enlarged when he had croupy cough; size of hen's egg on left side, very painful; numerous other lymph-glands enlarged, resembling small string of beads. Œdema of face and eye-lids noticed slight; none now. Past four or five days has rested comfortably at night, except that the glands on right side and the ears are painful, ameliorated by hot applications; worse early part of night. Fever absent; pulse 90 to 100, during sleep, more rapid as soon as he stirs. Tongue slightly coated; urine gradually increased in quantity until nearly normal; no thirst since fever ceased; albumin absent or nearly so, sp. gr. 1020, color good; plays in bed during the day. Respiration no more rapid than accounted for by fever; easy during sleep. Fair skin face barely flushed; dark hair and eyes; loving disposition. Tonsils not especially enlarged; adenoids visible in pharynx. Bowels fairly active. Fears entering an elevator or strange toilet-room since his sickness, fears having temperature registered or a poultice applied. Fears something will hurt him and wonders if others are not afraid of the things he fears. Past two days animal broth added to his diet. Takes plenty of nourishment and appears stronger in many ways. Has much earache or R. side, ameliorated by heat; face appears swollen about the cheeks; stomach and abdomen larger than normal though always had prominent abdomen; abdomen not hard or sore to touch, but child dreads being touched, in fear of being hurt.

Aversion to being touched: *Agar.*, *ant.-c.*, ars., calc., camph., CHAM., chin., cina, iod., *kali-c.*, *lach.*, mag-c., merc., mez. plb., *sanic.*, *sil.*, *thuj.*

Timidity: *Ars.*, CALC., *chin*, iod., KALI-c., *merc.*, plb., *sil.*

Enlarged glands; swelling of neck. CALC., *iod.*, KALI-C., MERC., *sil.*

Subject to earache: *Calc.*, *kali-c.*, MERC., *sil.*

Enlarged abdomen: CALC., SIL.

Grinds teeth: *Calc.*

Calc. 10m.

The subsequent reports entered on this record reveal that the remedy was equal to the demands. It altered the child in every characteristic, restoring order and nutrition.

The chief interest is in the method of selecting the remedy. *The characteristics of the child, revealed in the mental realm,* are the basis for study. From that basis it proceeds, selecting the symptoms that express the general character of the disturbances, and there is no tedious work before the list is narrowed to one or two remedies.

He who knows the characteristics of the remedies in our Materia Medica will quickly realize that the entire case is most similar to Calc.-c.

Subsequent treatment, of course, included the use of

this remedy in a series of potencies, as improvement progressed under its influence.

ASTHMATIC AND DROPSICAL

Case III.—Mrs. S., age 76, also an inmate of the *Memorial Home* came to my charge the same time as Mrs. F. She was dropsical and asthmatic. The urine was loaded with albumin, and, apparently, she was progressing to a fatal termination without interruption

She took Ars., Apis., Apocyn., Lach., with some relief. The latter seemed to give the only relief; finally, she was becoming very large; hands, face, limbs and abdomen all œdematous, while Lach. afforded relief I had decided not to tap. Though she had taken medicine at proper intervals, when there seemed a demand for a repetition, yet the time came when she seemed to get no benefit from the remedy. The suffocation after sleep was the special symptom guiding to Lach. 41m. was the preparation used. Early one morning I was advised as to her condition. She had suffered greatly during the night with pains in the feet and legs, and her feet were getting black. The matron thinking that she was about to die, gave her some whiskey without relief. *The great pain in feet and legs, skin turning black, perhaps threatening gangrene.* Ars. and Lach. had failed, guided me to Tarantula cubensis, which was given, 12x one dose. The pain subsided immediately, the dark color of the skin on legs became bright-red and in a general way, she felt improved and got up. Next night, she slept well until toward morning, when pain in lower limbs returned, Tarant. cub. 12x was repeated, with perfect relief. The medicine has been repeated by necessity about every day since November 20th.

December 1. There is now a fiery redness of the skin below the knee to the ankles on both legs, tender to the touch and covered with small blisters. Everybody that looked at it thought it was erysipelas. A serious transudation is going on from the surface of both limbs from the feet to about six inches above the knees, which runs down and drips from the heels and also saturates the absorbent dressings in a few minutes. A sheet placed on the limbs as an outer covering must be taken off every hour and another put on as the serum is so great in quantity. A sheet dried shows very little discoloration but is pungent to the smell. There has been no perspiration from any part of the body. The œdema appears to be going down.

December 15th. The œdema has gone from the face, hands and thighs. The abdomen has become nearly natural in size, and albumin has not been noticed in the urine since December 1. Urine has been very scanty. The legs are covered from knees to ankles with a profusion of flat ulcers which secrete a serous flow, and large yellow crusts are forming.

Decmber 20. Œdema gone out of feet and ulcers are still flat with red, and in the places blue margins and red and bluish interspaces on the skin. Yellow scales are forming. The patient is somewhat prostrated, but says she is more comfortable with ulcers than with the "bloat" as she nearly suffocated before. Since December 1, she has had an occasional dose of the medicine, as the pain in the legs became severe.

January 1, 1883. She shows signs of sinking, though she says she is feeling comfortable except the occasional sharp pain in the ulcers.

It is evident she is going to die, but will she die of exhaustion or will the dropsy return and death occur as usual from such condition? Such was my query.

January 9. She died of exhaustion.

BLADDER SYMPTOMS.—ERYNGIUM.

Eryngium aquatium 30, cured a lady who had suffered with the following urinary symptoms: For two years she was compelled to pass urine about every half hour night and day; the urine was scalding. There was burning during and sometimes after passing urine. She was greatly reduced in flesh from the continued painful urging and loss of sleep. She often lost her urine in bed because she became so exhausted it was impossible for her to awake in time to accommodate the call. The urine was not examined chemically but was high colored and strong smelling.

After taking the remedy during the day she arose only twice the following night, after which she slept well and rapidly recovered her strength and flesh. She was upwards of fifty years of age. No cause could be discovered for the irritable bladder.

I have seen similar bladder symptoms cured with this remedy (Eryngium aq.) when used in the 3x, 6x, 12x, 30x, in a surprising manner. *The continuous teasing, and dribbling, drop by drop, smarting and burning night and day*, I have often seen disappear under its use.

It is uncommon for the exaggerated sexual desire to be present, unlike Canth.

The patient is generally better in a warm place, unlike Apis.

BLADDER TROUBLE.

It is commonly asked by old prescriber: "Did you tell your doctor that symptom?" "No, he never asked me." Some years ago, being called to see a patient in counsel, it was said by the attending physician: "This is one of the most difficult cases to procure symptoms from that I ever saw." "What is the trouble?" "Well," said the doctor, "he calls me and says he is sick, has trouble with his bladder, and does not feel well generally and expects me to read his symptoms like a clairvoyant. When I ask him questions he replies, 'You are the doctor; you ought to know,' and so it goes." We went to the room to examine the patient, and both of us put questions indirectly for an hour or more, and there was no point gained except the bad temper that the patient manifested at every moment. Finally he jumped out of bed and ran into the bath room and slammed the door behind him. I concluded to follow him and observed him standing at the wash basin passing his urine. I, at once, asked him, "Why do you not sit to pass your urine?" He replied, "I have not been able to pass urine sitting for many years. I must stand always or it will not start." *Sars.* c. m. cured him in a few weeks, and there never has been a return of the bladder trouble.

BREECH PRESENTATION?

I had one peculiar case, but I am afraid to report everything. It was one of the cases of a midwife, experienced, well educated and of thirty years' practice. I had seen a number of her cases and considered her highly accomplished; she occasionally sent for me to share the responsibility, and this one was a tedious case. She had diagnosed a breech presentation, and sent for me with a note saying she expected a two days' job and wanted me to come and assure the family that if it should be three days it would have a favorable termination. I went to the house, made an examination, found a breech presentation and confirmed her diagnosis. The dilation of the os was nearly as large as a half dollar. I gave a dose of Pulsatilla and assured the family as she requested me with all conscientiousness and thought no more about the case.

The next morning she called at my office. The patient I learned had a good many pains, irregular and spasmodic. She was a Pulsatilla patient, and I paid more attention to the case by taking symptoms and seeing what remedy would help her through. The midwife then said: "Why did you not tell me I made a mistake in that diagnosis? I am an old fool to practice midwifery for thirty years and not know a head presentation. You knew it was a head presentation. That child was born head first." Did the Pulsatilla do it? It was born in a few hours after I left the house.

BRIGHT'S DISEASE

Child of C. N., a sprightly little girl two years old; symptoms; yellowish white discharge from left ear, profuse lacrymation from right eye, and some white, clear mucus flowing over the eye-lid and cheek that seemed to be blood. The under lid of right eye appeared like a water-bag, and the whole face was puffed and rather transparent; the right was much the worse of the two. The child looked sickly and cried much. The mother stated that it had not been well for several weeks. While thinking over Apis and Ars. I began to look for agg. by warmth, etc., when I was informed that the child could not endure any covering, and she was absolutely thirstless, which excluded Arsenic from further consideration. The mother believed the urine to be scanty but she was not quite certain, but says she, "Her water smells strong, like that of a horse." Nit-ac. 1200, and we soon cured the case, ear discharge and all, in the surprisingly short time of a few days.

This was not a case of acute Bright's disease following scarlet fever, but much like it. Every physician living in this malarial climate must have observed the same anasarca and otorrhœa following malaria attacks, home-treated or neglected. The dropsical condition follows all kinds of malarial attacks, and particularly this ear complication, associated with kidney disease. But will some astute pathologist inform me why nitric acid cured this case so promptly if on other grounds than that it was the similimum? These cases all die when not properly treated. They all recover promptly on a few doses of the appropriate remedy.

BUBO IN THE LEFT GROIN.

TARANTULA CUBENSIS.

Case I.—A young man came to me with a bubo in the left groin. He had been disappointed in that he had not obtained relief from the treatment used. His bones ached, his tongue was loaded, and his breath smelled badly. The tumification was hard and painful, *bluish and mottled, with great burning and sharp cutting pain.* It was discovered some distance around and the heat was intense. He took Tarantula cubensis 12x, and one powder dry on the tongue three mornings in succession. He returned on the third day after taking his last powder saying that he was poisoned. He complained of a wild feeling in his brain and a drawing sensation in the scalp and muscles of the face. He was in a great state of mental anxiety and said he felt as if he was going to lose his reason. Mental restlessness was marked in his countenance. He could not keep quiet even after I assured him that he was in no danger. His primary symptoms had nearly gone and the bubo had lost its bad color. The next day he was much improved in a general way and the bubo had nearly disappeared. I saw him again in three days and the improvement was going on rapidly. The chancre healed rapidly and in one month he told me he had never been so well.

CANCER CURES

(In private discussion.)

In cancer patients, when painful conditions arise, for instance, diarrhœa or urinary disturbances, caution in prescribing is necessary, that a remedy be not administered covering only the acute condition. Any prescription based on the more superficial, acute disorder, not covering the deeper, chronic, carcinomatous nature, will result in amelioration of the acute disorder only. Meanwhile suffering from the deeper affection will increase, and the progress of the deeper, malignant disorder will be more rapid.

Any prescription, to be of benefit to the patient, must have the nature of the chronic, as much as the nature of the acute manifestation.

The aim of the physician, first, last, and always, must be to find the remedy which most closely corresponds to the patient, and *prescribe for the patient, whatever manifestation that patient may suffer, when the prescription is selected.*

In cancer-patients, incurability depends upon the fact that few symptoms except those of the cancerous tissue-change are obtainable. The sharp pains, the ulceration, and the anæmia are symptoms of the ultimate disorder. Finding symptoms that preceded this period is necessary for gaining any curative results.

Ultimates do not indicate the remedy for the patient.

CANCER OF LIVER.

Dr. Lippe's daughter had cancer of the liver. Her distress was intense. As her father watched her, he noted that she rolled constantly from side to side. This reminded him of the description of Tarantula just published, which he had read a few days previously, emphasizing this feature. He administered Tarantula and obtained for the sufferer euthanasia that appeared impossible before.

CARCINOMA

Carcinoma relieves the sharp, burning tearing pains. With this remedy (nosode), patients have been kept comfortable, for many years, when cure was impossible and the cancerous development continued. The malignant progress was delayed, and sufferings usually accompanying the condition were avoided.

The preparation of Carcinoma which I have used, for years, was taken from a mammary cancer. The patient had continual seeping of clear, colorless, watery discharge from the open cancer. A small quantity of this fluid was saved and potentized, and has served satisfactorily, in many cases of advanced carcinoma.

In one patient in whom the cancerous tissue involved the neck, over the jaw bone, the diseased tissue had been cut out. When the patient came to me, the site of this tissue has been filled with tissue developed to the size of a goose-egg.

SELENIUM DIOXIDE

Selenium Dioxide was prescribed, and in two weeks, this new growth was openly sloughing. All the tissue that had developed after the operation sloughed out. Hopes were then entertained of accomplishing some permanent good. However, the ulceration continued progressively, and the patient died.

Selenium Dioxide is reported to have cured internal cancer, in the administration of the electics.

CANCER PATIENT CURED.

Mr. H. C. M. was a married man, twenty-eight years old when he appeared for treatment.

Oct. 1, 1903. Nose had a lupus growth across it, resembling a large red saddle. Malaria of nine months' duration five years ago. Checked by doctor with quinine. Irritable. Memory good. Sleeps reclining on back; inclination to place arms above head. Dreams depressing, latter part of night. Respiration slow. Heart pulse 60. No cough. Appetite and thirst small. Rheumatic pains in R. ankle, occasionally in shoulders. Steady pains in small of back. No pains intense. Agg. in winter, amel. in summer: itching and rheumatism. Skin dry; itching on cheeks and nose, and in winter on ears. Spots became hard, lumpy, then red and very itchy; similar itching on head and in rectum. Has never had pimples nor boils. Used to have warts:—burnt off. Feet always cold. Hair falling out. Tonsilitis recurrent. Perspiration copious from exertion. Urine light or yellow, frequent and copious. Rectal evacuation costive, daily, in morning. Sensitive to cold, not to heat. In childhood was sensitive to heat but always had cold feet. Urination frequent, difficult, urine nearly white, following the drinking of two glasses of beer when overheated ten years ago. Considers this the beginning of kidney-trouble and skin disorder. Nausea, riding in cars or on elevators. Psor. cm.

Nov. 7. Stomach—empty sensation. Itching over entire body. Rheumatism in joints; shoulder, wrists, elbows. Anus—moisture; itching. Kidney-region pain. Feet cold. Sensitive to cold. Psor. cm.

Dec. 16. Cold feet and sensitive to cold. No new symptoms.

March 4, 1904. Lupus has not broken out much this winter. Anus—moisture. Tired and languid; wants to recline. Constipation. Respiration sighing. Psor. cm.

April 23 and July 6. Psor. mm. Chief symptoms during this period were rheumatic pain in ankles, sensativeness to cold, nausea riding on cars, hair dropping out, and moisture about anus.

Oct. 1. (about.) Headache frontal. Stomach sour. Nose—lupus visible on crest and side of nose. Nausea, riding on elevated road cured by Psor.

Sulph. 10m.

Nov. 9 and Dec. 23, Sulph. 10m.

Feb. 15. Pains in small of back. Pain in region of

spleen. Headache frontal. Catarrh of nose. Slow to answer. Sleeps with covers over head.

Here the record ceases. The patient has remained cured many years.

CARBUNCLE ON THE BACK OF THE NECK.

Case III.—A lady aged about 30, suffered greatly from a carbuncle on the back of the neck. She had applied many domestic medicines and obtained no relief. The tumefaction seemed destined to suppurate. It was *mottled bluish* and the pain was *intense, knife-cutting* and *burning*. She was sick at the stomach to vomiting, and at night she was delirious. Her eyes were staring and there was some fever; the tongue was foul and the breath fetid. There was great *tension in the scalp and muscles of the face*. She begged for morphine to "stop that *burning* and *cutting*." Tarantula cubensis 12x one dose produced quiet immediately and the angry looking tumefaction failed to complete its work; it did not suppurate. The discoloration was gone in two days, and the hardness soon disappeared also. She regained her normal state very rapidly, and she said to me a short time ago that she had never had her old headache since that swelling left her, showing how deeply the medicine affected her whole system.

If a part is mottled (Lach.), bluish, growing dark, with those symptoms, Tarantula cubensis must be the most appropriate remedy.

CARDIAC PATIENT

In treating heart cases it is very important to be positive in selecting the remedy and then keep the patient on it, continuously. If not certain that the remedy selected is the correct one, the prescriber is apt to expect quick results, and not attaining them will be tempted to change. It is necessary to wait for evidences of improvement in such cases.

Miss C. M., 24 years.

Dec. 5, 1904. Gray hair (a family trait). Rheumatism in l. shoulder. Small goitre. Rapid pulse; mitral murmur, dilated l. side heart; O. S. doctors have given no relief and no encouragement. Endocarditis. Weight in heart, when tired. Back, pain in region of heart. Ribs, sore sensation in cardiac region. Constipation: no action, no desire for evacuation. Tongue, sensation fullness, at root, from exertion. Vision dim or rather strained sensation in eyes. This is felt also in heart. Flatulence in stomach. Cold feet; when excited; during conversation feet become cold and head hot. Excitable, company excites. Must recline during mens. period. Aversion to meat. Leucorrhœa white. Disposition mild. Not sensitive to cold except extreme cold. Puls. 10m.

Dec. 12. Additional symptoms: Respiration difficult, walking in the wind. Dislikes vinegar and pickles. Subject to hiccough. Darkness aggravates. Oppressed in the dark. Aversion to being touched. Improvement since last week: Bowels normal; Back pain imp.

During the next twelve weeks, prescriptions may be summed up briefly:

Jan. 5, PUL.: 10m;

Feb. 23, PULS. 10m.

March 29, PSOR. 10m.

In that period of time the record includes these changes:

General feeling of improvement; menstrual periods more comfortable; eyes improved; aversion to meat disappeared but returned; *Stronger*, rested in shorter time than formerly; craves outdoor air, which ameliorates; worse when warm spring weather appears; for several years has become worse at such time; not so much this year; very comfortable during mens. per. but worse afterward.

March 29. Desire to remain indoors, now. The most prominent symptoms in the record during this period. Complaints from excitement. If she has a good time, becomes sick afterward; feet and hands cold from talking with company. Dreads the dark. Exhausted after shopping; from ascending the stairs; languid; drowsy in the morning; averse to rising. Heat of head and coldness of feet after reading to herself; *Coldness after a bath*; *after a sponge bath*; *skin cold and clammy after a bath* (weak heart). Coldness of feet and hips frequently. Heat in vertex when standing. Leads a sedentary life. Heart palpitation after exertion; heavy sensation around the heart; weakness sensation; conscious of it; pain under left scapula. Vertigo one day when shopping. Mens. per. late (5 days). Nosebleed before M. P. Right ankle swollen (old symptom of many years ago, returned). Larynx sensitive to touch. Neck, glands sore in right side. During much of this period the symptoms were turning toward Psorinum but so long as Pulsatilla benefitted her, it was not wise to change the remedy.

During the following seventeen months, she received the following prescriptions:

June 2, PSOR. 10m.

July 24 and Oct. 20, PSOR. 50m.

Dec. 14 and Jan. 31, 1906: PSOR. cm.

April 10 and June 11, PSOR. Dm.

The most prominent symptoms during this period, varying in duration and intensity—the symptoms that characterized her when there was any discomfort or disturbance—as found in the record are:

Slight swelling of the parotids. (New). Complaints from excitement; chilliness; as previously mentioned. Coldness, with desire for fire during wet weather; chilly when tired, followed by heat. Perspiration after bath; cold; back of hands cold. Aggravation from hurry. Very apprehensive; fear on the street; of being run over. Aggravation from exposure to sun. Wakens with a start; dazed when waking from sleep. Agg. from fright, cold afterward. Sleepy in evening; after dinner; with sleeplessness, formerly could sleep. Tired, aching in limbs and back; Amel. walking in open air. Mens. per. 5—6 days late; nosebleed when per. is due. Hungry before M. Chilly before M. L. arm lameness worse after a storm. Lameness in r. knee; in shoulder and foot. Bruised sensation in arm and hip. Scapulæ, distress in; soreness sensation between scapulæ. Mucus in throat; odor of catarrh in nostrils. Mouth, offensive breath in mornings. R. ankle swollen, first for short periods; then continually; pitting on pressure. This is frequently mentioned at the same time that the patient reports herself splendid and improving. Uncertain sensation when walking on the street, after the July dose. Heart: consciousness of it after dentistry; after mental or physical exertion; heavy after exertion. Pulsation quickened, heavy, after reading to herself a few hours; when excited. Strained sensation in heart; fluttering in heart; sore sensation in l. side. Restlessness referred to stomach; physical exertion occasions fatigue in the stomach. Cold perspiration while walking one day. Cold feet. Weakness from bodily and mental exertion. Flatulence in stomach. Cheeks hot when tired; head hot when excited; heat in body; after rapid walking; heat flashes from much walking, amel, reclining (May '06). Agg. in hot weather, pressure in ears and throat. Neck discomfort from collar; fullness sensation. Vertigo.

Changes during this period of seventeen months include:

General improvement after Mar. 29 and frequently through the record. Stronger; can lift better. Symptoms all lessened. Face less purple than formerly. Gain in flesh on body and about waist. Mens. per. felt very well during period; very comfortable during period. M. on time; period one to three days early; mens. per. made scarcely any difference to her; attended social gatherings. Very active,

34

following accustomed routine during mens. per. Has been shopping much, enjoyed social gatherings, talking with people, attended concerts, and enjoyed all without discomfort or the heat in head she used to have following such meetings. Nosebleed slight. Better in warm than in cold weather. Out nearly every day without fatigue (Nov.). Sensitive to heat (summer of '06). Better when active; ameliorated by long walks; worked all day and was amel. by it. Pulse regular then rapid, otherwise heart appears normal.

It was about twelve months after beginning treatment that examination of the heart revealed no evidences of organic disorder, and since that time heart symptoms have been only functional.

After Psorium ceased to give results, no distinctive symptoms developing, Naja was prescribed. In many cases of heart weakness in children, where there are no distinctive symptoms, cardiac murmurs and cardiac disturbances being associated with nervousness, Naja has cleared away the cardiac troubles and changed the patients to robust children. On that basis the prescription was made, in this instance.

In 1906 she received NAJA 10m, Aug. 15 and Oct. 18. NAJA 50m, Dec. 18 and Jan. 21, 07.

In Sept. '06 she reported she felt the heart very slightly during the summer; she perspired freely and felt no fatigue; Desired open air, fond of walking in open air; chilly in morning.

Jan. 21, '07 she reported having "taken cold" which she said was just such as she had when she began with "heart disease." It was assumed to have been brought out by Naja and considered a good action.

In Feb'y. '07 she reported having had considerable excitement one evening without any heart symptoms.

In March '07 some liver disturbance with jaundice was the occasion of a prescription of NAT. SUL. 10m. The remedy was repeated in 50m potency and then there was no report for six months.

From Dec. 3 to June 20, 1908, there were two prescriptions of PULSATILLA cm, two of PULS. Dm, and one of mm, followed in Aug. by PSOR. mm.

During this period the record contains few symptoms, the chief ones being:

Nearly faints when first going to bed if reclines on back. Agg. in spring. Fear in dark, must have light in sleeping room. If wakens in the dark is frightened. *Sleepiness*. Nosebleed. Chilly before mens. per. Lameness l. arm. Heart: weakness sensation amel. by eructation. Soreness sensation in heart and fullness in throat, waking at night. Feet: puffy swelling. White line along upper lip.

The changes reported during this time are most interesting:

Generally feeling splendid. Fright when waking in the dark improved. Sleeps without a light in the room (June 1). Uses only summer clothing in cold weather. This is new for her and indicates how remedies will cure coldness. Mens. per. late. Reclines flat on back to rest, when tired.

1908. Well all summer; had long walks and much strength; Mens. per. normal, two days late.

After progressing, through a series of Pulsatilla, Psorinum and Naja, the patient turned again to Pulsatilla and that remedy carried her steadily toward health, leading again to Psorinum. Thus do the remedies take up the work, in alternating succession, while the patient advances steadily.

Frequent examination of the heart since the summer of 1908 have revealed no indication of organic changes, at any time.

CENCHRIS CASES
Diarrhoea.

Man of 60 years, Col. K. Diarrhœa. Pain before stool. Stool papescent. Cold, but not chilly. A dose or two of Cenchris 30th cured promptly.

Chill With Sore Throat

Mrs. R., æt. 52. Blond hair, blue eyes, full habit.

May 28, 1889. Had a chill a month ago, with sore throat after it, for which she took Chinin. Since yesterday afternoon, soreness of the right ovary and aching inside, as if gathered in a knot; she can move and walk but with much pain. Had a chill at 3 p. m. yesterday, shivering all over; could not get warm all night. Pulse small and frequent. *Perspiration* from slight motion. After taking supper, retching. Took Chinin, which gives her a headache and bad taste. Cenchris, 45m. 6 powders, one every night, dry.

June 5th. No better for the first two days, then *she was well.*

Pain in Right Ovarian Region

Mrs. H., tall, frail.

Dec. 6, 1887. After being married for three years, complained of a pain in the right ovarian region, like an ulcer, with a thrusting in pain; that she cannot move her leg two days before menstruation. Flow black, dirty discharge, followed a few days later with coagulated blood; later leucorrhœa of large brown and yellow lumps. Under the use of Apis and Sepia, high and highest potencies, she considered herself well by January 4, 1888. But the trouble came back in form of cramps in the right ovary. Apis high did good service again, but did not cure.

Dec. 30, 1889. The menses had come two days earlier. First day, bright red, then dark, lasting four days; not much. After it, pain in the right ovary, like a jumping toothache, for a day. The size of the painful spot had tapered down from three or four inches in diameter to about that of a finger tip. Cenchris cm.

Jan. 13, 1889. Had for the first time in her life a normal menstruation. There was only a slight intimation of pain in the right ovary. She feels good everywhere, and has gained.

The ovarian trouble came probably from injecting cold water immediately after coitus, which the ignorant young thing did, according to the advice of her mother-in-law, who thought her unfit to bear children.

CHILLS.

Case I.—W. B. says he has had several chills and that they are increasing in severity. The first he noticed of his departure from health was a peculiar burning of his skin, his face swelled and looked red, especially about the eyes. He thought it was erysipelas. The burning and itching were intense. It felt so badly that he could not resist pinching and scratching. His eyes closed from the rapid swelling and neck got too big for his collar; over the chest the itching and burning were almost maddening. He applied cold water to his face which gave him comfort and reduced the swelling so he could open his eyes. In spite of the itching and burning he must keep in a warm room. In spite of the local relief from cold the general state was made worse from cold. The urticaria went back and the chills came on beginning in the hands and feet. Chill 12 to 1 for several days, then 10:30 a. m. every other day. Chills begin by a dry cough which lasts until fever is marked. He climbed upon the heater and piled clothing over him during the chill and did not become even comfortably warm until the fever warmed him. Thirst only during chill, for large quantities of water. Bones ache during chill and fever. Fingers cold and dead during chill and the numbness wears off during the fever. Gushing diarrhoea during chill. Fever is not very marked and there is no sweat. During *apyrexia*, he must wear heavy clothing to keep warm; he is much affected by weather changes. Great restlessness day and night. The amelioration from warmth is a marked feature of his whole case. Rhus tox 1m. cured. No more chills.

The beginner might think of Apis in the above case on account of the urticaria and the thirst during the chill, but there was no suffocation attending the eruption, and the amelioration from warmth must exclude apis. Rhus. has no characteristic place for a chill to begin nor special time, but the gushing diarrhœa and aggravation from cold generally and more especially the chill beginning with a dry cough must point to *Rhus.* as the most appropriate remedy.

Where there is a gushing diarrhœa during chill or fever, and urticaria, Elaterium should be consulted. It is characteristic of Hepar to have urticaria during the chill, of Rhus, Ignatia, and Apis during the fever, Rhus, Hepar, and Apis during apyrexia, of Elaterium after the chills have been suppressed. But I have never seen the urticaria crop out incompletely during the apyrexia and seem to get relief by a gushing diarrhoea, in cases cured by Elaterium. It has been only a clinical observation.

CHRONIC ARTHRITIS.

Mrs. N., Age, about thirty-eight, has for about ten years been an invalid as a result of chronic arthritis of the left knee. When it was in the acute stage she was treated by Dr. Hammer, a well-known St. Louis surgeon. It was cupped and blistered but the disease progressed. She was treated by the best allopathic surgeons and still it progressed. The last to have control of it was our lamented Dr. Hodgen, who placed it in a splint, saying that if anchylosis could not be accomplished it must come off. "A stiff leg or no leg," was his language. Two months in a splint failed to accomplish anchylosis.

July 16th, 1881, I was called to the case. The knee was painful and extremely sore to touch, enlarged to twice the size of the well one and very hard. The thigh was emaciated and the ankle and feet were œdematous. The limb was wrapped and she was in bed. She could sit up but the limb could not be moved much, it was so painful from motion. There was great burning in the soles and top of the head. Sulph. 55000 one dose dry. Sac. lac.

The husband came to me the next morning, saying that Mrs. N. was much worse. She had suffered greatly during the night and had pain all over the body. I visited her and urged her to bear her suffering, that it would pass off soon. She took Sac. lac till August 20th, and Sulph. 81m was given, one dose dry. Slight aggravation followed, but she said she could bear it, as the first medicine which aggravated had been followed by such relief. September 1st. The pain has all subsided and she is moving about the house on crutches. September 20th, she sent for me. I found crepe on the door and learned that her husband had been sick a week and had died under allopathic treatment; that she had been up night and day attending him and was very nervous and the limb was much more painful. She took Ignatia for some days until the sad occasion had passed over a little, when I again paid my attention to the knee. October 8th she took Sulph. 81m and she thought it gave her rest, but not much improvement in the knee. She continued Sac. Lac. to November 12th. The joint has grown smaller, the foot is not so œdematous, no burning in the soles or top of head. Her appetite is good and she is gaining strength. In a general way she is much improved. Not seeing how matters could be improved by medicine, without better indications, I concluded to continue Sac. Lac.

December 3d. She complained of cold feet and that every change in the weather from warm to cold gave her pain in the knee and she had a craving for eggs. She had difficulty in keeping warm. Calc. 85m and Sac Lac for a month.

January 7th, 1882—Feeling very comfortable; slept well most of her nights; feet warm, and there was not much pain in the knee; swelling in knee going down; she is about the house on crutches; the sensitiveness is gradually going out of the knee. Sac Lac.

During all this time there has been limited motion in the limb, but the slightest motion has always caused pain, but she has been able to swing it off the bed, holding the foot up to prevent flexion and then with her crutches she has been going about the house with comparative comfort.

February 3d.—Calc. 85m. Improving slowly.

March 25th.—There is some motion in the knee without much pain; the joint is slowly growing smaller; no swelling of the foot; she now wears a shoe that mates the right, the first time for ten years or more. Sac. Lac.

April 4th.—No new symptoms; improvement has ceased. Calc-c. 85m and Sac. Lac.

May 3d.—No change from last date; no new symptoms; eating well, sleeping well; countenance looks well. What shall I do? Prescribe for the knee? No. I wait Sac. Lac.

June 3d.—Sour eructations that seem to burn the pharynx but do not come up into the mouth; knee more painful; nights restless; must move about, which seems to relieve; drawing pain in the knee; gnawing pain in the stomach. "A sour eructation, the taste of which does not remain in the mouth, but the acid gnaws in the stomach"

Lyc. "Incomplete burning eructations which only rise into the pharynx, where they cause a burning for several hours" (Allen) Lyc.

Lycopodium having all the rest of the symptoms, it was given 71m, and Sac. Lac. The knee became very painful and she was compelled to keep her bed for several days. Each day I visited her and she took Sac. Lac.

July 2d.—She is walking with crutches and has very little pain in the knee; no pain in stomach or eructation. Improving.

August 3d.—Improving. Sac. Lac.

September 2d.—Lycop. 71m and Sac. Lac.

September 6th.—Slight aggravation from the Lyc. Improving.

October 1st.—Improving. Sac. Lac.

November 8th.—Improving. Sac. Lac.

December 15th.—Lycopod 71m and Sac Lac.

January, 1883.—It is now eighteen months since taking this case. The patient is in good flesh, and the knee is the only thing that gives her trouble. There is still limited motion. The motion is not much painful except when forced flexion is attempted. She goes about the yard and out into the road. I furnished her a cane and advised laying aside one of the crutches. She has no fear of the knee being hit, which heretofore has been a great factor in the case.

May 1.—She walks with a crutch and cane. Limbs gaining motion continuously. No new symptoms, knee nearly natural. She can bear some weight on the left foot. Lyc. 71m dry and Sac. Lac.

July 8th—Rheumatism pains in both knees and such restlessness that she moves all night. Stiffness in joints, which passes off by motion; while in motion she feels better, Rhus. tox. 1m in water every three hours.

July 10th.—Improved. Restlessness all gone. Stiffness some better. Sac. Lac.

August 5th—Improving. Rhus tox 32m one dose, and Sac. Lac.

September 1st.—I found her walking with one cane. She moved over the house to show me how well she could walk.

October 1st.—Improving. Rhus. tox. 32m one dose, and Sac. Lac.

November 8th.—Rhus. tox. 32m one dose, and Sac Lac.

December 5th.—She walked with the aid of her cane two blocks to a street car, and came to my office without the aid of the cane.

January 7th., 1884.—Came to my office. She walks with a limp. Limited motion in the knee, but the soreness has gone. I asked her if she regretted going under constitutional treatment, to which she answered: "Ten thousand times, no."

I have referred to two distinguished allopathic attendants, simply to show that the best surgical skill had been applied, and that the value of the purely homœopathic method may be the better appreciated. Ten years she grew worse, and in two and one-half years she was cured. If it can be argued that she recovered without medicine, then the means that had been used were destroying her life.

CHRONIC DISORDERS PROMPTLY CURED
MALARIA FEVER

Mr. R., young man, 38 years old, was discharged from the U. S. army for physical disability from chronic malaria; had taken quinine in twenty grain doses for years to keep down recurrent malaria; he seldom went longer than six weeks before his chills would return; he suffered severely, but with a confused general condition. He had never permitted his case to develop into well-defined symptoms but he was pale and ached all over; full of chilliness

the afternoon and evening and heat all night. Chronic
digestion; can eat but few simple foods. Malaria con-
acted in Delaware over twelve years ago; has suffered
er since. Distended with much gas stomach and bowels.
urning pain. Restless during fever and must move con-
antly. Aching in limbs with fever. More sensitive to
ld than to heat; likes to be warm. Cannot concentrate
ind. Thirst only moderate. Wants everything very salty.
tool: urging drives him out of bed every morning. Feet
re so warm that he *sleeps with them out of bed* often in
ld weather. Sulph. 10m relieved all his symptoms and
e felt well for six weeks, then his symptoms began to re-
rn; he had been thinking he was well. Sulph. 10m was
peated and he did not return for 40 days because he
ought he could do without me, he felt so well. His
ymptoms began to return; Sulph. 50m. Has remained in
erfect health. He is an engineer and much exposed, but
is endurance is better that it ever was and he has added
esh and color.

GASTRIC DISTURBANCE.

Catherine W., aged 7. Every 2 or 3 weeks paroxysms
f vomiting, with high fever, red face, and thirst for ice-
ld water. Since infancy has had these vomiting spells.
he vomits yellow and green mucus, even pure bile. She
as taken much medicine and had several physicians.
aundiced eyes and skin. Constipation; has used cathar-
ics and injections. Stools usually undigested. Urine:
rickdust-sediment. Very chilly in cold weather but the
tomach symptoms are worse in hot weather. Lips chap
1 cold weather. Suffers much more in summer. The
varmer the weather the severer are the paroxysms. Cold
ands and damp feet. Skin mottled. Tongue heavily
oated. Temperature subnormal when the spells are not
resent. Excitable; cries, then laughs. Phos. 10m.

In five weeks one light attack. Phos. 10m.

Six weeks later she began to have signs of a return Phos. 50m.

Seven weeks later she vomited, after her mother gave her stronger food (as the child appeared very well.) Phos 50m. No sign of returning symptoms for two months and ten days. Phos. cm.

Two months later: Stool formed, undigested. Cold hands and feet. Mottled skin. Thirst for very cold water Phos. cm.

She is now a robust child, growing rapidly; no symptoms.

CICATRIX REMOVED BY MEDICINE

A young lady twenty-six years old, consulted me for some cicatrices on the left side of the neck, an indentation that disfigured her very much was there. She said with the exception of cold, damp feet, she was in good health The fistulous openings had been there, discharging several years, and finally closed under some sort of blood, or root syrup. Believing that her treatment had only temporarily controlled the trouble, I attempted to find what her remedy should be. From all I could glean, and she had very few symptoms, but the Calc-c. Symptom of "cold damp stockings" was there. She took one dose of Calc-c, 85m.

On the third day her neck began to be painful. She called to ask me if the medicine had anything to do with it Plenty of S. L. was given. The deep cicatrix suppurated and discharged several calcareous nodules and the neck healed with scarcely a scar where the one opened. A depression about two inches from this one is unsightly. She wished that had opened in like manner, but a little surgical skill may remove the other.

Lippe gives, Cicatrices breaking open; Carbo-v., Crocus, Crotal, Lach., Nat-m., Phos., Sil.

CLINICAL CASES
OLD SCHOOL DRUGGING

Miss W. L. C., aged thirty-five years, is a nurse, and has had free treatment many years, hence has had violent old-school drugging until she is scarcely able to earn her living. Deafness in both ears, agg. in left, from quinine. Perspires easily from exertion. *Quinine*; am-c., *ant-t., apis*, ARN.· ars., asaf., *bell.,* CALC., caps., carb-v., *cina.*, cop., dig., **ferr.**, ferr-ar., gels., hell., ip., *lach.*, merc., nat-m., nux-v., *ph-ac.*, phos., plb., puls., samb., *sep.*, stann., sul-ac., *sulph.*, verat. *Perspires on slight exertion*; Ars., calc., caps., carb-v., ferr., ferr-ar., *gels.*, lach., *merc.*, nat-m., phos., sep., stann., sulph., sul-ac., verat. *Impaired hearing*; Ars., calc., caps., carb-v., *ferr.*, ferr-ar., *gels., lach., merc.*, nat-m., phos., *sep.*, sulph., *sul-ac.*, verat. *Ears, roaring in*; Ars., calc., carb-v., ferr., ferr-ar., *gels. lach., merc.*, nat-m., phos., *sep.*, sulph., *sul-ac.*, verat. *Ringing*; Ars., calc., carb-v., *ferr.*, lach., *merc., nat-m., phos.*, sep., sulph., sul-sep., *sulph.*, **sul-ac.** *Impaired hearing, human voice*; Ars., phos., sulph. *Taste bitter*; Ars., calc., carb-v., *lach.*, nat-m., *phos., sep.*, sulph. *Catarrh of nose*; Ars., calc., carb-v., *lach.*, nat-m.· *phos.*, sep., sulph. *Desires fresh air*; Ars., carb-v., *lach., nat-*m., phos., sep., sulph. *Walking in open ac.*, verat. *Buzzing*; Ars., calc., *carb-v.*, lach., *nat-m.*, phos., air amel.; Carb-v., nat-m., phos., sep., *sulph. Warm room agg.*; Carb-v., *nat-m., phos., sulph.*

SULPH, 10m and on through a series of potencies, has made a radical change for the better; she is now able to earn her living.

EXOPHTHALMIC GOITRE.

Mrs. G. S. B., aged forty-eight. Married 24 years; mother of four children, three living; youngest child nine years old. Been sick three years. Exophthalmic goitre. Eyes not badly protruding. Gaining flesh. Very sensitive to heat. Stool daily; used to have diarrhœa after a full meal. M. P. last time was in the spring. Ceased every year for three months in summer. Profuse; painful first and last day. Weakness until next period. No hot flashes. No thirst, but drinks some water, not iced. Cheerful. Startled feeling on beginning to sleep; but not much now. Never strong; always tired. No hereditary trouble. Excitement agg. Enjoys intensely. Severe headache from eye-trouble; none now. Weak muscles. Small wounds bleed much. Desires hot food. Agg. in warm room. Must have fresh air. Wants to do things in a hurry and wants others to hurry. Other people's troubles are a burden. Sensitive mentally. Blind spells in summer. Can't think in the summer; weakness; depressed all summer. Winter, cheerful. Uses only light clothing day or night. Exertion agg. mental or physical. Diarrhœa from eating fruit: peaches, oranges, apples, bananas. Likes sweet and sour. Likes food well salted. Aversion to eggs. Activity of mind. Dwells on past disagreeable events. Sensitive to noise. Anxiety or fear when away from home; this had been true ever since had sunstroke when a child fourteen years old. Dreams vivid. Acute pain in left ovary while standing. Horror of blind spells. Depressed. Needs much sleep. Talking over her symptoms always agg. Pulse 140. Given up as incurable by her allopathic doctor. Lycopus 1m was given twice, at long intervals, followed by 10m 2 doses at long intervals, then 50m 2 doses at long intervals, cm 2 doses at long intervals; then the series was repeated, beginning with 1m.

This was many years ago, and she remains well; size of neck is normal; heart is normal and there is no protrusion of the eyes.

The patient was under treatment fifteen months.

ENLARGED GLANDS.

Miss J. Y., aged twenty-two. Family history good.

Enlarged gland left side of neck, tubercular. First started a year ago. Cut out nearly four months ago. Has now returned. Before operation, drowsy, sleepy, no ambition. Tired easily; better since operation. First menses at eighteen, normal. Takes cold from wet feet more than in any other way. Sleep good; usually wakens once. Appetite poor before operation. Does not care for corned beef, cabbage, nor stews. Very fond of ham and eggs. Prefers acids to sweets. Not especially sensitive to either heat or cold. Constipated; takes salts, etc. Usually no urging. Painless. Teeth decayed early. Feet, perspiration warm. Never thirsty unless eats salty food; drinks three or four glasses of water daily "Because people say it is good for you." Wants the water very cold, iced in summer. Patient came from Ireland at the age of sixteen; before coming to this country the patient often had weak spells with vertigo and staggering; amel. by fresh air. Feels better in this country. Perspiration in summer agg. on face; only comes when at work in a warm place. Eruption on face since coming to America; agg. in summer. Bloody discharge sometimes, at other times yellow. No special sensation in eruption. Menses every three weeks; flow a very bright red, no clots. Profuse first two days and lasts about four days.

TUBERC. 10m, 50m, cm, two doses of each, far apart, cured.

SEVERE PAIN BEFORE M. P.

Miss M. G., aged twenty-one. M. P.: Severe pain two hours before the flow begins; she faints. Cramping; soreness through abdomen. This trouble began a year ago. Every four or five weeks. Flow scanty; lasts one and a half to two days. Dark; clots first day; "black lumps of blood." Pain between shoulders. Headache sometimes over forehead. Likes to be out of doors. Walks a little, must sit down to rest; feet and sacrum get tired and ache. LAPIS-ALB. 10 m.

Two months later she returned with the following report:

Less pain at M. P. and periods four weeks apart; flow lasted three days; Few clots the second day. No pain between shoulders. Less pain in feet and sacrum. Lapis-alb. 10m.

In six months she returned with third report:

Been very well; no pain anywhere except between shoulders. Last period was late. Lapis-a. 50m.

MULTIPLE ULCERS.

Miss C. N., aged twenty-three. Multiple ulcers on left leg; four ulcers; began three years ago. Brown crust surrounded by very dark copper-colored skin; she has no history of syphilis, no loss of hair, no sore throat. Tapeworm six or eight years ago cured (?) by strong drugs. Cough dry. Desires cold and warm drinks. Not sensitive to heat or cold. Very nervous; drops what she holds in her hands, if spoken to. Sensation of a closely fitted cap on head. Feels best in open air. Kali-sulph. 10m and 50m, two doses of each, far apart, cured.

HEADACHE

June 16th. Mrs. W., Mother of Mrs. M. W. Headache for a number of days. Chill this morning, followed by high fever. Chills and fever three years ago; thinks they have returned. Aching in all the bones and muscles. Tongue coated, bitter taste. Nausea. Dry stomach cough. *S. L.*

June 18th. No chill yesterday, but a great pain in back and head. At 5:30 A. M. today had a racking pain in head. Chill began at 8 A. M. today, lasted three hours. Followed by fever, which lasted nine hours. Great pain in head during fever. Perspiration profuse, smelling like sour, musty water. Breath offensive. Tongue coated. No appetite. Urine very dark, passed every hour. Can hardly move her head. *Ars.* 103 m. and *S. L.* every six hours. One prescription cured.

ULCER

November 15th. Mrs. W., age 70. Ulcer in left ankle began with smarting, stinging pain, with a little spot size of a pea. Next day it broke and ran a thin, bloody discharge; flesh around spot was purplish red. The sore extended, and the discharge became thick and yellow, until it is now somewhat larger than a dollar. It is red and there are patches of yellow matter; looks something like a sponge. The cloths taken off it are slightly offensive. Ulcer burns, stings, smarts; sometimes has a jerking sensation through heel; she wants it kept cool, it is worse from warmth. Pain is something like splinters or buzzing. Limb from knee down sweats profusely; not so the other. Foot begins to swell when she gets up in the morning, swells until it is full and pains her much. About 3 or 4 P. M. she gets easier and can lie down. At night all the swelling goes down, and when she lies quiet with her foot on a level with her head she is easy. Upper side of arms from shoulder to elbow are very sore to touch. Using arms makes them ache, a "grumbling pain." Cords of neck are somewhat sore. Cannot put her arms back, and cannot reach out for anything, or the shoulder will catch her. Can put her arms forward and over head, straight up. Sometimes middle fingers of hand, generally the left, stand out in the morning so she can can scarcely bend them. Likes to sit with hands put together, the arms drawn toward each other and head bent forward; she cannot sit with her arms on the chair, spread apart. Has to fold arms and work herself over when she turns in bed.

35

Wants to drink almost every five minutes in the afternoon. *Puls.* c. m.

All symptoms were removed and the patient remained well until

March 21st, 1893. Rheumatism in right side; seems to be in hip-joint mostly. A steady pain all the time; sometimes more intense. Sometimes when attempting to walk, can hardly stand. Worse when sitting than when lying. Cannot lie on right side. Heat relieves somewhat; cold increases pain. Cold feeling through leg and foot. Flesh sore and slightly swollen. Came on suddenly three days ago, and remains in same place. Feels well otherwise. Appetite good. *Puls.* m. m. Cured.

DIABETES MELLITUS, CURED WITH PHOSPHORUS.

Case.—July 2d, 1890. Male, tall, well-formed, aged forty-seven. This illness has been coming on about three years; has lost thirty-five pounds in weight and is losing steadily. Ability to exercise steadily growing less. Sleepless nights. Two years ago had occasional attacks of diarrhoea, accompanied with abdominal suffering; after these attacks the sleeplessness increased. Sometimes the pain in abdomen keeps him awake nights. Dull aching diffused through abdomen; worse nights; worse when lying during day. Copious perspiration on slight exertion. Very nervous, must keep in motion. Stool light colored. Violent pulsation felt in body. Strong action of the heart and full rapid pulse, 95 to 100. Had "grippe" last winter and has been losing much faster since. Greasy cuticle on the urine.

Brickdust in urine, not always. Excitement often brings on a sensation as though the head or skull is divided above the ears, and lifted up and down. Can sleep in one position as well as in another. Heat overcomes him quickly but he is not sensitive to cold. Weak from exertion of body and mind. Must arise in the night to pass urine. Quantity of urine four to five pints. Specific gravity of the urine, 1030 to 1035. Fermentation test gives sugar twelve to fifteen grains per ounce. Rumbling in abdomen. This patient has visited several allopathic physicians who had given him many strong drugs, especially Podo., Strych. He had not received any homœopathic advice. Thirst for cold water. Smarting of anus. Has been told he had fissure of anus. A few days later after a careful study of all remedies related to the case he received Phos. cm, which was followed by a sharp aggravation of all symptoms.

He improved steadily without further medicine until October 31st, when his symptoms began to return. The sugar disappeared from the urine within a month, and has not since appeared.

October 31st same year Phos. mm. He is in perfect health, doing active brain work, and his endurance is as great as ever.

DYSMENORRHŒA

Mattie E.——,age twenty-three. Since the first menstrual nisus, which occurred at thirteen, she has suffered great pain at every period, which has been every three weeks. Pain in the uterus and down the limbs. Before and during she has suffered from an empty, hungry, all-gone feeling in the stomach (Sep., Murex, Ign.) ; she cannot stand long on the feet, the pain is so much aggravated; cold, feet, great dizziness when going up stairs, voracious appetite.

The fact that this difficulty dated back to puberty guided me to Calc-phos. She never had any more pain. This young lady was compelled to avoid any engagement that might come on her sick day, as she was compelled to keep her bed most of the first day. Her expressions of gratitude have often cheered me, and her praise has brought me much business.

So important is Calc-Phos. in the painful affections
of the uterus connected with puberty, and resulting from
bad habits or neglected advice at that time, that I feel
like emphasizing this feature of it. It is a common practice in rural districts for girls at puberty to wade in water
and do many careless things, thereby laying foundation
for dysmenorrhoea and sterility. The complaints growing out of these causes find their remedy in Calc-phos. in
a very large number of instances.

DYSMENORRHŒA

Miss X____, twenty-four years old, had suffered from
dysmenorrhoea since puberty. She always kept her bed
during the first day. Menses a few days too soon and
profuse, lasting five days. The pain was labor-like, and
there was some bearing down in the vagina, with a sensation as if the parts would protrude. She often felt as if
her menses would come on at different times during the
interim, and sometimes a sexual flame annoyed her. Generally she was robust and free from complaint. Calc-phos.
cured this lady in two months.

She was an orphan, having no mother to advise her,
therefore exposure at the time that she most needed to
exercise judgment, brought on the suffering that lasted
ten years before she obtained the appropriate remedy.
This patient had submitted to local treatment without
palliation. She had been told that internal medication
could not benefit her.

DYSMENORRHŒA

Miss Susie C____, twenty-two years old, consulted me
for dysmenorrhoea. Her menses came very much too soon,
and lasted from seven to ten days. The flow was dark
and clotted the first three or four days; the severe pain
was at the beginning; she got some relief after passing
membranes. She complained of aphthous patches in the

mouth and sometimes on the labia. She always had a leucorrhoea several days before menstruation, white-of-egg-
like and ropy. Her pains were often labor-like, constricting (Cactus), extending into the back and up the back
(Gels.), and down the thighs (Cham.), and sometimes to
the stomach, causing vomiting. She would always weep
from music (Natrum) and grow sick and become frightened when going down from any high building in an elevator.

She got Borax 3m at proper intervals. The result
was satisfactory. The second period was painless and normal. The relief in this case has been permanent.

EPITHELIOMA.

1885. Mr_____, clergyman. Epithelioma of several
years standing on the left upper lid. The scale that comes
off about once in three or four weeks is dark red. It
fissures and bleeds in the spring of the year. Sometimes
it pulsates. The lid is thick and indurated. No constitutional symptom obtained. Lachesis 4m cured in six
months.

CHRONIC LIVER.

October 10th, 1893. Mrs. M. W., Age, 36. Weight, 200
pounds. Gouty constitution. "Chronic liver." Enormously
enlarged liver. Great soreness in region of liver. Warm-
blooded woman. Red face. Gets up with bad taste in
mouth. Has taken everything (and will now obey.) Formerly used a rubber cushion to prevent pain in coccyx,
cold hands. Very cold feet. Hyperæmia of brain. Fullness
in head. Urine scanty at times. Menstrual flow scanty. No
pains. *Natr. sul.* 20 m. One dose and *s. l.*

November 8th.—Pain in side much better. Old
symptoms returning. Before menses leucorrhoea with
fishy odor. (Old symptom.) Has always been much heated

in summer, but never perspired. *S. L.* Milk always failed with her children.

December 10th. Soreness and swelling in region of liver has entirely disappeared. Fullness in head and pain in back part of head is bad all the time. Fullness in eyes; feels at times as if there was a cloud over them; this disappears after closing eyes two or three times. Dreadful taste in mouth, worse in morning. Drinks very little water. Perspires more than she ever did; arms warmer; legs and feet cold. Gout in right foot. Heart very quick at times, often when she only rises to walk across the room (always walks fast); notices it more in the evening. Is generally a good deal swollen before menses. Always feels better the two weeks after menses. Soreness in breasts only lasted three days before menses and was not so severe. Bowels regular, though more constipated than she has ever been. Urine very scanty, light color, except for about ten days before menses, when it is the color of orange juice. Not so much of the fishy smell to leucorrhoea. *Natr. sul.* 20 m. One dose and *s. l.*

January 18th, 1894. After the first three powders vertigo, worse closing eyes. Fullness in back of head and eyes. Red spot on cheek no better. Nose, legs and upper part of arms cold. Rheumatism in back of legs. Pain so severe at times that she cannot lift legs or straighten up. Severe pain across lower part of back, as though hundreds of needles were going in. Must keep clearing throat all the time. Dryness in nose and back part of throat. Dreadful taste in back of mouth. Urine darker before menses, clear and profuse after. Odor of stale crackers. Menses last three days. Pain in back came very suddenly as she was stooping over. Dreams in latter part of night. Sore throat on awakening this morning, l. side yellow. *S. L.* 30 powders.

February 26th. Swelling over liver and around waist

for three weeks. Shortness of breath. Color of urine changed; like thick orange juice in morning, natural in afternoon. Sharp pains about heart. Sharp pains from sternum to l. breast. At times sensation of weight in region of l. breast. Pain in lower part of back. Bearing-down pains. Leucorrhoea for six weeks. Has not had it before for twelve years. Dull, heavy pain in l. leg from hip to knee. Pain in l. ankle, as though knife had cut through; lasts about three hours and is so severe she can't step upon foot. Gout in fourth toe of *left* foot, formerly in *right* foot. Head worse than for four years. Intense fullness in back and fore part of head and eyes, worse at night. Top of head sore to touch. Eyes feel as though they would shoot out of head with burning pain. Breasts very sore. It is within a few days of menses. Dryness in throat and nose very bad. Feet and legs cold all the time. Deaf in l. ear for six weeks. *Natr. sul.* 50 m. *S. L.* 30 powders.

April 3d. Fullness in occiput—dreadful. When tired, cloud in front of eyes. Dry mouth; bitter taste. Dryness in nostrils. Crawling like a worm in throat. Feels like sighing. Sore pain in breasts during m. p.. continues after. *S. L.*

May 14th. Bad taste in mouth. Fullness in head, worse at night. Heavy feeling in liver. Pain in hip bones, particularly the right, worse lying on them. Return of gout in *right* foot. Menses on time, but flowed only two days. Urine is better. Hawks up thick, offensive matter from throat. Nose and throat still very dry. Red spot on face remains. *Nat. sul.* 50m. *S. L.* 30 powders.

September 14th. Rush of blood to head. Burning hands and face. Pain in left side of the back (lumbar). Soreness at end of the spine. Soreness in liver. Frequent urging to urinate. Menses regular, lasting only two days.

Before menses a fishy smell to urine; menstrual flow offensive and greenish. *Natr. sul.* 50 m.

October 2d. Urinary symptoms amel. Leucorrhœa thin, white. Feels wretched all the time. Head full of blood, face purple, spot on the right cheek worse than it has ever been. Pain over eyes and at base of brain. Sight seems blurred. Soreness in region of liver. Offensive taste. Great desire to clear throat; dryness extending up into nose. Stiff and sore all over. Excessive nervousness. Fluttering at heart. All symptoms agg. from 6 A. M. to 1 P. M. *Natr. sul.* c. m.

October 16th. Sensation of fullness in head and body, with cold hands, feet and nose. Menses on October 9th, three days late, flow lasted only two days, but from that time till now there has been little discharge of blood all the time; she took *Puls.* one dose as head was so bad and she hoped this would bring on menses; it did not make her feel any better. Pain in back. *S. L.* 30 powders.

March 17, 1896. Entirely free from symptoms until recently. The last remedy helped her much. Very nervous. Palpitation. Pulsating all over with twitching. Great flatulence. Eructation of wind and food, of all things eaten. If she has eaten a little she feels as if she had eaten a full meal. Bad taste in mouth. Tongue parched and dry. Menses very regular, offensive odor. Pain in back of head when tired. Legs so nervous in evening that she cannot keep still. Breasts sore when she takes off the pressure at night. Feels oppressed before menses. *Lyc.* 43 m.

April 18th. For the first ten days after medicine she could jump out of her skin. Good action of remedy. Left hand and arm numb. Pain in the pit of stomach. Bloated abdomen before menses. Dreams much. White tongue. Offensive taste. Palpitation. Skin not so dry. Perspires. Burning hot on warm days, with pricking, tingling. Burning like coals of fire on top of head. *S. L.*

May 25th. Symptoms returning. *Lyc.* 43 m.

Dec. 1st. Burning pain in stomach. Mist before eyes before m. p. Pain in sacrum after m. p. Offensive taste. Difficulty in hearing. *Lyc.* c. m.

Dec. 12th. Very sore throat, red all over, yellow spots on both sides, worse on right side, hurts on swallowing fluid; no fever; heaviness in head and fullness; right ear aches. Second finger on right hand very sore. Has used flaxseed poultice without relief. *Sac. lac.* in water.

January 23, 1897. Burning pain in stomach. Mist before eyes before m. p. Throat still troubles her somewhat. Numbness in left hand. *Lyc.* c. m.

April 9th. Burning above the navel. Feels worse after coffee; weak feeling. Symptoms returning. Has been very well since last remedy until recently. *Lyc.* c. m.

Patient now perfectly well. No aches or pain.

ECZEMA-MEZEREUM

August 24, 1884.—Mrs. C., aged forty-two. Eczema of twenty years' standing. Eruptions on back of hand and wrists half-way up to elbow; itching, aggravated by scratching; small, burning vesicles, drying down to crusts, itching and burning after scratching, and becoming moist after scratching. Violently worse from the application of water; considerable burning in the vesicle.

Eruptions on back of hands, Arg.-m., Asar., Berb., Mez., Phos., Plat., Plumb., Stront., Thuj., Zinc.

Particularly eczema, Mez., Phos.

Burning vesicles, Bov., Caust., Graph., Merc., Mez., Mur.-ac., Natr.-c., Nat.-m., Nat.-s., Nit-ac., Phos., Sep., Spig., Spong., Staph., Sulph.

Eruptions, itching, made worse by scratching, Amm.-m., ANAC., Arn., Ars., Bism., Bov., *Calad.*, Cann.-s. Canth., *Caps.*, Carb.-an., CAUST., Cham., Kreos., Ledum., *Merc.*,

MEZ., Mur-ac., Natr-c., *Phos.*, Phos.-ac., PULS., Sepia, Silic., Spong., Staph., Stront., Sulph.

Itching, burning after scratching, Anac., Arn., Ars., Bovista, Calad., Canth., CAUST., Can., Kreos., Led., *Merc.*, *Mez.*, PHOS., Puls., *Sep.*, SIL., Staph., Stront., SULPH.

Eruptions itching, becoming moist after scratching, Ars., Bov., CARB-V., Caust., Kreos., Graph., LACH., Ledum., LYC., Merc., MEZ., *Petrol.*, Rhus-t., Sep., Staph., Sil., Sulph., and many others not related to the general case.

Eruptions aggravated from washing, AM.-C., ANT.-C., Bov., Calc., *Canth.*, *Carb.*, Caust., CLEM., Dulc., Kali-c., Lyc., *Merc.*, *Mez.*, Mur.-ac., *Nitr.-ac.*, *Phos.*, RHUS., *Sars.*, SEP., *Spig.*, Staph., Stront., SULPH.

Mezereum 20m—One dose dry and Sac. Lac. The burning and itching passed away in a few days. The skin became soft and normal in less than four weeks, and has remained healthy. She never had been entirely free from the suffering caused by the eruption.

How much superior this expectancy is to doses so large you are sure to have medicine in! Why don't they bring on their cures?

Perhaps it is because this agnosticism makes them doubt that they have made any. It seems here to please some of these doubters. I was told that anybody could report cures, that such reports were not to be admitted as evidence. I therefore presented a paper on the sixteenth section of the *Organon* of Samuel Hahnemann as an argument without cures. I hear of no answer that has offset those statements of facts; again I am coming with cures to corroborate the doctrine—these principles. Hence I have so fully presented a very simple case of a most natural chronic disease where washes and ointments and *alternatives* had been used for twenty years, and in all antagonism had never been met. The true specific for the disease was met in Mez. 20m. *Cito, tuto e jocunde.*

HEADACHE.

Mar. 17, 1894.—Mrs. Alice T------, age 60. 1121 R------ St. Large, fleshy woman. Gray hair. Headache —"comes on me like a shadow"—between scalp and brain. Has had these headaches for ten years. Feels as if going out of her mind. worry, trouble. Must hold on to something. *Followed prolonged nursing and loss of sleep.* Sensation of opening and shutting of occiput. Pains rolling, pressing, crushing, as if head would burst. Vertex and occiput— as if bound. Had to roll head and vomit. Pitches toward right side when walking. Can hear what is going on when asleep, even snoring. Cannot relieve herself by weeping. It is a burden to keep eyes open. Could not sleep at all for several months. *Cocculus* 30m. March 24. Improved. Headaches seem to go down over her like a shadow, look- ing or reaching up. *S. L.* March 31. Improvement. *S. L.* Apr. 7. Improvement. *S. L.* Apr. 14. Headache again. From this date until May 12, 1894, she continued to re- ceive S. L., when she considered herself cured, and as late as March, 1895, there had been no return of the symptoms.

GALL STONE COLIC CURED

Mrs. F. B. W., aged thirty-seven years, had been ex- amined by her brother-in-law, a surgeon among the allo- paths, and another surgeon, and was to prepare for an operation for removal of gall stones, the week following her first consultation here. When told that it was possible for her gall-stones to be dissolved, without an operation, by the action of homœopathic medicine, she reported to her family and the surgeon-brother said that only a quack would promise or presume to dissolve gall-stones with a remedy. Accordingly the woman's husband appeared at the office with denouncement of him who offered encouragement to the wife that she could be cured without an operation. However, when the query was presented: "If your wife should be treated with a remedy, so that she would be free from gall-stone colic and the gall-stones should disappear and she should be strong, who would be the quack, the doctor who gave the curative remedy or your brother?" he unhesitatingly decided in favor of the prescriber of the remedy. Accordingly his wife began with homœopathic treatment.

Nov. 2, 1904. Has had a long siege of typhoid fever. Headaches, followed by vomiting of bile, recurrent, for years. Pain starts in r. eye, extends over forehead with a dragging sensation in occiput. Face purple. Mother had gall-stones and grand-mother died of gall-stones. Gall-stone colic, in August. Pain > by heat. Sleeps with shawl over her head. Very nervous; easily startled; apprehensive. Sacrum-pain extends to thigh on r. side. Intensely fastidious. Cold feet: hot water bottle in bed at night. Headache at menstrual per. for sixteen years, since her boy's birth. M. flow thick, clotted, dark, only one day. Fecal evacuations light, when sick; then dark, as recovers. Must restrain herself or would commit suicide. Pulse slow at times. Nat. s. 10m.

Reference to the repertory, with the following symptoms:

Inclination to commit suicide; *startled easily*; *sacral pain extending to thigh*; *feet cold in bed*; *m. flow clotted*; *m. flow dark*; *m. flow thick*; *vomiting during headache*; *vomiting bile*; results in the following totals for the most prominent remedies: Merc. 14; Nat-c. 9; Nat-m. 14; Nat.-s. 12; Sulph. 20. From these the selection was made.

Nov. 12. Nat.-s. 10m.

Jan. 3 and Jan. 24. Nat.-s. 50m.

By February symptoms of gall-stone and suicidal symptoms had entirely disappeared.

HÆMOPHILIA—LACHESIS

History.—Has been a bleeder since birth. Just before he was born his mother had a tooth extracted, and the bleeding from the gum could not be stopped for a long time. Every scratch or little cut he had would keep on bleeding until he was almost exsanguinated and then the wound would heal. Had smallpox when a year old. At 12 years of age he sustained a small cut on forearm, the hæmorrhage from which could not be stopped. Suturing was attempted in Pennsylvania Hospital, but this only increased the bleeding points. Was in hospital for 5 weeks, and when he was "bled out" the wound healed. Fracture of right thigh bone and delayed union—8 weeks before any union was observed. Every slight bruise followed by extensive ecchymosis. Epistaxis continued for 3 or 4 days once. Rheumatism for the past two years, since the development of which the bleedings have not been so troublesome. Just before coming here he has been in bed for two months suffering from "inflammation of bowels" and hæmorrhage till he was "bled out."

June 2, 1896. *Present symptoms.* Rheumatic pain in knees and elbows; can hardly stand. Swelling of the knees. Pale from bleeding. Bleeding from gums constantly. Small wounds bleed much. Small bruise makes him black and blue. Great thirst for water; hydrant water satisfied. *Lach.* 41m., one dose.

July 29.—Felt first rate until July 2d. Rheumatism returned to elbows—*left* first. *Lach.* 41m., one dose.

Aug. 22. Improving constantly.

Dec. 7. Stiffness in knees and elbows. *Lach.* 41m., one dose.

Jan. 30, 1897. Some stiffness returning. *Lach.* cm., one dose.

Sept. 6. No symptoms.

Oct. 5. Some bleeding. Rheumatic swelling in right elbow; only lasted a short time. *Lach.* cm.

Dec. 15. Bleeding again. *Lach.* cm.

March 19, 1898. Bleeding again. Rheumatic symptoms returning. Stiffness in elbow. *Lach.* mm.

July 16. Only some stiffness in l. elbow.

ULCER ON THE LEG—PULSATILLA.

Mrs. W., age seventy-three, writes: "The first breaking out of the ulcer she felt a smarting and stinging pain in her left ankle; there was a little elevation the size of a pea; the next day it broke and discharged a thin, bloody pus; around it was a purplish red color. The sore kept extending, also the discolored surface; then came a thick, yellow discharge of pus. The ulcer is now somewhat larger than a silver dollar. The surface of the ulcer looks like a sponge and very red, covered with yellow, lumpy matter; the outside is almost on a level with the sore, I should say flat. The cloth that comes off (with mutton tallow) is slightly offensive; the ulcer I can scarcely smell; it burns, stings, and smarts; sometimes has a jerking sensation through the heel. She pulls her skirts up to cool the limb, which is better in the cool air. The warmer it is the worse it smarts and burns. Sometimes she describes the pain as something like splinters. From the knee down the leg sweats so that the hose is constantly wet. The well one is not so. As she gets up in the morning the foot swells until it is full and pains her very much; about three or four P. M. she gets easier and can lie down with some comfort. When she elevates the foot it feels much better, and does not swell so, and she is quiet free from pain."

She has also some rheumatic symptoms that I suppose you want to know. There is great soreness from the shoulder to the elbow, and also in the cords of the neck. If she fans herself or uses her arms she has great pains in these parts. The upper arm aches with a grumbling, burning pain, she cannot put her arms back; both sides are alike. She can hold her hands over her head, but cannot reach out for anything. The fingers are swelled and stiff in the morning; the left hand is worse than the right. She often holds on to one arm, then the other; when she turns in bed she has to fold the arms and then work herself over. She is thirsty and feverish in the *afternoon*.

Puls. cm one dose, was immediately mailed to the patient, who lives nearly three hundred miles from this city.

Several watery stools followed, and all her symptoms were made worse, but she has many times taken a homœopathic remedy, and she remarked to her daughter that she was now going to recover again.

This leg ulcer is an old relic of barbarism with her, as she had had it cured several times allopathically. Some years ago I healed it with Sulph. very high, but it had to come again. The ulcer and the concomitants all departed in due time, and she is a picture of health now. The ulcer has been healed a year now, and she has not taken a dose of medicine since the Puls. mentioned. I am informed that at the end of six weeks the ulcer was healed.

When compelled to prescribe on a letter written by a lay woman, many things are wanting, but in the above we have the picture as given—no more and no less. The remedy was sent and the patient, after all her family had settled down to this as her last sickness, made a good recovery. This is not the exception, but the rule after such prescription. If experience is appealed to or theory or *cures*, the inductive method must give us safest practice.

ULCERATED THROAT.

Lady, thirty-four years old, mother of two children. Face marks much sickness, though flushed. Letter states: "I have always been troubled most with left side of my throat, but at present it is the right. A small lump will come and then enlarge until it reaches the tonsil. Then ulcers will come and fill both sides. The roof becomes very red, and there is dryness and choking. Dry choking compels coughing; difficult swallowing." I further learned that this sore throat with ulceration has been coming just before menstruating for several years. It commences on one side and goes to the other. There has always been great swelling of the outside, sometimes the whole neck. The ulcers do not disappear until after the flow ceases; then a gradual subsiding; scarcely more than ten days of freedom from suffering. Leucorrhœal discharge, white mucus before menses. She got Mag-carb. 45m, one dose, at the close of menstrual nisus. She has never had a recurrence of the trouble nor any sickness in its place. She has remained free from throat trouble now over two years.

URTICARIA APPEARING ANNUALLY

Mrs. S., about forty years old, wife of a prominent clergyman in this city, consulted me for annually appearing paroxysms of urticaria, or whatever you may be pleased to call it. On the 13th day of May every year for seven years she had been seized with a burning and itching of the skin that would seem nearly to drive her to distraction. I saw her in one of these attacks in bed with her entire surface and her eyes closed with œdema of the lids. The hives were so confluent that not a spot of healthy integument could be seen. The whole paroxysm lasted twenty-four hours. She seems to be in terrible distress and exclaimed every moment. "I shall die this time surely." She seemed suffocating and was throwing off the covers. It seemed from her movements and speech that her skin felt as if on fire. There was no perceptible thirst and time was precious, and I am satisfied that I made waste by my haste in giving her a dose of Apis 200, which had no effect. But the paroxysm passed off and another year rolled by, when she called on me, as I requested her to do, a month before she expected paroxysm. I then learned more of her symptoms. I learned that when the eruption was out distinctly in nearly all of the attacks she had found that heat calmed her terrible distress and ameliorated the itching and burning. While she craved cold and had even thrown the covers off she was made worse by it, but when she had retained presence of mind and covered herself warmly with clothing she soon became quiet and the paroxysm terminated with less suffering.

This being the case, Apis could not be her similimum, and I could now understand clearly why I had failed to interrupt the paroxysm and bring about a feeling of contentment so usual in such cases. I have quieted such patients very frequently in an hour, and plainly as a result of a homœopathic remedy, but this case furnished me no evidence of curative action of my selected remedy. With the symptoms as given and the new modality, I gave her one dose of Rhus rad. 200, and bided my time ten days before the expected paroxysm. Within a few hours after taking the remedy she declared that her "spell" was coming on; but it was only the shadow, the paroxysm never appeared again. She missed it two years and she is in better health than ever. She remarked to me one day, "Doctor, your powders have made a new woman of me." She had been treated allopathically, physiologically, eclectically, pathologically, and with all very badly. This may not have been urticaria. Some of the wise heads of the old school told her it was from eating strawberries, and she refrained from these luxurious

36

fellows and still did not miss the paroxysm. One told her one thing and another disputed him. What was it? I don't know, neither do I care. Perhaps some pathologist could inform me as to the scientificity of my prescription. I simply know that when comparing the pathogenesis found in the Symptomen Codex I found a picture of the disease to be cured, and that is enough for me. The highest potency at hand was administered and never repeated. The slight aggravation usual to such work followed, and then I was contented to await results.

I am contented with such results, and so will any man who knows how to apply the law—the similimum, the smallest dose, the dynamized drug. In this way only can we progress, and in this way shall we become the most useful to our patrons.

UTERINE HEMORRHAGE

Mrs. _____, age thirty-one, weight about one hundred and twenty pounds. *Chronic illness, uterine hemorrhage.*

January 19, 1890—Menorrhagia, large clots mixed with bright red liquid flow, *copious.* On the day of her marriage she was seized with uterine hemorrhage, from the excitement.

Any severe shock or mental disturbance brings on uterine hemorrhage.

Has a sickly face and is subject to sore throats on taking cold. Sensation of enlargement of the base of tongue. Feet always cold and damp. Stockings always feel damp.

Sour taste in the morning.

Sour eructations.

Constipation, going many days without desire for stool.

Glands of the neck enlarged and sore when she has

taken cold or disordered the stomach. Tickling in larynx and throat. Unable to endure exertion.

Sadness, weeping, perspires much and easily. Calc. 13m. Dry choking cough.

March 13th, Calc., 13 m. April 22d, Calc. cm, June 29th, Calc. cm, *cured.*

PAIN IN HEELS

Pulsatilla—Mrs. P., aged forty-two, has been a most able sufferer for several years, trying to have comfort through allopathy. Symptoms: Pain in the heels like the pricking of tacks or nails; hot flushes, followed by chilliness; menstrual flow black and clotted; puts feet out of bed to cool them, they burn so; she must put her shoes on before she can walk, "heels ache so;" vertigo mostly before menses; she has been deaf since childhood, from scarlet-fever; constipation, character not ascertained; open air is grateful, craves open air; warm room is oppressive, she suffocates and must go out into the air; church oppressive; watery discharge from eyes and nose; purplish appearance of the skin of the heel; sprained feeling in the ankles, weak ankles.

May 23rd—Puls. 51m, one dose, and plenty of Sac. lac.

June 30th—Puls. cm and Sac. lac. She needed no medicine until April 13th, the next year, when she consulted me with the following symptoms: Rattling cough; loses her urine when coughing; feels stopped up in a warm room; menses every two weeks, profuse, dark, offensive; urine offensive, strong; sharp pains in rectum; toe joints very sore; hot flushes; limbs tire easily when walking. Puls. cm. one dose.

April 26th—Felt so much heat in vulva that she was compelled to apply a cold cloth; no appetite; sleepless; burning heat all over body; throws covers all off the bed; "I feel no two days alike," "I am so fidgety." She got more Sac. lac.

May 3d—Says she is well; plenty of Sac. lac. June 20th—Loses her urine when coughing. July 10th—The same symptom continues to bother her. Puls. cm. finished the cure and she remains well.

CLINICAL NOTES
RATTLING IN CHEST—KALI SULPH.

Kali-sulph.—There is no remedy so competent for rattling in the chest when that state has followed an acute attack of inflammation. When a child has passed through broncho-pneumonia and seems to have recovered and after every change in the weather to cold the child coughs and rattles in the chest, then it is that this remedy cures.

RATTLING COUGH—KALI SULPH.

A boy four years old was brought to my office for treatment. He looked well, but coughed several times with a rattling cough. "He never expectorates," says the father, "but he always has that rattling. It is worse in cold weather. He eats well and seems well, but always has more or less rattling."

Kali sulph. 200, one dose, dry, cured the case. In one week the rattling that had been there all winter was gone; the weather changes do not affect him now.

DOUBLE PNEUMONIA—KALI SULPH.

A little girl baby fourteen months old had a very violent double pneumonia last winter. Having been called to the case rather late, it was with great difficulty that the baby was saved. But, finally, it convalesced and looked well. During the cold spring weather it rattled in the chest and coughed. Otherwise it was healthy and plump. Some two months after the acute attack it was rattling when the weather changed to cold or damp.

Kali sulph. 200, cured immediately.

I prescribe Kali sulph. 200 for rattling in the chest, with or without much cough, in the absence of distinct indication for other remedies—in sub-acute or chronic cases.

RINGWORMS

A child two years old. Plump and well nourished. Ringworms on chest and face.

Dulc., Hell., Nit-ac., Phos., Sepia, Tellur.

The child craves meat and refuses everything else, ravenously clawing at the meat-plate, stuffing its mouth full to choking if permitted.

Craves meat; Abies-can., Aloes, Aur-met., Ferr-met., Hell., Lil-tig., Mag-c., Meny., Merc-s., Merc-v., Nat-m., Sabad., Sulph.

Child keeps up a chewing motion during sleep, grinds its teeth. Ars., Bry., Cic., Cina., Hell., Pod.

Child rolls its head during sleep; Hell., and others.

Hell. 1000, two powders—one at night, the other in the morning and Sac-lac.

The ringworms disappeared promptly.

SORE ON LOWER LIP

Mrs. H. age 28, married, came to me for treatment. She had a sore on the red part of the lower lip as large as a hickory nut. It was dry and covered with a scab; it was hard as horn; it had been several months forming and was quite painful. The sub-maxillary gland was enlarged and hard. The lymphatics were enlarged on the right side of the neck and she had enlarged tonsils. The history of tuberculosis was in the family and she had been told that this was an epithelioma. Several dry scales had been removed and as soon as one had separated a new one had formed.

She got Merc. proto-iod 100 (home-made), one dose every four days. It healed in five weeks—perfectly, I withhold my opinion as to diagnosis. I have neglected to mention that it had been deeply cauterized before calling upon me for treatment.

PAINS IN RIGHT OVARY

Mrs. R., a married lady, age 36, was taken violently ill with pains in right ovary. It was time for menstrual nisus. Her suffering was very intense and she called her usual allopathic attendant; Morphine hypodermically administered failed to give her the desired relief. She grew worse for four days. Dr. B., one of our medical students—boarding in the house at the time, was asked to try his hand, but he advised them to send for me.

When I arrived her suffering had not abated. The pains were all over the body and the family were fearing a fatal termination, with no confidence in Homœopathy. But allopathy had failed, and something must be done.

She was restless and thirsty. There was sweat and coldness. The pains were even worse in the sweating condition than before . Extremities cold. Fetor of breath and sour perspiration. Lifting of the covers chilled her.

I prepared Merc-sol. 6000 in water and left the young man to administer it. In two hours she was sleeping soundly—the first rest for four days. No more medicine was required. She took Sac-lac for a few days and was dismissed.

TEARING AND STINGING IN RIGHT OVARY

Mrs. M., age 27, married, was taken with violent tearing and stinging in the right ovary. She called a homœopathic physician, who gave her Apis, Lyc, Bell., Lach., but without benefit. When I saw the case she was suffering most intense pain all over the body. There was great thirst, hot perspiration, which did not improve the pain; fetor of the breath, vomiting bile, restlessness, and her screams were heard by the neighbors.

Merc. sol. 6000, one dose, dry, brought sleep. She had been subject to these attacks, but never had had so violent a one before. She has never had one since.

In looking over the symptoms of these two cases, where can a remedy be found that could cover any part of the case but Merc.? Apis was excluded (although there were stinging pains) by the fact that she must be warmly covered and no relief from perspiration. Where Apis is indicated, patient will throw the covers off; the cool air relieves. The pains did not go from right to left, as in Lycopodium; there was not the heat, burning, throbbing, and aggravation from jarring the bed, like Bell.; there was no lifting of the covering, nor left to right, so peculiar to Lach. But Merc. was the similimum, and it cured—as the appropriate remedy always cures.

GLEETY DISCHARGE

A young man (twenty-eight) called on me for treatment. I found a gleety discharge, entirely painless, gluing the meatus in the morning. He had contracted gonorrhœa several months before, and it had nearly stopped discharging. Five years ago he had an attack of gonorrhœa which resulted in producing a stricture for which he had been operated on. I could only pass a No. 8 bougie at this time.

The symptoms upon which to base a prescription were: Slight painless discharge, gluing the meatus; sickly, sallow face; constipation, sour stomach, general debility.

He took Sepia cm, one dose, dry; then Sac. Lac.

The next night he sent a note, saying he was very sick; to please send him medicine; that the discharge had come back.

I sent him Sac. Lac., requesting him to come to the office as soon as able.

He called in a few days, he said the medicine sent him gave great relief. The discharge was profuse, thick and yellow. Sac- Lac. was given, and advised to call in a week.

Next call; Discharge yellowish green; some pain on micturition; night sweats; bone pains; worse during the perspirations; had a chill during night.

Merc. sol. 6000 in water every three hours for twenty-four hours and Sac. Lac.

One week later; Symptoms all improved; discharge diminished.

Merc. sol. 6000, one dose; then Sac. Lac.

One week later; Discharge nearly gone; feeling well; Possesses as large a stream of urine as ever. He took one dose a week of Merc. sol. 6000.

At the end of the three months passed a No. 14 bougie. No discharge. He is in good health. The bougie passed without effort. The two remedies had completely cured the stricture and the treatment was painless. Could anything have been more satisfactory?

PARALYZED IN INFANCY

Miss N., aged 19, was paralyzed in infancy, from which she partially recovered. The arm is normal but the lower limb is small and weak in the joints. *Face flushed*, body well nourished, short and stout. Has suffered mentally and was placed in an insane asylum for *many* months. Came out heart-broken and feeble-minded. Extremely excitable and full of apprehensions. If she talks or sings much she becomes hoarse. Catarrhal symptoms of nose and pharynx; constant accumulation of mucus in pharnyx and larynx. Often there is dryness and sense of burning in nose when inhaling air. Sense of soreness deep in ears, left worse. Constantly taking cold. Throat symptoms worse mornings, much mucus tasting sweetish. Menstruation ceased for four months, but has returned recently. Leucorrhœa like white of egg before menses. Slight exertion causes her to become *heated up all over*, increasing the redness of the face, and the ebulitions. Slight excitement is followed by wakefulness. Cold, sweaty feet, sometimes a little offensive.

Her mental symptoms come on after the excitement of the theatre and she becomes sleepless; then full of fear, especially at the piano; was constantly on the lookout for something to happen. The symptoms during her insane months not obtainable. Since she has been with her family she has heard voices constantly. Very hot head and face and wakeful nights.

Watching the case for several weeks without medicine, developed further symptoms: *Leucorrhoea instead of menses*; craves spices, something salty. Two hard corns painful, the pain nauseates her; shooting pain in the abdomen comes with the desire to urinate, urging to urinate, but the urine does not flow; she feels as though her limbs are separated from the body; no feeling below waist line; sour eructations; sensations as though her warm feet were cold. Violent sexual dreams and sexual excitement. Sensitive to cold. She feels that she is going to be taken back to the asylum.

Phosphorus 45m. one dose, cured every symptom in six weeks.

SUNSTROKE

Case I.—*Natrum Sulph.*— Mrs. A. A. B., aged 48.
Gnawing pain in back of head, extending down spine, brought on from grief and protracted anxiety.
Thin, sallow.

General mental sluggishness.

Throbbing in back of the neck.

Has had much trouble with back of head and neck since an attack of sunstroke many years ago.

Bowels constipated, no stool for days, no urging; but the head symptoms are improved after a stool.

Dreadful bitter taste in the mouth.

The headache is mostly in the morning and gets better after moving about a while.

The other symptoms have been better and worse for years.

Coming in wave-like attacks, but never well.

Cathartics once gave relief, but nothing seems to give her any comfort now.

She was given a few powders of Natrum sulph., 500, with instructions to dissolve one and take of it frequently at the beginning of every spell of growing "bilious," as she called it, and to hold the rest of them. She has never taken but the first, she is holding the others.

All the symptoms that remained through the interim of the more severe attacks have departed, and she is perfectly well.

DEAFNESS

Case II.—*Pulsatilla.*—Miss E. B., aged 35.

Deafness, cannot understand except when watching the motion of lips.

Can only speak in a whisper.

Deafness and aphonia of many years' standing, but has been whispering for four years.

Accumulation of yellow, thick phlegm in throat, especially in the morning.

Burning feet and ankles.

Warm room suffocates and flushes face.

Fast walking causes nausea, faintness and flushes the face.

All kinds of bodily exertion heats her up and suffocation follows, with purplish red face.

Fast motion is quite impossible.

Brown spots on the face.

Constant swallowing.

May 9.—Pulsatilla 15m.

July 15.—Voice mostly recovered; hearing only slightly improved. Can take active exercise without flushing. Ankles become very weak, they turn when walking, otherwise steadily improving.

No medicine.

Sept. 13.—The only symptoms left are deafness, which has not improved, and weak ankles.

Pulsatilla cm. (H. S.).

Oct. 20—Ankles became strong; "except the deafness am perfectly well."

She has remained perfectly well, but the deafness does not change.

HEADACHE AND PAIN

Case III.—*Sepia.*— Mrs. J. R. A., aged 33.

Tall, slender woman, mother of several children. Dry cough only in daytime. Has been poorly since birth of last child (two years). Headache on vertex, throbbing, feels as though head would open on top, worse from any noise, *perfectly relieved by sleep.*

Headache comes before menses.

Pain in left side of nose to left eye, very sharp, almost constant when the headache is present.

Burning on top of the head, then comes a sensation of throbbing, as with little hammers on top of head, sometimes within the skull.

No appetite.

Chronic constipation with no urging to stool for a week, then a very painful, difficult stool.

Dull aching pain in region of spleen.

Leucorrhœa quite constant, thick, yellow, sometimes white.

March 29.—Sepia 50m, one powder, dry, all symptoms removed and she remains cured.

PULSATILLA CASE

Case IV.—*Pulsatilla*—L. M., lady, single, age 28. Has always been sickly.

Reaching up with the arm brings on a peculiar pain that runs from the pelvis to the throat. This pain also comes on after exertion, especially after climbing stairs.

After walking any distance or climbing the stairs she has a desire to urinate.

She has horrible dreams of robbers. She dreams of her lover who disappointed her.

She wakens from sleep in tears, even sobbing.

She has had a dark, yellow, thick leucorrhœa since puberty.

Constipation alternates with diarrhœa.

Aching in the lumbar region of the spine.

Despondent before the menses.

Inability to sustain a mental effort.

Headache, with severe pains on one or the other temple that makes her blind.

She is very fidgety and generally nervous.

Melancholy and tearful.

Cannot lie on either side, only on the back.

Menstrual flow dark, clotted, offensive.

She is greatly prostrated from any warm air, warm room or slight exertion.

Aching in the back that compels her to lie with her arms under it, as the pressure relieves.

She feels a desire to go to bed and sleep in the daytime.

Oct. 22, 1884.—She took Pulsatilla 51 m, one dose.

Nov. 19.—She had improved in every way and improvement ceased. Pulsatilla 51m, one dose. She has been perfectly well ever since. Every symptom removed by Pulsatilla, two doses. An invalid was restored to usefulness. A more useful lady cannot be found.

MENSTRUAL FLOW SCANTY AND ENLARGED ABDOMEN

Case I.—Short, plump, married woman, aged 36. For several months her menstrual flow has been but a mere stain, and the enlarged abdomen made her suspect she might be pregnant. Her menstrual habit has always been profuse. Her ankles are œdematous and her hands slightly swelled. Marked nausea when hungry. When in one position long becomes stiff in all the limbs. Great weakness from simply walking up a flight of stairs. Great prostration during menses, and so tired and heavy all the time. Sudden spells of overpowering sleepiness. All her morbid feelings are made worse in a warm room and greatly improved when she is in the open air. Must urinate frequently day and night, copiously during the night. Sense of soreness, perhaps in the region of the uterus; on "sitting something pushes up that is painful." Great sense of heat in the dorsal spine. Hot flushes from spine to face. Brown spots on abdomen. The slightest exertion causes profuse sweat. "To-day I could not eat my dinner; every time I swallow my hearts jumps so;" Feet go to sleep.

"There is a yellow, sandy deposit in the urinal, hard to wash off; soap suds will not wash it off."

She received Lycopodium 43m, a single dose on the tongue.

Three weeks later she reported; "The swelling of the abdomen has gone, and I can breathe easily." Sac. lac.

Four weeks later she reports: "I do not think I am quite so well. I have been going back again for a week." The difficult breathing had returned, and the feet are beginning to bloat; the abdomen is again distended with flatus.

Lycopodium cm, one dose.

No report for two months. Word was sent that all the symptoms had disappeared.

Some three months later was sent for in haste. She had passed a quantity of limpid fluid from the vagina, so suddenly that she was alarmed. It looked like a muco-purulent fluid that had been followed by the disappearance of a lump in the left side of the abdomen the size of a fist. There was no more of it, and no more symptoms. Evidently a pyosalpinx. Upon re-examination, several of her old symptoms had returned, and it was thought proper to give her another dose of her old remedy.

As she had made a great constitutional gain, Lycopodium c. m. was given, a single dose, dry.

She reported some three months later for the first time, thinking herself well up to within a few weeks. The painful pushing up feeling on sitting down has returned.

Menstrual flow scanty and clotted.

Pain in ovaries before menses.

Abdomen distended and hard with flatulence.

The uterus is sore to a jolt in the street car.

The whole abdomen seems sore to the concussion of riding or stepping.

Frequent urination during the night.

As soon as there is any urine in the bladder she must pass it.

Nausea all day.

Eating often to relieve the hunger and nausea.

Cannot endure clothing about the waist.

Pain in the uterine region at the beginning of menstruation that passes off after the flow begins.

Sick stomach from riding in a carriage.

Must make haste when the desire to urinate comes or she will lose it.

Petroleum 45m., one dose, dry.

She sent word some weeks later that all her symptoms had gone, and that she would report if they returned.

It was nearly four months when she called to report that she had menstruated once, perfectly normal, but the next time not quite right, and the last time she was very sick.

Great tenderness in the region of the uterus, compelled to keep her bed; clotty, scanty, coffee-colored menstrual flow.

Jar of the bed made her suffer very much.

The mammae and nipples extremely tender.

Pains ceased when the flow became free.

Pains through ovaries, and in the back (sacrum) before menses, until flow became free.

She had been troubled with pains all during the month as if her menses would come on.

Seems that the very sensitive uterus pushed up when she sits down.

Belladonna 50m., one dose, dry.

She is perfectly well and says she is much stronger than ever in her life. She says, "I am now a perfectly healthy woman."

Ferrum iod, gave me a very interesting study in comparing it with remedies in this case, but I could always feel safer among the remedies that I have so often tested. I neglected to say that there was never any albumin in the urine.

WHISKY DRINKING, ETC.

Case III.—Mr. ____, aged 52, been addicted to whiskey drinking for many years. States that he had a copious flow of blood from the bowels some four months ago. He considered himself well up to two years ago. During these two years he has declined steadily, "growing weaker all the time," he says. At present the exertion of walking a few blocks to my office caused suffocation; in fact it was some minutes before he could talk, he was so out of breath. After the loss of blood, above mentioned, his feet began to swell, and at this time both limbs to middle of thighs were very œdematous. Has had two or three nondescript chills. A few days ago he had a sudden paralytic weakness of left arm and leg, which passed off in three hours, leaving a numbness in the left hand and rending pain in left side of head and face. No appetite, and there are bloody mucous discharges with the stool, which is otherwise normal. "I feel as if in a dream all the time."

Loss of memory. His wife came with him for his safety and to tell his symptoms for him. Thinking hard enabled him to recall many of his symptoms, and simple incidents. When I would let him talk he would keep saying, over and over, "If I should run I would drop dead."

His face was covered with varicose veins and very red. A general venous stasis prevailed. Feeling on top of the head as if he had been hit with a hammer. (The wife said he often mentioned the last symptom.) Must pass urine several times in the night; urine thick and cloudy after standing, but is clear when first passed. Has had much worry from financial losses during the last ten years, which had made him resort to whisky. He has always had a very red face. He cannot pass urine while sitting at stool, but it flows freely when he is standing;

albumin in the urine He has taken much medicine during the last two years. Always very strong.

While this case seemed to be very unpromising, and the wife was promptly informed that the case would most likely prove fatal. I was urged so strongly by her, that I took considerable time and settled upon a remedy. Sarsaparilla cm., one powder, in water, eight doses spread over two days, and plenty of Sac. lac. No aggravation seemed to follow, and at the end of a month he was so much improved, and still improving that he continued to take Sac. lac. which restored him to a very comfortable existence and he is temperate and works for his living and supports his family, which was previously done by his wife with her needle.

CONSTANT HEAT OF HEAD AND FACE.

Case II.—Almost constant heat of head and face. Pulse slow, sometimes as slow as 45. Cannot endure any mental exertion. Sweating of palms. Appetite voracious. Stitching pains in the heart.

Naja 45 m., one dose, cured.

PAINS AND GENERAL WEAKNESS.

Case IV.—Tall, slender young man, aged 21, blonde, writes out the sickness he wants removed, says, he has been a great sufferer from pains and general weakness, all caused from masturbation when a lad, which he has been able to abandon. From his long letter the following symptoms were considered useful: For several years he had been disturbed by pustulous formations all over his face and forehead. Bluish red discoloration of face and neck comes and goes, which a doctor said was erysipelas (?). One year ago in the heat of the summer he over-worked in the harvest field, and was sick with what was called "typho-malaria," fever, and it was three months

37

before he could go to work. The following winter he coughed all winter and the cough has not left him. In the following spring boils came out all over him. Almost constantly feels a constriction of the chest. Headaches come about weekly. His back is always covered with pustules. Common food distresses his stomach as soon as eaten. Trembling from exertion and becomes tired easily. Gloomy and thinks his habits ruined him. Says his head hurts so from constantly thinking about his failing health. He cannot keep his mind off his health. The face is painful in cold air, and the nose is so painful inside. His seminal losses were only occasional and I soon concluded that the cursed drugs he had taken and the advice he had had were worse than his youthful sins.

The cases coming by letter are often not what we want, but what best can be obtained. He took Sulphur 55m, and made good improvement for some time, always thankful for much improvement.

Finally he got another dose of Sulphur cm, that continued him in the curing way.

His cough was troublesome finally and he could not lie on the left side, and the cough was worse from the cold air; taking into account his shape he received Phosphorous 45 m. and improved again; the cough ceased for a time.

Finally he wrote me a lot of symptoms that I could make nothing of, except he seemed to have lost much he had gained, was losing flesh, and had an appetite that he could not satisfy, "The more I eat, the thinner I get," he writes. He took Iodine 58m., one dose; Oct. 15th, another; Dec. 21, same potency. March 8, he got Iodine 20 m., and he has never needed any medicine since, and can work very hard and is a picture of health. There were no new symptoms after he took Iodine, and when the symptoms would return and continually grow worse, he would get another dose, which shows that the first dose cured for two months, and the next dose exerted curative action about two and a half months, and the last dose finished the work. He never failed to notice the positive curative action of a dose of Iodine. It acted without aggravation. Amelioration would begin in a few days after a dose, and steadily his symptoms would diminish and his strength correspondingly increase. It will be well to remember that this young man had taken drugs with no benefit, and when the similar remedy was administered he responded promptly. He knew nothing of the system of Homœopathy only as he was advised by a cousin that lived in the city, to correspond with her physician. This hard-working young man was bowed down with fear, produced by reading the cursed charlatan literature sent out to deceive the young, so that they will squander their money on advertising doctors and patent nostrum venders. Homœopathy restores them when they are sick, and removes their fears when they are not sick, and the family physician should be the only adviser of all the young in his vicinity. He should be the friend to all the children, and so hold their confidence that he first of all will be consulted in those matters.

SWELLING FACE AND NOSE.

Case V.—Girl, age 13. Considerable swelling of face and nose, bones of nose very sore to pressure, pain in bones of nose, unable to breathe through nose. Two other children had disease of nasal bones and fetid discharges. Father had died with suspicious symptoms. The mother could tell nothing, but the case appeared to be specific. Every question to the girl was answered by a shake of the head or "don't know." She was remarkably stupid. There was much sweating about the head, and from the extensive bundling up I concluded that she was chilly.

There was no discharge from the nose, but the great shining tumefaction seemed to look as though pus must be forming somewhere. The nose was swelled to unsightly appearance. She got silica 5m. May 8th, and a few days later a copious discharge of bloody pus came from the nose and for some weeks the discharge continued as a laudable pus and the child improved.

July 5th. She reported with a most offensive discharge, thin and ichorous. The bones of the nose greatly affected and very tender. The swelling had gone under Silica. She received a dose of Aurum 75m.

August 1st. No discharge and there seemed to be no trouble. No medicine.

She remained away until Oct. 15th, when she reported, discharge returned, thick, bloody and very fetid. Sometimes the blood disappears, then it is yellow, but always thick, Aurum cm., one dose.

Nov. 6th. There was no improvement. Kali bich., 45m.

Dec. 8th. There was no improvement. The discharge was very excoriating, thick and yellow. Arsenic iod. 30th, in water, one day, and Sac. lac.

Jan. 4th. Soreness all gone from nose and the discharge is thin and white, and she begins to breath through the nose, Sac. lac.

Feb. 12th. She can breathe nicely through the nose; no soreness in the bones of the nose when pressed between thumb and finger, discharge scanty and only slightly offensive, Sac. lac.

March 10th. Discharge increasing, becoming thicker and yellow, some pain in the bones of nose and a stuffed feeling. Discharge burns the lip. Child fully as stupid as ever. Arsenic iod, 45 m, one dose, dry, and Sac. lac.

April 13th. Girl seemed quite well; there were no symptoms.

Her uncle said to me some six months later that the girl had made a great change and was becoming quite bright and womanly. No nasal trouble.

The thick yellow discharge cured by Arsenic iod, is a verification of that symptom in a proving made by myself, wherein this nasal discharge was like yellow honey. I have many times cured this symptom with Arsenic iod. The proving was made with the 200th potency, and now verified with the 45 m. It may here be said that the discharge in the proving was gluey and like yellow honey. This is a very valuable characteristic of this almost unknown remedy.

CONSTIPATION.

Case VI. Long standing constipation. Stools large, hard and difficult to expel. She goes four to six days with no desire for a stool, and then she strains until covered with sweat to pass a stool. The left ear is deaf and the left Eustachian tube is closed. Sanicula 10 m, cured without repetition.

SEASICKNESS—TABACUM

There is a most astonishing resemblance between *seasickness* and the proving of *Tabacum.* I have always guarded myself against routine practice and advised everyone else to keep away as far as possible from routine practice, but a great many times I have been consulted, where without any symptoms at all, somebody will tell me, "Every time I cross the herring pond I get sick. Cannot you send me something?" And I have had some most astonishing results from Tabacum used for seasickness in a routine manner, without any symptoms.

One man in particular I know, who had crossed the ocean a good many times, having a business office in New York and one in London. He always dreaded to go.

He said: "I am sick from the time I go on the boat until I get off. I can eat nothing. I do nothing but vomit and vomit food from one end of the trip to the other." His fortune is invested in such a way that he needs to go two or three times in the year across the ocean. Now I provide him with the infallible protections, and when he gets out and feels his dizzy spell coming on he takes his powder and he can take his meals all the way over. The one powder has always done it, and he keeps on hand some powders of *Tabacum* 70 m.

I have used it many times for the sickness from riding in the cars. You can understand the Tabacum sickness if you will get on the rear end of a boat and watch the waves as they go away from the vessel. The boat goes up and down, and pretty soon the stomach goes up and down and everything goes up and down. Well, sitting at a car window and watching the scenery as the car goes along produces a similar deathly nausea. *Tabacum* often relieves this nausea from riding in a train. *Petroleum* and *Cocculus* sometimes helps seasickness, but *Tabacum* is a broad remedy that seems to cover most of the symptoms.

NUMBNESS IN FINGERS AND SOLES OF FEET

Case II.—Mr. T____, aged 35, a travelling man, with syphilitic history, came back from one of his western trips, with the following symptoms: Numbness in fingers and soles of feet, with much awkwardness of all his motions. The staggering was marked and he walked on a wide base. He could not distinguish between small objects with his fingers. His manual movements were irregular and would miss his purpose. His movements thus far were not more irregular by closing the eyes. His staggering was no worse when walking with his eyes closed. The reflexes, tendon patellæ and ankle joint were abolished, and he had to wait a long time for his urine to start. Fulgurating pains coursed through his limbs and back and he was in a general way going down in bodily health. He says he has had these symptoms three months and they have grown stronger every day. His visual apparatus has been defective a long time but there are no new symptoms traceable to the probable nervous state. Every seven days he got one powder dry on the tongue—Alumina met. 200, no other medicine. A change for the better took place after the second dose. He took four doses in all. Every homœopathist conversant with our literature must see a resemblance between this case and the one cured by Bœnninghausen. While the symptoms in both cases are analogous to signs of sclerosis of posterior root-zones, yet, the essential features are wanting. But the action of the remedy, as applied for a purpose, is just as demonstrative. While it, in my judgment, is evident there was no sclerosis, it is highly probable that a disturbing factor was at work in the tracks of co-ordination, the posterior lateral columns; and in time a grave pathological change would have been established.

RHEUMATISM IN MUSCLES AND JOINTS

Case III.—Rheumatism, aching and soreness in muscles and joints, compelling him to move after a few minutes and find a new place in which he seems more quiet. Rhus 1m. Next day no improvement and no change in symptoms, except growing worse generally. The pain in the ankle joint feels as if sprained, joints and muscles sore to touch. He says, "I move all the time; when I get into a new place I feel better but very soon the bed in the new place feels like iron and I must move. The moving I am compelled to do not from an innate restless pain but from the hardness of the bed as it seems to me." It must be observed that Rhus tox could not cure this case, yet at my visit the language was calculated to deceive. Arn. must be the most appropriate remedy. The soreness which gradually grows worse by the pressure of the bed and the peculiar soreness as of a sprain precluded any other remedy. Arn. 1 M. was given in water. The pain and soreness were gone at the end of three days. Sulph 6 M., one dose finished the cure. He was out of the house on the eighth day.

RHEUMATISM IN LOWER EXTREMITIES

Case IV.—Mrs. P., aged 35, rheumatism many months in lower extremities, after failure to cure with strong remedies, Quinia, Salicylic acid, Colch, and Iodide potassium, concluded to try liniment. Strong applications were made with relief to the lower extremities. I was sent for, the messenger saying that Mrs. P. was dying. I found her sitting upright in bed with great pain in the cardiac region, quick, sharp, irregular pulse, smothering breathing, clothing all removed from neck and breast, choking and gasping, covered with perspiration and very pallid. She got Lachesis 41m. in water. Immediate relief followed, and was able to lie down; although she was relieved from the more distressing symptoms, it was evident that she was in great danger as the pain in the heart remained only slightly abated. The danger in these cases need not be mentioned here, and I will only say, it appeared to be as usual a dangerous case of rheumatism endocarditis from metastasis. She took Abrotanum 6th and 12th. Recovery was gradual from the beginning with the remedy and finally complete. She says that she now enjoys better health than ever

CLINICAL REMINISCENCES
HEADACHE (SICK) LAC-DEF., LAC-CAN.

1886, July 10th—Mrs. R. S., widow, aged thirty-five. "I have had sick headaches many years." Had peritonitis, had typhoid fever, and was down in bed four months. These headaches have been coming ever since, now five years.

Headache back of eyes.

Sunlight brings on the headache.

"If I go without eating I have headache."

"If I eat too much I have a headache."

"Excitement brings on the headache."

"I have lain three and four days in a dark room, not able to endure any light."

Milk brings on the sick headache.

Eating never relieves the headache.

"When sick with typhoid fever I was fed on milk until I vomited whenever they brought it to my bed."

"I am never free from headache, but I am able to be at my desk about one-half of my time, much of which I suffer intensely." Seldom vomits, but much nausea.

"When I vomit it is of the food eaten, sour and bitter."

Here are the symptoms. What is the remedy?

It was evident that I had no ordinary case on hand, as two good prescribers had failed to help and told her so. Many whom I do not regard as careful physicians had treated her also. If the remedy must out, here it is: Lac-def. cm.

July 16th.—She returned. "Just finished one of the most violent headaches ever had. So sleepy while writing my letters that could hardly hold my eyes open. Had to quit work two afternoons and go home. I am greatly discouraged when the headache is on." Sleepy while writing is new. Sac. lac.

July 23d.—No headache since last call.

July 30th.—A short headache, but feeling better. Lac-def. cm. dry, one dose.

August 2d.—Headache came, lasted two days, but has heretofore generally lasted a week. Improving generally. Lac-def. cm.

August 10th.—Improving.

August 26th.—Improving; has just finished a headache, but went three weeks.

September 11th.—Headache in two weeks. Symptoms about as usual. Sulph. cm. one dose.

September 12th.—Headache is on full force, started in left eye, sunlight makes it worse. "I felt the headache this time from delaying my dinner." Gnawing, hungry feeling, not relieved by eating. Everything I eat makes me worse but fish." Cold brings on headache. Headache worse from weight of hat. This headache began in left eye and has extended to occiput. "The thought of milk makes me sick." No palliative was given, but watching the symptoms seemed to be the only way of finding the remedy.

September 13th.—Reports that the afternoon of yesterday, the 12th, headache went over to right eye and side of head, but now it is back in my left eye. Lac-can. mm was given, and immediate relief followed, and it was three months before another headache came, and it was very short and did not compel her to leave her desk.

February 10th.—She had a slight headache and took another dose of lac-can. cm. She has been compelled to lay aside all her clothing and procure larger size. Can eat anything, and enjoys life like other people.

HEADACHE (WEEKLY)

Periodical conditions often trouble a young prescriber and sometimes an old one. A young physician once brought me his patient who was suffering from periodical congestive headaches which came on every seven days. Many remedies had been given but no change had been made in the case. The rubric in the repertory that had been consulted was "weekly headaches." The patient was then more carefully examined and it was found that regularly

Sunday evening and night he suffered from this headache. The modalities were confusing and contradictory but after a careful questioning as to what he was in the habit of eating on Sunday that he did not eat at other times it was found that he ate plentifully of "roast of beef" for his midday meal and at no other time. It was soon seen to be not a periodical headache, but one that came after eating beef.

Staph. covered all his symptoms and cured.

HEADACHE PERIODICAL—AFTER EATING ICE CREAM

A middle aged woman suffered from Sunday periodical headaches and none of the remedies in the rubric for weekly headaches helped. It was subsequently discovered that she had these headaches always after ice cream and then it was seen that *Puls.* corresponded to her other symptoms and that remedy cured her.

All the facts in the case should be gathered before prescribing. Hasty conclusions are as dangerous as any form of negligence. Our remedies will cure when they are similar to all the symptoms in the case.

Some years ago it was necessary to listen second hand, through a well-disposed woman, to the complaints of her sick sister. The sister was under the care of an eminent Old School specialist for some deep seated uterine trouble, which was called, in a letter from the doctor to his patient, endometritis. Local treatment had gone on many months and still the sister failed. Then came the story: "Oh, Doctor, you should hear her complain of these awful headaches at night. She says there is a feeling as if she had a stone on the top of her head and she cannot rest or give me any rest from that pressure until the gas is lighted; then she goes to sleep. The odor of the room is awful from her feet."

This good woman took one powder of *Silica,* which she was to give her sister on the sly. The patient never needed a light in the room at night again. It cured.

Here was a supposed periodical headache, but it was a headache *worse in the dark.* It was supposed by the eminent specialist to be due to *endometritis,* but as a fact the woman was sick; her uterus did not make her sick. What a profound thought, when the doctor tells his patient that the uterus makes her sick.

A PERFECT CURE OF ERUPTION, ECTROPION DIARRHŒA AND FINALLY OF THE MAN

Some years ago, when gunning in the southwest, it was rumored among the people that a city doctor was in the land, and I was waited upon frequently for remedies, as they rarely had such a chance among the ranches. One young man who came to me excited my pity. Having no time to take his case with care, no paper upon which to write out his symptoms, it was possible only to make a good first guess and hope for the best.

Describing the young man from memory could be but a mild picture of the real case. He was a constant taker of all drugs for "the blood" that he could procure cash to buy. He had taken all the roots, barks and leaves that grew in that wild country. His face was red and chapped, lips and eyelids checked with fissures. Green discharges from his eyes, which looked hideous from ectropion. Green thick discharges from the nose. The extremely thick skin of the inside of the hands was chapped, cracked and bleeding. Acrid tears had burned roads down the cheeks. During the last five years he had morning diarrhœa. In spite of these sufferings he had a good appetite, and kept his place in the saddle as a "cowboy." It was while in the saddle I gained this information, and then remarked, "Are you happy, and do you enjoy life?" "Doctor, you do not know how hard I have worked to keep from blowing my head off with this thing" (a six-shooter hanging at his belt). Before he made this remark it had not dawned upon me what his remedy was. In fact I could see only *Sulphur* in what had appeared. Now *Natrum-sulph.* came in view, and from my case a 500th potency, one dose, was put upon his tongue. I never expected to see him again, but he asked me for my address. I gave it to him, and some time after he wrote for more of that wonderful medicine. It was never changed. Some two years later he ceased to ask for it. His last letter showed a perfect cure of the eruption, ectropion, diarrhœa and finally of the man.

This case again shows the importance of mental symptoms in the cure of deep-seated conditions. Eversion of the lids has been cured by *Sulph.* but not before by *Nat-sulph.*, although *Nat-m.* has shown curative action in this relation frequently. *Nat-sulph.* will do more when handled properly in the hands of a Homœopath than Schussler ever dreamed of.

ECZEMA.

June 13, 1910. Mrs. G. F. H., aged forty-two years. Eczema of vesiclular form. Vesicles filled with thin, yellow fluid. Copious on inside of hands and fingers. Lips cracked. Has had stomach or intestinal trouble for years. Cannot eat strawberries or veal without diarrhœa. Can eat peaches and oranges. < pork; tomatoes; sweets; pies; pudding; fresh bread; apples; bananas; pears; fats. Craves quantities of rich candy and very rich cake. (One sister is insane; eats much candy. Mother craves candy.) Sensitive to heat; warm room, warm air, summer heat. Perspires easily from exertion, warm room, walking. Desires cold air. Fond of open air. > walking in open air. M. periods always too soon. Flow copious; sometimes clotted. Constipation and diarrhœa alternating. Neck—aching in back. Kali-sul. 10m.

June 29. Blisters are about gone. Cracked lips improved. Eructations empty >. Sac.-lac.

July 15. Blisters entirely disappeared. Eructations—though some improved. Abdomen sore sensation. Constipation <. Sleep poor. Kali-sul. 10m.

Oct. 4. Has felt well since last report. Nervous ache at base of brain. Eructations. Kali-sul. 50m.

Nov. 9. Rectum bleeding two weeks ago, not now. Eruption on one finger. Vertigo when sitting in church; when walking. Itching resembling rhus-poison. Abdomen —sore, burning sensation. Flatulence; eructations. Nausea >. Kali.-sul. 50m.

Dec. 28. Abdomen—weighty, burning sensation. Stomach disturbed by Christmas-dinner. Vertigo with ache in vertex. Kali-sul. cm.

No further treatment needed.

"FIBROID RECURRENT" CURED BY SILICEA IN HIGH POTENCY.

Frank H., a compositor in the Globe-Democrat office, St. Louis, came to my office to have a tumor removed by the knife. It had been removed twice and was called a recurrent fibroid. It was the size of a hen's egg and very hard, located in the left side of the neck, not connected with the parotid, though growing a little below it. I advised him to give me time to prepare him for removal. I took his symptoms and found that he was better by wrapping up over the head. He was timid in going into a new enterprise, though abundantly able to perform the task. He lacked confidence in his own ability, yet when he had begun he would do well.

He took Silicea 5m., April 1st, 1883. Six weeks later he called, and the tumor was reduced one half, Sil., 72m., dry, one dose. S: weeks later almost gone. January 23rd, 1884, Sil. 72m., one dose. The tumor had disappeared.

This prescribing has been commented upon by a large number of friends, who think the one dose business a mystery. He got no Sac. Lac., as I had his confidence. I did not prescribe for the tumor, but for the patient. My prescription could not have been different had the tumor not been present.

The tumor was not included in the totality of symptoms, as it was not a symptom, it furnished no part of the guide to a remedy. The symptoms expressive of the whole state existed prior to the tumor, and it was the language of this pre-existing state that I read, as out of this pre-existing state, grew the tumor. I must interpret the language or expression of cause, not effect. The man who is guided by pathology can use the knife. To use the knife is but to acknowledge one's ignorance of a method by which he can avoid cutting.

HEART AFFECTIONS REMOVED

Roy S. M., aged twenty-three years.

Sept. 15. Spasms of the mitral valve. Fainting spells 4 or 5 times a day, without loss of consciousness but with weakness: rather spells of sudden weakness. Face flushed when studies after eating. Thoughts vanishing. Forgets of what he was thinking when figuring; a blank appears. Perspiration when reciting· forgets what he was to recite, though he knew it before. Sensitive to heat and warm weather. Wants window open. Better in motion than in rest. Sadness intense. Irritable—weeping paroxysms. < from sight of blood or an accident. Much thirst for iced drinks; Heartburn > by them. Heartburn after eating fats or sours. < coffee and "postum." Eructations· sour; of undigested food· Flatulence from eating fruit. Late beginning sleep; wakens early. Spine—sore spots. Legs—paroxysms of weakness. Erections waken him and urging to urinate, if sleeps on back. Psychopathic

constitution; lost consciousness when under influence of a
mesmerist, and return to consciousness was long. Diarrhœa
after drinking cold milk. After eating. Sensitive to
noise: confusion. Dreams while awake. Tension of muscles.

Eructations of food: *Aesc., arg-n.,* ars., *calc-c., calc-s.,*
carb.-s., *carb.-v., caust.,* CHIN., *con.·* FERR., FERR.-PH., *kali-
bi.,* kali-s,. *lach., lyc.,* mag.-m *mag.-p.,* merc., *mur.-ac.,*
nat-m., PHOS.· PH.-AC., SULS., *sulph.,* sul.-ac., thuj.

————— SOUR: Aesc., *arg-n., ars.,* CALC.c., *calc-s.,*
carb.-s., CARB.-V.· *caust.,* CHIN., *con., ferr., ferr.-p.,* kali-bi.,
KALI-S.,*lach.,* LYC., *nat.-m.,* PHOS., *ph.-ac.,* puls., SULPH.,
SULPH.-AC., thuj.

Sensitive to noise: *Ars., calc.-c., carb.-s.· carb.-v.,*
caust., CHIN., CON., *ferr., ferr.-p.,* kali-s., *lach., nat.-m.,*
PHOS., ph.-ac., *puls.*

Diarrhœa from cold drinks: ARS.· *carb.-v.·,* chin.,
phos., ph-ac., puls.

Heartburn: *Ars.,* CARB.-V., *chin., phos.,* ph.ac., PULS.

Faintness: ARS., CHIN., *phos.,* ph.-ac., PULS.

Vanishing thought: *Puls.*

Desires windows open. PULS.

Open air ameliorates: PULS.

Motion ameliorates: PULS.

Coffee aggravates. PULS.

Cabbage aggravates: PULS.

PULS. 10m.

Oct. 19. "Was feeling fine until medicine gave out."
Better in general spirits. PULS. 10m.

Nov. 5. Better in general. < onions, greasy food.
Craves cold drinks. Cramp after cold drinks taken. Confusion when nervous.

Nov. 20. Vertigo few times. PULS. 10m.

Dec. 18. Symptoms returning. Nasal catarrh; blows it
much; stuffy at night. Yellow mucus. Dreams troublesome. Of seeing dying man. PULS. 50m.

1913. From a sickly child and weakly young man, he has developed perfect health with more than ordinary physical strength.

The general condition and the local symptoms and functional derangements must yield to the power of the properly selected remedy. The characteristics of the patient indicate the remedy; it requires only a trained prescriber to find it and keep to it.

HEART TROUBLE FOR SEVERAL YEARS

Mrs. J. L. H., 38 years of age.

June 23, 1910. Very nervous, trembling. Had boils when young and carbuncles more recently. Heart trouble for several years, for which she has had allopathic and osteopathic treatment without improvement. "Hypertrophied." Mitral murmer; Pulse rapid. Palpitation lying on left side; sleeps on back and right side. Cyanotic when born. Thirst for cold water. Generally better in summer than in winter. Ankles swollen some. Phos. 10m.

July 6. A violent aggravation followed.

Aug. 8. Gaining rapidly; no nervous trembling; can sleep on left side; feeling quite well; no symptoms past two weeks.

Oct. 1. Was kept on Phos., receiving 10m August 31. Chief heart symptoms have decreased or disappeared. Nervousness prominent; weeps when telling her symptoms; tired constantly; wakeful from active thinking; *conversation tires her*; *noise excites her*; trembling hands; easily worried. Swelling of face, lips and ankles at times. Prolapsus with dragging sensation in uterus. Ambr. 10m. was given on the basis of the character of nervousness and sensitiveness to company in connection with the other features after the heart symptoms were dispelled.

Ambr. 10m repeated Oct. 1 and 28.

Ambr. 50m. Dec. 1. During this period the record

includes—Abdomen distention more or less. Desire for cold drinks. Headache after mens. period. Heart—burning sensation in that region; Palpitation worse lying on left side. Respiration difficult in a crowd. Tonsilitis in Nov.; subject to it; during that period—Heart pulsations rapid, with dyspnœa and protruding eyes. Hurried sensation. Subject to cold-sores.

Feb. 9, 1911. Had appendicitis after Dec. 1, carried to recovery with Phos. followed by Arsen. Her would-be friends did what they could to persuade her husband to have operative measures used, but without avail. When the dragging sensation as of prolapsed uterus was most troublesome the would-be friends urged having the uterus fastened to the abdominal wall, but Homœopathy held the case.

Mar. 8 to Oct. 9 the symptoms of the patient in her usual disorders were not satisfactorily or completely reported so that not much progress in the chronic condition was evident.

Feb. 15 to Oct. 9 pain in the appendix recurred twice, temp. 102, each time promptly dispelled by PHOS. which was given in 50m, cm, dm and mm potencies, twice in succcession in each potency, each time holding for four or five weeks.

Dec. 1911, to Feb., 1912, Phos., 1m was used three times, each time followed by improvement as revealed in mental condition and general strength. Each time her medicine was needed the *aggravation from noise, crowds and confusion, the restlessnes and craving for air* returned, though the menstrual periods became more comfortable and regular, and some progress could be detected.

Mar. 30, 1912. Aggravation from noise is found throughout the record. Made her irritable; Averse to company; wants to be quiet; Made her lose consciousness for a few minutes; Worse from people's talking; Rustling of paper or escaping steam annoys; Cannot stand confusion nor crowds; Sudden noise makes her sink, lips become white, frigid and swollen; Makes her feel faint, dog's barking, beating of rugs, piano (for awhile appeared better from music but later the noise of it aggravated her intensely, violent "nervous spells" occurring). During these months needed much space, much air· and had—Functional heart symptoms or "nervous spells" especially when things did not pass smoothly, harmoniously. Coldness, numbness, with slow heart-pulse; sudden dizziness; weakness; pale or bluish face and fingernails; circulation poor; sensation as if would faint; heavy ache about the heart followed by exhaustion and weak pulse. Despondent, especially when waking in morning. Aversion to being touched. "Bloating:" abdomen, ankles, face. The association of heart symptoms and intense aggravation to noise lead to the prescription of—AURUM 1m. Repeated May 6, in 1m and June 6, in 10m potencies. The changes in her condition during these three months are different from all the preceding: Color, circulation, sleep, strength—all improved; "Bloating" steadily decreasing; Thirstless; Menstrual period progressively improved; Aggravation from noise less constant. Felt so good that she overexerted visiting with friends and having a general good time, following which symptoms were temporarily worse.

In the course of this record other remedies were given without evidence of any action. Phos. removed the physical diagnostic symptoms. The functional symptoms have yielded to Aurum.

Aur· 10m, 50m, cm, dm—two doses of each, have been used in succession, as her physical tone was reduced. Each prescription held usually four or five weeks.

April, 1913, she was strong, robust, having been entirely free from cardiac disturbance since the summer of 1912.

The only symptoms have been extreme sensitiveness to noise, excitement, and confusion which Aurum has always relieved immediately.

A POOR HEART RESTORED TO USEFULNESS

Mrs. H. M. R., from Mass., age 20. Sept. 16, 1890. Enlargement of the left heart; has had this trouble since she had Scarlet Fever. Palpitation over entire chest and pulsation felt in extremities; < after eating. Sharp pain compelling her to sit up. Cannot lie on right side, but can lie on left side. Lil.-Tig.

Sept. 17. The prolapsus with bearing down, for which she has been treated has been somewhat relieved. Choked sensation when preparing to do anything. Wakens choking, dreams of choking. Anxiety when preparing for church often brings on diarrhœa or headache. When excited, pain in hypogastrium and ovaries, > by urination, for which there is urging; she must urinate or she will have pain. Copious colorless urine when excited. Any kind of talk that interests her in a cause of excitement. Very enthusiastic. Back of neck pain with stiffness. Extends up into occiput. Followed by headache in forehead behind eyes. Arg.-n. 40m. Sach. Lactis powders.

Sept. 30. Reports herself decidedly better in every way. Can lie on the right side now. Sach. lactis powders.

Oct. 8th. Restless, anxious, tearful, hysterical, < from meeting people and from 1 to 3 a. m. Palpitation, heartbeats strong and visible, must have clothing loose.

Oct. 20. Generally condition is better, though some paroxysms of almost all the old troubles. Gaining in strength and endurance. Occasional palpitation. Occasional sharp pain caused apparently by flatulency. Boring pain especially at night. More difficult to lie on right side. Slight paroxysm of choking before begins to sleep. Anxiety not so noticeable but followed by the desire to urinate, as reported. Stiffness is back of neck and head but less pain. Numbness of the left side considerable. Headache with heat. Menstrual period less pain.

Oct. 29. Not so well for the past week. Heart pain almost constantly, a boring pain. Thinks it has been caused by over-exertion. Had one of the severest paroxysms of the sharp pain that she has had; it was of longer duration than usual. Palpitation and trembling sensation as if something were fluttering in the region of heart. Exhausted after she went to church Sunday. Too nervous to attend a meeting Tuesday. Excitement intense and an unusual desire to urinate, even in the night. Stiffness in the neck and headache less. Arg. n. 40m.

Nov. 18. After taking last powder she began to improve; this improvement lasted about a week, then her M. P. came and she has not been well since. She suffered more pain than last month, and heart also troubled her at the time. Very little sharp pain, but considerable pain in heart. No faintness. Left side aches constantly, and is worse in the night; sensation of soreness in the morning. Very little choking in the night. Less anxiety. Some urging to urinate with dragging pain. Pain in back of neck severe at times, but not constant. Much headache with heat in head. About two weeks ago her jaw became so painful that she could not eat, the trouble is at the joint. Often in chewing the bone appears to slip out of the socket, usually there is no pain but at the time it pained her it was quite swollen in that region. The pain has gone out now, but the slipping continues to occur. A number of pimples on face lately, more than usual. Heart pain intense. Sach. Lac.

Dec. 1. All the old symptoms have been much less noticeable since last report, but has discovered two new symptoms. Headache almost constant in the top of head and down the back into the base of the brain. Nausea accompanies this headache if she attempts any mental work. Has also been troubled with neuralgic pain coming quickly and suddenly disappearing. Bladder: much dragging pain at times low in the abdomen. Frequent desire to urinate. Urine often quite thick and cloudy in appearance. Physical exertion produces only a temporary effect, but mental exertion uses her up completely. Any anxiety or worry causes that dull aching in heart, and a general nervous depression. Sach. lac.

Dec. 17. A general improvement in all the symptoms. No attack of sharp pain, but slight palpitation. The dull pain comes with excitement or worry as usual. No faintness and less nausea. Some pain in the back of head and stiffness of the neck. Uncomfortable when lying on right side but does not produce pain. Pain in ovaries and urging to urinate are the most prominent symptoms at present. Suffered extremely at menstruation, more than for years.

Jan. 20, 1891. Heart feels dull. Aches even up under arms. The old symptoms are all lighter, but she has undergone a wonderful constitutional gain. Chokes when she sleeps, even in daytime. Urine thick with brick or pink colored sediment. Decided improvement of heart. Numbness in left lower limb when sitting. Dull pain in back of head. Has had no medicine for two and one-half months. Arg.-n. 3 cm.

Jan. 29. Some palpitation. Chokes when going to sleep. Old symptoms: sees figures dressed in white come and clutch the heart; ghosts, but knows they are dreams. Nightmare; makes noises in sleep. Menstruation, pain during—Amel. by the flow (usual). If pain is not relieved by the flow fainting or vomiting and diarrhœa, copious sweat. Flow thick and dark clotted. Flow returns after ceasing if she overworks. She thinks she once had a right-sided inflammation in ovary. Sach. lac.

Feb. 25. Health has been pretty good since returning

home, although she had several acute attacks caused by some undue excitement. The ache in left side around region of heart continues. Sometimes the dull pain extends into arm and leg producing numbness.

May 14. Has been quite well up to now. Has had a return of several of her unpleasant symptoms. Aching and numbness in left side. Unpleasant sensation in heart. Stiffness and pain in back of neck. Arg.-n. 3 cm.

June 26. Health very good since last report. Heart very well during the day but sometimes at night it pains. Has had much backache. < on the left side which is very tender. At intervals in the last few weeks she has had a severe twitching of right eyelid and a wooly sensation along the edge of the lid, making clear vision impossible, < by using the eyes intently for a while. Constant application to almost any kind of work causes headache and backache.

Aug 20. Remarkably well until within the last two weeks. The last attack of pain has left her completely exhausted, and she does not seem to recover her former tone. One or two sharp attacks of pain in heart; much of that dull ache which she had when in Phila., with an unusual amount of numbness extending over entire left side. Head aches in the entire left side. Pain in the lower part of the brain is sometimes intense with much stiffness of the neck. Has a frantic feeling at times which she can hardly explain, as if head would burst and she should be insane or idiotic. Choking in throat the last few nights. Anxiety and excitement, with the old pain in the ovaries and urging to urinate returned. Arg.-n. 3 cm.

Oct. 4. In almost as bad a condition now as when she first went to you for treatment. She has been overworked this summer and likewise has been subjected to an intense mental strain. She has felt that her heart was going back on her for some months, and at the time of M. P. she has suffered considerable. The past few weeks she has been suffering constantly, and has become very weak and depressed. Palpitation. She notices this whenever she meets anyone unexpectedly, or otherwise startled, but it is slight compared to the flutter apparently within the heart, which comes without any apparent cause, and is always followed by intense weakness. Sharp pain, compelling her to sit up, occurs only occasionally. Worse when lying on right side; always worse when lying prone, she keeps moving back and forth but finds no satisfactory position. Choking very seldom, usually in the night. Anxiety extreme. Excitement, pain in ovaries, urging to urinate, all very marked. Pain in back of neck with stiffness, suffering also from swollen glands in neck and a fierce headache. Symptoms are identical with the ones previously reported. Arg.-n. 40m. Sach. lac. powders one each night.

Oct. 9. Very much better since last medicine. Heart much better. The pain comes occasionally but soon passes. No stiffness in back of neck. Choking in night, at times, is the most prominent symptom now.

July 5, 1902. After taking the last medicine she was so much better that she thought it unnecessary to report. Since that time she has been as well as usual, heart troubling only when physically overworked, or under extreme nervous excitement. The heart is still enlarged, at times it presses out the ribs quite prominently, but it gives very little trouble.

This case-report is worth more than a casual reading. To the careful student, it reveals the very remarkable restoration of strength, comfort and activity in a woman, rapidly declining and about hopelessly helpless from long-continued illness and cardiac weakness. The reader must image the picture sketched by the several reports, to realize the result accomplished. It affords a good text for study of the remedies prescribed, and carries many lessons.

An important observation is the effect of a return to the lower potency, beginning the series again, when, after ascending the series, the higher potencies cease to be active.

Many of my patients' records indicate that the patient has steadily improved after each potency to the highest, with symptoms becoming fainter, and he himself growing stronger, mentally and physically improving on each potency for three or four months.

RHEUMATIC HEART.

Mar. 21, 1908. S. E., thirteen years old. Heart: rheumatic myocarditis. Apex beat too slow. Violent aortic beat. Mitral regurgitant murmur. Enlargement l. side. Pain at times. Pulse 120. Strong pulsation in neck. Rheumatism in legs and knees. Began when four years old. Rheumatic fever six years ago. Pin-worms. Catarrh. Thirst for cold drinks. Mouth —bad taste when waking in morning. Teeth covered with blood in morning. Urine copious. Perspiration often at night. Must have much air at night. Room must be cool. Reclines on l. side; with head high. Headaches in temples, over eyes, vertex. > in cool air. Cheeks red. Ledum 10m.

April 18. Appearance much improved. Improved generally; catarrh and all symptoms. Rheumatism appears and disappears in legs and arms. Pulse 88. Ledum 10m.

May 11. Sleeps with mouth closed, now. Pimples forehead and around mouth. June 9. Rheumatism now and then, slight. Eyes improved. Stomach, funny sensation—pain—after eats few mouthfuls. Stools three a day, beginning after breakfast. Urine frequent; must sit long for it to start. Aur. 10m.

June 29. Itching in throat. Pulse 80; irregular. Heart strong pulsation.

July 13. Urine offensive odor, as of something spoiled. Less delay in starting. L. side pain at times; stomach? Heart pains. Aur. 10m.

Aug. 24 and Oct. 10. Aur. 50m.

Jan. 11. Aur. cm.

Mar. 29. Mitral regurgitation. Sensation as if beats 4 or 5 times, then stops. Rheumatism. Vertigo. Blood in mouth and on teeth in morning, when awakens. Throat, sensation of lump when swallowing. Bowels normal. R. leg cramps. Aur. 10m. Repeated May 8 when symptoms worse after taking cold.

June 30 and July 28. Aur. 50m.

Aug. 25 and Oct. 6. Aur. cm.

When the remedy was repeated in May, 1909, there was Cough with expectoration nearly all blood, from "taking cold." In June, the patient had been bathing three times a day in the Lake and had pain about the heart. Other times, pain in heart or rheumatic pains returned but a general improvement continued, and she became a strong, hearty, robust girl.

ILLUSTRATIONS OF COMPLEMENTARY RELATION-SHIP.

Menstrual headache in the occiput.

Pain pressing, bursting, violent; < motion, turning head, bending head back; < lying on right side; > standing or sitting. Must lie on left side or back. Face pale, cold and dry, haggard. Eyes *wide open*. Winking < the pain in the back of head.

Eyes seem to be forcibly held open.

Drawing or tension in eyes.

Wild look on the face.

Feet icy cold to knees.

This patient usually menstruated copiously bright red. She took *Puls.* some weeks ago for some nervous symptoms. At the next period the flow was scanty. black and putrid.

Carb. V. 500 cured the headache at once and improved the general state.

This case serves to show how it is that a partially indicated remedy seems to cure many symptoms, but leaves the patient's condition in confusion; and also how it is when the real complementary remedy follows. In the above case Carbo. v. complemented Puls. and left the case in a good state of order. Symptoms must be treated conservatively, must be nursed so that the complex of symptoms will be a good index to the next required medicine.

A hard, loose cough appeared after a long study, to call for *Puls.*, but after the remedy was given it was seen that it had only created confusion, as the *patient* was losing, growing weaker, having sweats, and the loose cough had become dry and most distressing. *Stann.* cured promptly, yet it could not be made out from the first study. This is another instance given to show the antidotal relation as well as the complementary. It often requires two remedies given in this way to cure. The first only seems to arouse. If the patient is left after the first remedy, or if he quits his doctor at that moment, or if his doctor be too ignorant to grasp the situation, I have no doubt of fatal termination. It is a critical time and must be known at once and duly met.

INFANTILE PARALYSIS.

Nov. 25, 1910. R. P., 9 years of age. Sickness began 12th of Aug.: fever, followed by paralysis. Paralysis left deltoid; (Caust. cm.) left arm and leg. These limbs jerk in sleep and waken her. Chilliness; complains much of cold. Feet burning sensation; puts them out of bed. "Never saw a more restless child," mother says. Excited when playing and hands are constantly in motion. Tearful when cannot have her own way. Tired from walking any distance. Caust. 10m.

No further treatment. Child reported cured.

INJURY TO HEAD.

A number of years ago in one of my own families. a family I had been in the habit of prescribing for, a little boy about four years of age, while sliding down the banisters one day, lost his hold and came down pretty fast, striking his head on the tiled floor. I was absent when sent for and a surgeon living near me was called in in haste and remained in attendance, as they did not like to stop him, so that I did not see the case for two or three days. Immediately after the fall the child became unconscious and remained so. A clear white watery discharge started from the ear, and this, the surgeon said, was cerebro-spinal fluid which was pouring from the fracture in the base of the skull that lead to the ear; that was his opinion. The child remained unconscious and the surgeon gave no hope for recovery, saying that the child would surely die. Finally I was sent for and found the cnild very pale, unconscious, with stertorous breathing, and that discharge was flowing, drip-dripping like clear water from the ear in to the pillow, and the water that was flowing out of the ear (I do not say where it came from) was forming little vesicles. It seemed to be acrid enough to form vesicles. The ear was red, and wherever the discharge came in contact with the skin the part became red. That was all there was about it. I could not see any more. My first thought was to give *Arnica*. But I did not. I gave him one dose of *Tellurium*. In two hours the child vomited. That discharge gradually ceased, recovery took place and in two weeks the child was perfectly well. What did the *Tellurium* have to do with it?

There was a discharge from an injury. *Tellurium* without any injury produces just such a discharge as that, and we know that the *Tellurium* discharge is not cerebro-spinal fluid, at least we have no reason to suppose it is. The first action of the remedy I observed was the child's vomiting, showing reaction. It is laid down in all the books that after concussion if vomiting takes place it is considered a reaction and the case will probably recover.

INVOLUNTARY STOOLS—PHOSPHORUS.

A lad eight years of age had been treated allopathically for five years, without any benefits, for losing his urine and stools in his pants. His mother informed me that she has often whipped him, thinking that he could prevent it. When she would go for the whip he would seem to be worse, and immediately soil himself from the fright. The stool passes without any warning, or it comes on too soon for him to accommodate himself. It seldom occurs at night or in the forenoon, but in the afternoon he passes several stools and always passes urine with stools. He takes cold easily, and when he gets a cold he has a high fever and delirium, and sometimes becomes croupy. The color of the stool is brown and the smell is very offensive. Urine stains the linen dark brown and has a strong smell. For the choice of remedy:

Involuntary stools and urine—Acon., Ars., Bell., Bry., Calc., Camph., Carbo-v., China, Cina, Colch., Con., Dig., Hyos., Laur., Mosch., Mur-ac., Nat-m., Phos., Phos-ac., Puls., Rhus-t., Sec., Sulph., Verat.

The afternoon aggravation is characteristic of Bell. Every time the child takes cold he had a high fever, and delirium is also characteristic of Bell. The general features of the case being covered by Bell., he was given two powders 4m, with instructions to watch and make a fuller report of his symptoms.

One month after taking the medicine, the mother writes:

"My son is very much better, but not entirely cured. He had had only two involuntary stools since taking the medicine, both between 12 m., and 4 p. m. He urinates involuntarily two and three times every afternoon, between 2 and 5. Never in the morning or in the night. He says he had not the slightest desire until he begins to pass stool, and then he cannot control himself, when he does feel an inclination he cannot control himself, but is obliged to go at once. His urine stains his clothes a reddish brown and is very offensive. He says when he has an involuntary stool he has a pain start from the base of the spinal column and run up his back to the brain, in top of his head, and remains there for an hour. He almost always urinates with his stools, and only has the above pain when the stool alone occurs."

The peculiar pain running up the back is a symptom characteristic of Phos., and as that is the most peculiar symptom it was taken as the guiding symptom of the case. (See Gregg's Illustrated Repertory). "Darting pains, during stool, from the os coccygis through the spine as far as the vertex, the head being drawn backward by it" page 77, plate 5. Phos. also had paralysis of the sphincter ani. (Bell., Gels., Hyos., Graph., and others.) Phos. had a brown stool, and it is offensive. It has also aggravation from excitement and fright. Looking over the first symptoms with many others, the involuntary stool and urine. The child takes cold easily, and it settles in the respiratory apparatus, which also strengthens the choice. The P. m. agg. I cannot find under Phos., but so small a condition cannot contra-indicate the remedy, in view of the fact that none of the other remedies correspond to the peculiar symptoms so well as Phos. Phos., 5m., one dose at night, cured the case promptly.

KALI PATIENTS.
STOMACH TROUBLE.

Dr. A. H. A., thirty-six years old, has had stomach-trouble for six or eight months. A specialist called it "Ulcer of the stomach." He has had the stomach washed out, and has taken much strong medicine, and now appears hopeless, as no progress has been made.

Nov. 2, 1902. Aversion to breakfast—(with nausea). Weakness in morning before breakfast. Sometimes before lunch. Stomach—sinking sensation before breakfast. (Kali-bi.) No thirst. Sternum—sore sensation as if deep within; < from exertion (Kali-bi.) Neck—muscular soreness. Trachea—sensation as of a string pulling, when clearing the larynx. Chilly patient—extremely sensitive to cold. > when at rest. Constipation last summer, not now Feet perspire; Cold at nights when going to bed. Sensitive to drafts. "Catches cold" easily; Affects nose and throat. Scalp—dandruff. Kali-bi. 10m.

Nov. 16. Improved generally. Sternum—some soreness. Larynx—tightness. Sac. lac.

Nov. 30. Improved. Neck—sensation of cord drawn down on r. side to chest. Sac. lac.

Dec. 14. Improvement—general; Chest and sternum. Nose and throat trouble when wakens in morning. Soreness when swallows. Kali-bi. 10m.

Jan. 25 and Mar. 3, 1913. Kali-bi. 50m. Reported from time to time improved.

He is now a robust man with no symptoms, and is a great friend of Homœopathy.

LEPRA-VULGARIS—WITH CLINICAL NOTES ON PULSATILLA

CLINICAL NOTE ON PULSATILLA.—In lepra vulgaris the diffuse form of psoriasis, when it occurs in large patches about the size of the palm over the abdomen and other parts of the body, with heat and redness, and itching worse at night in the warmth of the bed. *Pulsatilla* has worked wonders. It goes to the bottom and cures it in an orderly way. This is a feature that is not brought out in any of the books. From the observation of this fact I have been able to cure the mange in dogs at once with *Puls.* when the disease took this patchy form. We see the depth of action of this drug also in its ability to antidote the effects of *Sulphur*. When *Sulphur* has been used externally and internally to suppress itch, Pulsatilla will antidote it and bring back the itch.

In all skin diseases, however, let it be your aim to fit the remedy to the constitution of the patient and not to the character of the eruption alone. Always leave the consideration of the skin to the last. When the reverse is done and the remedy suits only the eruption, while the skin symptoms are benefitted, the patient is invariably made worse.

MAMMARY TUMOR CURED WITH CARBO-AN.

Mrs. H. has had several children; she is about thirty-five years old; she has always had much difficulty with all her confinements. The last one was comparatively easy, and yet it was tedious, owing to an elongated cervix. With the first she had an abcess in the mammæ (r) and it was badly treated, so that the cicatrix has always been a source of trouble. Preparatory to her last confinement I prepared her as best I could, guided by her symptoms. The child is now some two months old and she is suffering with a hard lump in the right mamma. When I first observed the threatened trouble after the milk began to form, she took Graphites without benefit; also Phytolacca, but only temporary relief followed. The milk mostly dried up and she now has a nodular lump with retraction of the nipple, and there are lumps in the axilla; she complains of burning and stinging in the lump and her menstrual flow has come on. She says she has always menstruated during lactation. The flow is dark and clotted; when she goes to sleep she perspires freely; she seems greatly prostrated after a moderate loss of menstrua; she is somewhat cachectic.

For a choice of remedies we might arrange: Burning in Mammæ.—Apis., Bell., Calc., Carbo-an., Iod., Led., Mez., Selen., Laur., Phos., Lyc., Tarent-c. Stinging in Mammæ.— Apis., Berb., Carbo-an., Con., Kreos., Graph., Grat., Ind., Iod., Kali-c., Laur., Lys., Murex, Nat-m., Phos., Rheum., Sang., Sep. Nodosities in Mammæ.—Bell., Carbo-an., Coloc., Con., Graph., Lys., Nit-ac., Sil. Cancer of Mammæ. —(Minton) Bell., Carb-an., Coloc., Con., Graph., Lys., Nit-ac., Sil. Perspiration during sleep.—Carb-an., Cic., Chin., Dros., Euph., Ferr., Jatr., Merc., Nux-v., Phos., Puls., Selen., Thuj. Great exhaustion after Menses.—Alum., Carb-an., Chin., Ip., Phos. Menses During Lacation.—Calc., Sil.

Neither of the last remedies correspond to the balance of the symptoms. But it will be seen that Carbo-an. and Phos. cover the case, and the menstrual flow, which is dark and clotted, is not so characteristic of Phos, as Carb-an. The exhaustion after the flow is more marked in Carb-an. than in Phos., though both have it in a marked degree.

"The flow weakens her; she can hardly speak; blood dark; (Guiding Symptoms) under Carb-an., Carb-an. 3m, one dose dry was administered. Four weeks, burning and stinging all gone; glands in axilla nearly gone. After the dose the cutting pains became worse for a few days. Medicine repeated in thirty-nine days. The lump has disappeared.

NATRUM SULPH. IN SYMPTOMS ARISING AFTER AN INJURY TO THE HEAD

This case, involving the most intense suffering, was

30

the result of a violent accident, that of being trampled upon by a spirited horse. While visiting the farm of Chancellor Nicholson of Dover, Del., he invited my attention to his farmer who was suffering at that time from the following symptoms:

Rheumatism in left side, no pain elsewhere, worse in hands to wrists and knees to hips. Pain like a knife sticking in him, had not had such an attack for a long time. Agg. in bed, can't sleep for the pain.

Does not feel sleepy, gets mad because he cannot sleep.

Gets stiff all over when sits or lies down.

Amel. from pressure or moving about.

Having learned that Mrs. Nicholson had given Rhus about the 30th potency after the accident, and that it had worked well, and the symptoms seeming to agree, I gave him one dose of *Rhus.* mm on Oct. 27, 1897. This had only a temporary effect, as will be seen by the following letter from the Chancellor:

SYMPTOMS OF R. R. E. Dec. 1, 1897

Since the days of his apprenticeship in a Vienna Brewery he has been a very poor sleeper.

Immediately after taking your last powder he slept for four or five nights, "better than in all his life," say four or five hours of good sleep each night. Since then has not slept at all. Says positively that in the whole time, day and night put together, he has not been asleep two hours. His eyes wide open all night long except when he holds his hands over them. Has waking dreams all day. Sees and talks with his father, and with me. Sees what he reads all over the world, particularly military scenes, such as battles in Cuba, etc. (He served through Franco-Prussian War in the Bavarian cavalry.)

Is very nervous and startles at any sound during the

night,—"not scared exactly, but nervous all over down to the tips of his fingers." This is something very novel to him.

Has nearly the whole time what he calls a "zumming in his ears," usually not very loud, "like a bumble-bee in in a hollow board." If he gets up very slowly and carefully he escapes this. With the loud "zumming" a pain comes across the top of his head from ear to ear running back to the point where the hair centers.

Pain in his head comes when he lies down, on the side he is lying on. On account of this he always lies on his back with his head propped high. This pain goes away when he sits up or stands. His forehead always feels very heavy, and frequently at the top of it, on the left hand side, he has a sharp throbbing pain for a little while. About eighteen months ago my big colt trampled on his head about this place. His memory has been bad ever since then and he has had great suffering with his head at the injured point especially.

He sweats very easily and profusely, which makes him feel cold and take cold very frequently in his ordinary outdoor work.

His breast is now very sore to the touch in the region of the ribs and breast bones, the muscles apparently.

He seems tireless in his work, says he feels no fatigue when he works all day long and is full of restless energy. Have noticed frequently of late a wild look in his eyes.

The terrible sleeplessness in the one symptom upon which he himself dwells, and which he tells me "his wife says is driving him crazy."

He drinks coffee three times a day, but says that if you direct him to stop it he will not miss it. Has very little appetite. Is habitually a small eater and the sight of any large quantities of food on the table is so repulsive to him that it makes it impossible for him to eat anything.

If these symptoms do not clearly indicate a remedy, please let me know and I will send him up to you, provided you think his condition serious.

On these symptoms I sent, to be taken once, one powder of *Natrum-sulph.* 20 m.

On December 28th the following report was received:

"Effect of last powder is amazing; patient sleeps well and looks like another man. The wrinkles are smoothed out and his eyes are mild and youthful. Two days after the powder he was worse, but he later became sleepy and then sleep came normally."

OVARIAN TUMOR CURED WITH LYCOPODIUM

June 1, 1888.—Miss A. W., aged thirty, Irish housemaid. Pelvic tumor, about which opinion varied. Abdomen resembled pregnancy of nine months. Her friends refused to go upon the street with her because of her appearance. She consulted several surgeons, and some declined to operate. The tumor could not be moved, seemed to fill the pelvic cavity. Its origin could not be traced; tumor was very hard. It being immovable, very hard and painful, were the reasons why one surgeon could not operate. No vaginal examination was made by me. She came to my office because she had heard that a local examination would not be made. She dates her discovery of it to five years ago. For two years she has felt much pain in the pelvis. Swelling of the pit of the stomach below the abdomen became distended. Feet œdematous. Constant headache; cold milk causes pain. Cannot take cold things; everything must be warm. Nausea and vomiting. Everything eaten makes her sick and causes vomiting, vomiting after every meal. Constipation, no desire for stool for many days. Always feels a constriction about the waist from pressure upwards of the tumor. Distension in stomach after eating so little. Menses regular, with cramping pain, has always relieved it by whiskey. Starts suddenly from a noise. Restless, and sleeps badly. Teeth decayed young; they are dark colored. She says she felt a lump in the right side as large as a child's head, which was the first she felt of it, about four years ago, it was then very hard. Pain in this lump in the side has been felt from time to time. Feet burn; must remove the shoes to cool them. She says feet feel like there was mustard on them. Lycop. cm.

July 23d.—Up to a few days ago she had no vomiting, and the pain is much better. She is again feeling worse. Lyc. mm.

August 2nd.—Called to see if medicine was expected to make her worse. S. L.

August 9th.—Called to say the aggravations had passed off and that she was much better.

September 25th.—Continued to improve up to a few days ago. Symptoms returning. Vomiting after eating and pain in the stomach. Lycop. mm.

October 28th.—Symptoms all passed away until a few days ago the pain came back in the pylorus, and again she received Lyc. mm.

November 27th.—No symptoms. S. L.

December 13th.—Reports no symptoms. S. L.

January 7th.—The tumor has diminished some. No bloating of feet. Can move the tumor and can discern that it belongs to the right side of the pelvis.

January 26th.—Symptoms returning. Lyc. mm.

February 16th.—She is growing smaller about the abdomen and gaining in flesh and color. March 7th.—Improving. No symptoms.

March 28th.—Still improving.

April 25th.—Stomach symptoms returning. Lyc. mm.

June 3rd.—Has been entirely free from symptoms until recently. Feet swelling again; cannot drink water

nor cold milk; cannot take cold things; everything must
be warm. Headache in forehead and eyes; pain in lumbar
region; bowels constipated; now goes three or four days;
feet burn. Lyc. mm.

June 15th.—Symptoms all better.

August 15th.—All symptoms have returned. She returns when the symptoms return. Lyc. 2 mm.

October 7th.—Reports herself cured. The tumor can
be discovered by close examination. She had not been able
to find it, therefore she thought she was cured. She remarked that the last medicine did her most good of all
the medicine taken. She remains in perfect health.

PARALYSIS.

Lad, age six. Paralysis of left arms, œsophagus, and
pharynx. Difficulty in swallowing. Liquids come out of
nose. Solids cause much choking. Nasal voice. Limited
motion in left arm. Cannot grasp with the hand. Pale
sickly face, waxy and shiny. When talking he throws the
head back. Choking when eating. Bowels constipated, no
action. Ineffectual frequent urging. Trouble progressing
rapidly. The attack began only a few weeks ago. No history of any kind discovered in the family. Family supposed to be psoric. Lad was poisoned by Rhus three years
ago, self-cured. Talks and cries out when sleeping. Cannot abduct the arm, but can flex it feebly. The paralysis
of left is almost complete and the right is showing signs
of weakness in abduction. Rash comes out on the body in
heated air. Plumb. 42m. Cured in six months.

THREE PECULIAR CASES.

PELVIC CELLULITIS

Case I.—Mrs. L, age 36, had been in bed with pelvic
cellulitis. She apparently had been a sufferer, notwith-
standing ample medical attention. There was much tume-

faction of the abdomen and great tenderness of all the pelvic organs, and the tenderness extended to the abdominal tissues and viscera. There was enlargement of the uterus and ovaries with erosion of vaginal portion of the uterus and anterior wall of the vagina. Hot douches per vagina and hot hops constituted her only possible comfort, when her abdomen had cooled from the absence of the hops, pain became unbearable, so she lived and so she was dying. Every change to cold increased her suffering.

Her bowels were constipated, her menses came too soon and her feet were always cold and felt damp. The evidence of her suffering was ample. Her mental state was gloomy. The hop poultices and hot injections were discontinued and she was placed in warm clothing. Calc-c., 85 m, one dose, was given.

No more medicine was needed. She was able to work in four months and is now perfectly well. Three days after taking the medicine her menses came on with profuse flow and increase of pain; at the proper time the flow ceased and all the tenderness and previous suffering passed away.

PERIODICAL ATTACKS OF CHRONIC SPASMS

Case IV.—Phosphorus: Mrs. G., widow, 42 years of age, was afflicted with periodical attacks of Chronic Spasms. I called at the house one day and removed a tumor from the hand of her mother, and the excitement brought on the most intense spasmodic jerking of the whole body. *Whenever a thunderstorm is raging she has these attacks,* said her mother. They last two or three hours. I administered Phos. 5m. dry, one dose. Thunder does not affect her now. She never had another attack. Her whole constitution and mental state have changed. She considered herself an invalid and expected no relief.

PROLAPSUS.

Case V.—Sepia: Mrs. K.—a married woman, 28 years old came to me from the country, with what a gynecologist had called a prolapsus. She was a tall, slim woman, otherwise in good health. She was wearing a Hodge pessary. She could not walk or stand long without her "ring." She came to the office in a carriage. I removed the ring and gave her Sac. Lac. At the end of a week I had noted the following symptoms:

The urine passed slowly, and she must wait a long time for it to start. Sepia., Lycop., Arn., Hepar., Zinc, Cann-ind. She was greatly constipated, and always felt a lump in the rectum, even after stool. Sep. She complained of a hungry, empty feeling in the stomach. Sep., Murex., Ign. Hydr. and many others.

She always had a bearing down in the pelvis, as if the uterus would issue from the vagina, Sepia, Murex· Lil-t., Nux., Natr-m., Puls., etc. She must press on the vulva with a napkin for relief, Sep., Murex, Lill-t. She often crosses her limbs to prevent the uterus from escaping. Sep. Tall, slim and sallow, Sep. She got Sep. C. M. one dose, dry, and Sac. lac. It is three years since this case called, and she has never needed a physician since. She was an invalid before. The one dose cured her.

PROLAPSUS

Case VI.—Lil-t. The above lady went home and sent me a similar case. She called it "a case just like mine." She was a short stout woman, dark hair and eyes. She had worn a Hodge pessary for a year. She was unable to be about at housework, without the pessary. I removed the pessary and informed her that she would need to visit my office every day for a week or so. She was given Sac. lac., and every day I noted symptoms, until at the end of a week I believed I had the symptoms that expressed the individuality of the disease. The most marked feature was her mental state. The remedy that would cure this case must have mental symptoms of prominence in its picture. She complained of a wild feeling in the head, and feared she would lose her reason, Lil-t. Bearing down in the pelvis as if the uterus would protrude, Sep., Lil-t., Murex, Natr-m., Nux-v., Puls, Pod. and others. She must press on the vulva with the hand to prevent the parts from protruding, Lil-t., Sep., Murex. There were some flying pains going through the pelvis and down the thigh like those found in Lil-t. She took Lil-t. 30 for a day in water, and then Sac-lac. one week. She had then improved so much that she had walked over the Zoological garden, which she had not undertaken even with the pessary *in situ.* She was sent home with a few powders of Lil-t. 200, to use as per instruction, viz., to be used when she felt a return of the difficulty. One year later she wrote me that she had taken one of the powders, and was keeping the others with great care. For this last case I was presented with a check for $50, over and after the full payment for my services. The husband said it was the cheapest doctor bill he had been called to pay. One gynæcologist had receipted a bill for $200, and this was but a small part of the "*sick expenses.*" It may not pay as well to practice pure homœopathy but it is the honest way.

PHARYNGITIS

A woman of fifty-three years called in January, when she was scarcely able to go out-doors, suffering with sore throat which she had for six weeks, under old-school treatment.

Jan. 20. Had "grip" six weeks ago. Pharynx soreness since then, better and worse; Began on left and extended to right, side. < swallowing solids; > warm liquids: Externally, swollen enormously and very red. Voice and hearing lost. Larynx and side of neck pain, with dry hacking cough. No rest in the morning. Desires cold drinks but cold aggravates the throat. Constipation· for months (chronic symptom). With the exception of the aggravation from warmth, all features of the case were prominently Lachesis, i. e., it was predominantly a Lachesis case. Lach. 10m.

Jan. 25. Throat, pain on left side much worse after first dose. < cold water. Burning sensation at night from inhaling cold air. Thirst constant for cold water. Bowels now normal, first time for months. Wakeful: hears clock strike 10, 11, 2 and 3. Head pulsating; Cracking sensation at base of skull when turning head. Sach. lac.

All throat symptoms ceased at the end of a week.

The favorable action of the remedy was evidenced in the aggravation occurring on the first day and the improvement in rectal evacuations. The wisdom of continuing the same remedy was quite clear when the disorder of six weeks' duration was entirely eradicated within a week.

RHEUMATIC PATIENT.

Aug. 15, 1910. Mrs. M. W., aged fifty years. Rheumatism, both ankles swollen. Nearly helpless from it for a year. Many O. S. doctors and much drugging without relief. > by cool, < by heat; > in rest; Extended from right to left. Bowels sluggish. Strong appetite. Guai. 10m.

Aug. 22. Ankles better than for a month. Knees lame. Thighs, cramp in outer side; shooting pains, inner side.

Sept. 5. Can tolerate warm bath.

Sept. 19. Swelling and pain in R. foot and ankle.

Oct. 3. General improvement. Rheumatism in ankles and feet. Guai. 50m.

Nov. 14. After beginning the higher potency, slight

agg. then relief. Rheumatism now worse again; feet and ankles swollen; hands stiff; knees lame. Guai. 50m.

Dec. 10. Steady improvement until recently. Left thigh, cramp again upward. Guai. 50m.

Jan. 9, 1911. Improved less, recently. Guai. cm.

Has been free from rheumatism and in good health, ever since.

This patient presented few symptoms, but a strong characteristic: *rheumatic pains < from warmth, > from cold.*

Three remedies are characterized by this feature in rheumatism: Guaiacum, Ledum and Pulsatilla. When this symptom is reported in a patient of general Ledum type, Ledum will cure; when it is found that the patient is a Pulsatilla type in general, Pulsatilla is prescribed. In this instance, the patient was neither Ledum nor Pulsatilla, hence Guaiacum was selected, with beneficial, curative results.

SERIOUS DISORDERS REMOVED
A CARDIAC PATIENT

When Mrs. A. C. C. first presented herself at the office she was thirty-one years old and very nervous.

Jan. 16, 1909. Very tired. Headache begins in forehead and extends to occiput. Almost continuous past three months. Confused with it. Menstrual period seven to fourteen days late. Flow scanty; very dark or watery. First part clotted, dark. Odor putrid. Has been of this character from the beginning. Vagina ulcerated sensation during coition. Clothes bands around the waist occasion pain. Aching through all the body; sharp pains; < when rising in morning and in forenoon. Eyes—sore sensation; pain in motion. Worked hard all summer. Thirsty continually; drinks small quantity, frequently. Appetite best for breakfast. Chilly usually. Feet always cold; never too warm. *Heart—pains*; *stops beating, then the sharp pains appear*. Pain < hurrying. Aches and tumbles, from exertion and ascending stairs. Nausea and vomiting if eats one mouthful too much. Easily excited. From riding in cars. Likes warm room and warm clothing. Disturbed by little screams of the baby. Very nervous from noises. Flatulence very slight. Desires sweets not acids. Very active; unable to sit still a minute. Quick-motioned. Sleeps easily; can sleep any time of day or night. Naja 10m. Sac. l. powders one each night.

Feb. 11. Better in general. Head aches only when tired; eyes less pain; less chilly; no heart-pains. Weak. Sensation as if heart ceased beating. Empty sensation in stomach. Naja 10m. and Sac. l. powders.

Mar. 23. Much improved generally. M. flow dark and thick, more copious. Vagina much less of ulcerative sensation during coition. Naja 10m.

Apr. 28. Menstrual period only a few days late. Discharge scant, dark; less putrid. Soreness in vagina nearly entirely disappeared. Never weighed more than 107 lbs. until now; weighs 129 lbs. Naja 10m.

MENTAL DERANGEMENT

July 23, 1904. Mrs. E. M. D., aged forty-five years, has been distressed by an adopted daughter. Finger ends sensitive, does not want them touched. Spine, sensitive spots—one in dorsal region, one in coccyx. Head sensation of a steel band over forehead. Used to have menstrual headaches. Constipation. No children. Sensitive to heat. Feet, ankles and sometimes legs, cold. Tearful. Sleep ameliorates. Friend reports: She is very suspicious of her husband and a neighbor woman, without cause. Father was insane about a year. Imagines her daughter the cause of her troubles. Many imaginations; scolds her husband; abuses people without occasion; will not work, takes no interest in her home. Talks constantly. Headache mornings, when waking. Perspiration during night. Weary. Lach. 500.

July 30. Grating in joints; an old symptom, continued one day. Stirring here and there (old symp.). Sleeping well. Less tearful. Pulsating in stomach. Perspiration in sleep, day and night. Head hot to touch. Conscious of her uterus. Sach.

Aug. 13. Appetite reported improved a week ago, for the first, also more interest in her work. Perspiration on back and shoulders after first taking Lach. Twitching of eyes. Loneliness; forsaken sensation. Trembling; tremulous after doing some housework. Anxious; was always anxious. Abdomen, sore sensation (O. S.). < respiration. Generally < before a storm. Constipation; has used enema every day. Feces slip back. Feces knotty. Silica cm.

Aug. 20. Hot flushes (O. S.). Less nervous tremor and less headache. Abdomen sensitive to clothing. Must recline on back to sleep. *Bowels much improved, daily normal evacuation in the morning.* Sach. l.

Sept. 21. Improved; less perspiration; can sleep while reclining on the side; much improvement in general; bowels regular until recently. Neck stiff for a few days. Roaring sounds in ears, > boring in ears (O. S.). Exertion aggravates. Heart sensation of pressure over it. Head creeping sensation on vertex. Sach. l.

Sept. 29. Head "feels so much improved." Spine nervous sensation. Gaining in general.

Oct. 14. Sil. cm. Followed by an aggravation.

Dec. 14 and Feb. 11, 1905. Sil. 10m. During this period was general improvement: in strength; cold feet; gain in weight; appetite and stomach improved; constipation; heat flashes; Prominent symptoms: Ears ringing noise. Head, heat in vertex; sensation of drawing back, when waking. Pain in vertex < exertion and fatigue, <noise. Pain in occiput when laughing. Scalp itching; dryness; biting sensation. Pulsation, when waking. Chilli-

ness; creeping sensation in night. Small of back tired when waking. Pain between scapulæ. Must sleep on back. Suspicious of neighbor.

Mar. 22, 1905. Feet heat at night, extends them outside the covers to cool. Hungry about 10 or 11 a. m., must eat. Cold, damp air penetrating. Chilliness and perspiration, when waking at night. Scalp dry scale. Tired easily. Sulph. 10m.

July 5 and Oct. 27, Sulph. 10m.

Dec. 9, and Jan. 18. Sulph. 50m.

April 16, 1906. SULPH. cm. Record indicates improvement between these reports; steel band sensation absent, not much pain in head; bowels orderly; heat flashes only when tired; enjoys being out-doors. Shooting pain in hip, and r. thigh sometimes sore to touch in bone. One day pain and swelling in r. heel; disappeared, and appeared in r. elbow, then in l. elbow. Head: sensation of a million small things in scalp or in brain in vertex; sometimes it extends to sides of head and front, or in entire crown; > by scratching. Whirling sensation in vertex when waking from nap, not in morning. Less of the large spongy sensation. Tired tremor through body, extends to vertex when worried. Soreness sensation in thorax, in walls and l. mammary region. Perspiration followed by chilliness. Eyes redness; sensation as if upper lid covered over the lower; sensation as if eyes turned the wrong way; sensation of sand associated with agglutination in morning; sensation of crack in eyes when trying to sleep.

May 25. Jealous and suspicious; permits her thoughts and speculations to weigh her down. Sulph. was continued until 29th of June, 1907, used twice in mm. and twice in 3 mm. potency, while the following symptoms were the prominent ones reported: Head spongy sensation; heat in vertex, > by pressure; sleeps with cold cloth on it; pain in vertex when quickly turning the head; pain in back of neck with headache and when becomes cold. Sore spot.

Confusion and dizziness when emotions excited. < heat of sun; remains in dark room on hot days. Abdomen pain in region of spleen. Numbness in feet and hands when not lying on them. Urine dark; red particles not difficult to remove from vessel. Perspires easily, lameness or other aggravation from suppression or cooling. Feet hot at night. Sensation: as if nerves twisted off, while reclining; pains in wrists when overtired; numbness in fingers. Nasal dryness; sometimes dripping. Much sneezing. Through all the period general improvement, gain in flesh and decrease of these symptoms.

June 29, 1907. Urine, brick-dust sediment occasions rough surface in vessel. < from over-eating; hiccough; cankers in mouth after eating sour food. Stomach, burning sensation after eating strawberries. Calc. 10m.

Mar. 5, 1908. Cramps in calves of legs when goes from out-doors to house; sitting, or standing, less when walking; at the worst, cramped while lying in bed by > continued motion of turning. Head pain in vertex < pressure (?). < by talking of others; company. Perspiration easy, on slight exertion—between mammæ and around body, not on face. Had many small, flat warts in childhood. Must wear exactly same weight clothing every day or is chilly. Heat flash followed by perspiration and then chilliness, from worry. Heated from walking. Numb, dead sensation in hand or arm, when wakens. Dreams all night about company. > in open air. Thighs stiff from continued sitting. Ferr.-Pic. 10m.

April 19. "Last remedy did everything for her.". Head —sore, sensitive spots relieved immediately. Ferr.-pic. 10m. May 21, Ferr.-pic. 10m.

Aug. 31, Oct. 29, Dec. 15, Ferr-pic. 50m. During this period, steady improvement with the chief symptoms: Fatigue from company; head pressure of a band; pain back of eyes from extreme heat; fullness; sensation as if would become unconscious; each side of center of vertex. Weeps after unpleasant events or if reprimanded or blamed. Cramps from cold, damp weather; small twists all down calf. Wakens at night with cold feet; at times cold to waist. Heart pain from vexation.

Feb. 18 and May 29, 1909. Lecithin 10m.

Aug. to Mar., 1910. Stomach soreness at entrance if drinks little hot tea. Tension on waking. Mouth-sores if eats acid. Craves water as cold as can get it. Milk must be cold. Head sensitive on vertex, nearer front. PHOS. 10m.

May. 6. "Head better than in years." Phos. 10m.

June 10 and July 30, Phos. 50m.

Sept. 27, Phos. cm. Improvement continuing.

Nov. 7. Abdomen soreness across it, > holding it up. < reaching; going up-stairs. Heart sometimes darting pains. Nostrils bloody scabs. Murex 10m.

Jan. 21, 1911. Head sensation of animals eating inside, knitting inside. Heat, top and sides. Heavy, top and sides. < mental disturbance. Wakens with pain—shooting. Sensation of band. General health better than in ten years. > open air; motion. Heat when waking in afternoon. Lyc. 10m.

April 5. Lyc. 10m.

Aug. 4 and Nov. 18, Lyc. 50m.

Jan. 16 and May 3, 1912. Lyc. cm. Improvement through the two years continued with mild return of symptoms when repetition of remedy needed.

To describe the condition of this patient in the early months, even through the first year or two of her treatment is impossible, so to convey an adequate idea of the disordered condition of her mind. By the hour, she would talk on and on in a monotone, with no inflections of voice, detailing her complaints and the annoyances of her family affairs, if one would listen. To reason with her was an absolute impossibility: there was no reasoning faculty apparent in her.

Then other members of the family would report the strange things she did. By the hour they would recite her vagaries—many unthinkable things. She said the family made her so nervous she just must go away from them. At the time her family and her neighbors reported how she would leave the house immediately after an early breakfast and not return until late afternoon, neglecting everything in the house, shirking all responsibility.

Now, two years later, at the last date on the record, not only is she filling her place in the home as a splendid house-keeper and cook, but she is her husband's accountant and book-keeper, attending to the details of a large business employing dozens of men and many teams. In her husband's absence she directs the men and keeps oversight of them and their horses with extreme efficiency.

She is devoted to Homœopathy, interested in its philosophy, and wonders why others are not believers in it.

SEVERE MALADIES
ACUTE MANIA

R. T. aged twenty-three years, had gonorrhœa which was treated allopathically for four months before it was controlled. Habits of secret vice. Was sent home from college for treatment.

Mental condition, diagnosed by a specialist "Dementia præcox"; Weeping; Forgets everything; Answers no questions, makes unintelligible, slight mumbling; Hears voices; Thinks he is a criminal; Thought he was Christ; Thought he was to be buried alive; Hears officers coming to arrest him; Mind appears to be gone; Hands and feet clammy. Violent—had to be tied and held in bed. Face red; continually flaming red. Head—pain in occiput > in

40

middle of the day. Ears—pressed-in sensation. Constipation. Wakens with a start. Noise <. Light>. L. pupil appears larger than right. Medor. 10. Given to test the case to determine if it were a case of suppressed sycosis. No response followed and the case was thus determined not due to suppression. Under observation day and night by day and night nurse.

Mar. 23. Hears voice from a distance: of father: of mother: of policeman. Voice called him a liar; voices said he was dead; told him to "run for it;" of mother, told him to say "Lord" very loud. Thinks he is damned; that people are laughing at him. Somewhat religious phases of delirium: commanded by one of the voices to say the Apostles' Creed. Breath fetid, ever since he came home, now better. Fecal evacuations were black when first returned home. Voices: Bell., cann.-ind., carb.-s., cinch., *cham.*, crot-c., *elaps.*, hyos., *kali-br.* lach., lyc., med., phos., stram.; many more not related to him.

Religious affections: *Bell.*, carb.-s., *cham.*, HYOS., kali-br., LACH., *lyc.*, *med.* stram.

Weeps: *Bell.*, CARB-S.,*cham.*, hyos., KALI-BR., lach., LYC., *med.*, stram.

Mania: BELL., HYOS., KALI-BR., *lach.*, LYC., STRAM.

Insanity: BELL., HYOS., *kali-br.*, *lach.*, LYC., STRAM.

Answers incoherent: Hyos.

Irrelevant: *Hyos.*

Confused speech: Bell., *hyos.*, lach., med.

Incoherent speech: Bell., HYOS., kali-br., LACH., STRAM.

Confusion: BELL., *hyos.*, kali-br.* *lach.*, med., stram.

Delirium: BELL., HYOS., kali-br., LACH., STRAM.

Delirium raving: BELL., HYOS., LYC., *stram.*

Chill: *Bell.*, *hyos.*, *lach.*, *stram.*

Summary: Bell. 24; Hyos. 27; Lach. 20; Stram. 21.

Hot head: Bell.* hyos., lach., stram.

Cold feet: BELL.* *hyos.*, LACH., STRAM.

Clothing < *neck*: Bell., LACH.

Occipital pain: BELL., *hyos., lach.,* stram.

Starting on waking: BELL., HYOS., *stram.*

Light <: *Bell., hyos., lach., stram.*

Noise <: BELL., hyos., *lach.*

Summary: Bell. 44; Hyos. 38; Stram. 34.

Though Bell. stands highest in the anamnesis, the bodily heat of the remedy is lacking and the case may later demand Hyos., as the mania is not active enough for Stram. Bell. 10m.

S. L. two hours in water.

Mar. 25. Struck his nose twice; Bell., hyos., stram. Thinks he is about to be arrested: Bell. Just ascertained that he has lost all shame. No other change. Hyos. 10m.

Mar. 26. Thinks his medicine is poison. Breath less offensive. Hears scarcely any noises. Sach, lact.

April 4. Voices say he is dead and he wants to know when they are going to have the funeral. Wants to dig his own grave. Wants to be buried. Thinks his coffin is in the house or cellar. Rubs his nose much, it itches. Thinks the medicine is poison. Collar fits too close. Lach. 10m.

April 9. Thought that he was dead only once; voices less. Feet and hands cold. Sach. lac.

April 12. Struck his attendant several times. Quarrelsome; wants to fight. Thinks he is a criminal. Appears worse on Lachesis. Hyos. 10m.

April 13. No more fighting since last remedy. More quiet; appearance improved; face less red; nose itches less, does not rub it constantly, as he did.

April 18. Laughs much. Hears voices of the family and of the nurse. Thinks he is a criminal. No initiative: waits for commands before acting; when told to eat he eats; to go to bed, he goes to bed, stands until told to sit and sits until told to stand; when told to do anything he does it, almost mechanically. Irresolution. Does not talk; appears unable to answer. Sach. lac.

May 2. Heat in head marked; > by cold. Aversion to hot soup. Intense fear. Nervous. Voices. Delusions. Irresolution. Phos. 10m.

Remedies heretofore used removed the violence and the intensity of the mania, so that he could eat at the table with the family. He was constantly under the observation of a carefully observant nurse, who at this time noticed that he could not take hot soup. In connection with the other symptoms, it was evident that Phosphorus was closely related throughout the case. Hence the prescription.

May 28. Much improved; no delusions; seldom hears voices. Now very nervous. Aversion to being touched. Likes cold water. Phos. 10m.

This case was finished by a repetition of Phos. in 50m. potency, a month later. By the middle of June, the mental symptoms had disappeared and he had gained much flesh. Since that he has been normal and robust, traveling about the city as would any one else.

TOTALITY AND INDIVIDUALITY.

SYCOTIC EXCRESCENCES.

CaseI.—Thuja: A lady who suffered from sycotic excrescences became reduced from repeated hemorrhages. When she would go for some time without the loss of much blood her totality of symptoms was similar to Thuja, but an exhaustive flow would add several symptoms to the original picture and mask the individuality of the true chronic disorder. One symptom in particular was a cold feeling in the left side of the head, another, cold damp feet. These would make a young man naturally think of Calcarea, but a closer study must result in a conclusion that Calcarea could only result in a failure to cure until Thuja had removed the sycotic nature of the disorder. The cold sensation is not found under Thuja, but the case made a good recovery, because it was similar to the ruling feature of the case. Now because Thuja removed the individuality of a case with the cold left side of the head, it is no sign it will remove that symptom. It only shows that the individuality of a disease must be known; such information is best acquired by observation in the wilderness of symptomatology. The pathologist might score this as a victory for himself, but he only has learned it from a careful individualization of symptoms.

When the evidence of a chronic miasm is suppressed by a remedy corresponding to the acute or last appearing symptoms, after which the individuality of the chronic miasm will be manifested by its true expression or symptoms. These little things were well known to the great Hahnemann, and are taught in the *Organon* and *Chronic Diseases*.

No Homœopathist can make a truly homœopathic prescription when the individuality of a disease is unknown, or only partly known. The individuality can only be known by observing and knowing all the symptoms. When a woman calls for treatment with a pessary in her vagina, she will most likely fail to obtain a correct remedy because her symptoms are masked or changed so that the totality does not express the individuality of the disease. The pessary should be removed, and the disease permitted to express itself in the language so well known to every true Homœopathist. After a week the symptoms will most likely express individuality, in its totality of symptoms, and then an appropriate remedy can be found. There is no other way known. These things were all known to the great Hahnemann. The ignorant pretenders use the supporters and smile at the *Organon*, and go on with their failures; they seem to glory in their ignorance of the true healing art.

The physician who does not individualize uses Mor

phine to stop the pain and reports his ignorance to the society, having the audacity to ask what remedy he should have used. The question asked, no less than the failure, shows that he is not acquainted with the teachings of the *Organon*. Each case must be studied with a view of its own individuality. The physician who is not competent to direct the appropriate remedy is not acquainted with the individuality of his case; and with such ignorance of his case, how can even a more competent physician inform him what an appropriate remedy might be? The questioner could not prescribe for his own case as a general thing if he would individualize correctly. These are the ones who are wise enough to direct remedies on their knowledge of pathology, only to fail, and then have the audacity to ask for the right remedy to be pointed out.

TARENTULA CASES.
ROLLING FROM SIDE TO SIDE TO RELIEVE THE DISTRESS.

Rolling from side to side to ease the distress is a characteristic of Tarantula. A man with inveterate constipation, who had used physics until they would no longer serve, was encouraged by his daughter to wait for further action until the proper remedy could be recognized, as advised by the doctor. In his distress he rolled from side to side, on the bed, wailing "Oh dear me, oh dear me!" Tarentula quieted him; two days later he had a normal evacuation, and thereafter had no difficulty.

THREATENING TUBERCULOSIS.

Tall, slim young man, age eighteen. Very spare. Tuberculosis parentage. Temperature 99½. Cachectic aspect. Pulse 100 to 110. Varying. *Right knee sore*, painful when letting limb hang down. Has been ill with inflammatory rheumatism many months. Seems declining. The paucity of symptoms and generalities persuaded the giving of Psor. hoping to develop the case.

Psor. 42m cured the whole case, and the young man remains well and is thriving perfectly.

Several homœopathic remedies had been given and still he was declining, was an additional reason for Psor.

The cure of the young man is of itself good work, but the important lesson is the relation of Psor to the knees and probably the right, which was speedy, and the aggravation from letting the limb hang down.

TUBERCULAR GLANDS
TUBERCULAR GLANDS OF THE NECK

Mrs. J. S., 28 years of age.

April 24, 1905. Tubercular glands of the neck—some have suppurated. A surgeon said she must have an operation, immediately. Not sensitive to cold. Thirst for cold water. Has always worked actively. Tuberc. 10m.

May 9. No new symptoms. Breath fetid odor. Sensitive to cold. Feet "cold as ice" in cold weather. Gland under the chin gives sensation of softening in the centre. Tuberc. 10m.

June 1. Improvement is very marked. Sach. lac.

June 30. Feels very good, though glands on neck not entirely absent. Tuberc. 10m.

Aug. 8, Sept. 20 and Dec. 20. Tuberc. 50m.

May 15, 1906. Pregnancy developed in July. Improvement continued throughout. Has had no medicine since Dec. Glands enlarging again. Headache. Teeth ache at night. Perspiration and chilliness. Tuber. cm.

June 13. Some evidence of improvement; glands not so large, yet four or five are quite prominent. Has been feeding the baby at the breast, having plenty of milk. Head improved; no perspiration at night. Sensitive to cold. Thirst for cold water. Rectal evacuations not every day. Generally amel. in motion. Tuberc. cm.

Oct. 20. Tuberc. mm.

Dec. 17. Lumps becoming smaller.

Feb. 2, 1907. Tuberc. mm.

March 12. Lumps increased in size, from cold, two weeks ago. Sore sensation when turning neck. Tuberc. 10m.

April 11. Sore lumps in neck. Feet swelling. Head-ache constantly. Appetite poor. Tuberc. 10m.

April 15. Feet and ankles painful swelling. > when feet elevated. Red spots where swollen. Rheumatic condition. Emaciating. Weak; walking difficult. Cold at night. Perspiration as soon as sleeps, continues until midnight. Back and front of thorax. Cough at night. Sleepy. L. flank pain. Headache constant. Hands cold. > when quiet and can recline. Appetite poor; no thirst. Never fond of meat. Fond of milk and eggs. Calc. c. 10m.

May 15. All symptoms of last report have disappeared. Sach. lac.

June 13. Feet pain, aching. Gaining flesh; feels very well and strong; not coughing; appetite good; hands not so cold. Calc. c. 10m. Sach. lac. each night. Glands in neck tubercular.

July 20. Tubercle in neck improved. All symptoms improved. Tuberc. 50m. four powders to be followed by Sach. lac., one each night.

Oct. 4. Glands, one on each side of neck, open and close; red. Feels very well. Feet cold at night and all winter. Stomach and appetite good. Tuberc. 50m.

Jan. 23, 1908. Feels well; some old lumps in neck; face, good appearance; gaining flesh. Tuberc. 50m.

Later report says she is in good health with no lumps in the neck.

Mrs. C. W., aged forty-three, reported that her mother and one brother died of consumption,

TUBERCULAR GLANDS IN LEFT SIDE OF NECK

Dec. 30, 1907. Tubercular glands in left side of neck. These had been examined by allopaths and condemned to operative treatment. Very sensitive to warm room; must have fresh air at night. Feels well indoors or outside. Appetite good; bowels normal. Active, attends to her own housework. Feet cold; hands cold easily. Appearance of face, sickly; dull red color. Tuberc. 10m.

Jan. 27, 1908. Had a cold she called Grippe, two weeks ago, cured with Ars. 10m. Tuberc. 10m. Repeated also Feb. 24.

Apr. 6. Gland in left side neck began to be sore about three days ago. Remedy acted over forty days. Tuberc 50m.

Apr. 21. Swelling of lump continued a week, with some suppuration; two days ago began to dry up and now presents better appearance than it has at any time. Sach. lac.

July 7. Swollen gland became normal in few days, and in a month the lumps were so small they could scarcely be felt.

May 5 and June 4. Tuberculinum 50m was repeated. Had been having company and was very tired. Abscess at root of tooth, now. Glands swollen. Tuberc. cm.

Aug. 6. Instep—aching pain before menses, was reported two weeks after last report and has continued troublesome during and after walking. Tuberc, cm.

Aug. 31. Instep—aching continued in both feet so that she walked on the sides of the feet, when reported ten days ago. Has cold effects, now; Neck—a very sore spot, a lump too sore to be touched, slightly under the chin. Tuberc. cm. 4 powders; 1 each night and morning; Sach. lac. powders to follow, taken the same way.

Oct. 6. Swelling and suppuration of the old spot. So tired, constantly. Tuberc. mm.

Oct. 20. Feeling fine. Aching in insteps and soles returned.

Improvement continued throughout the year; the lumps disappeared from the neck and the pains disappeared from the feet. A cough in November was cured by Bry. 10m., and later the same month Tuberc. mm. was repeated.

In May and June, the system was weakened by overexertion which to some extent interfered with the action of the remedy. Hence it was repeated at closer intervals than would have been done, had the course of its action had no interruption.

In August, when the remedy was to be given in the cm. potency for the third time four doses were administered in succession at twelve-hour intervals, to push the action of the remedy.

The progress of the case throughout is delightful, even to read. Without operation, the glands of tubercular nature disappeared from the neck and gouty pains appeared in the extremities. As these disappeared, the patient was cured of tuberculosis and of gouty tendencies simultaneously, and became a robust, hearty, stout, strong woman.

TUBERCULAR GLANDS OF RIGHT SIDE OF NECK

Mrs. N. D. J., thirty-four years old.

Apr. 25, 1191. Tubercular glands of right side of neck. These were cut out. Rigg's Disease. Bilious disorders—subject to vomiting of bile. Hands and feet cold. Apprehensive; disposed to worry; weeps easily. Prefers cold to heat. Better in motion than in rest. Tuberc. 10m.

May 9. Another lump discovered. Craves coffee. Worse in damp cloudy weather. Sach. lactis.

May 22. Tuberc. 10m.

July 5. Stronger and generally much improved.
Tuberc. 50m.

Sept. 13. Feels perfectly well; glandular swelling disappeared completely.

For a better appreciation of these records, the reader should study the provings of, and the indications for the remedies prescribed. (See "Tuberculinum" in March Homœopathician, "Calcarea carb.," in Kent's Materia Medica, and other presentations of these remedies, elsewhere.)

Patients with such glandular disorders present themselves to the physician with few or no other complaints. They seek a removal of these, and having slight suffering elsewhere, at times offer no characteristics such as the prescriber seeks as a basis for remedy selection. Then the remedy most similar in its effects to the nature of the disorder must be used.

In the first case of this series, improvement occurred for a year, under the influence of the same remedy· repeated at intervals as return of symptoms demanded. In this time pregnancy, parturition, and lactation aroused no increased disturbance, but the improvement continued throughout. This should encourage others to expect benefit from treatment even when serious conditions are present.

The change from progress to decline, after the first year of treatment would appear alarming except that the prescriber learns to welcome any symptoms that develop as a guide for treatment, the symptoms forming the image of the remedy which the patient requires. Developing symptoms indicate the power of the system to express the internal disorder; reaction of the patient to the remedy thus demanded measures the ability to recover. In this instance the reaction was all that could be desired after the administration of Calc. carb.

When its influence appeared to cease, localization of the disorder in the glands occurred, with more activity there. Then again the remedy most similar in action to the process of local degeneration—no other characteristics of the patient being present—continued the work of restoration.

The records of these cases are but outlines for the study of the doctrines, but for the ambitious student who wishes to master the application of the doctrines, they form a sufficient text.

VOMITING BLOOD IN DROPSY.

Case II.—Mrs. F., æt 84, at *the Memorial Home*. Some months before I assumed control of the Home this old lady had an attack of vomiting blood. The matron declared there was over a gallon; the physician then in charge said he never saw so large a quantity of blood vomited, and expressed his opinion that it was from the lung as he did not see the act of vomiting, disputing the matron who saw the vomiting. The treatment was directed to prevent another hemorrhage from the lungs—large doses of astringents. The old lady continued to decline, and when the attendant acknowledged his impotence in the case, and the friends of the old lady outside the Home made complaint, I was requested to assume the duties of medical attendant of the Home, and this case with others came under charge. The matron explained the situation and I immediately suspected that the hemorrhage came from an ulcer in the stomach. The dropsical condition prevented a satisfactory examination, but the subjective history confirmed the diagnosis.

But the important thing is the dropsy. Her limbs were enormously swollen and her abdomen no less so, and her stomach could not tolerate nothing but a little milk. The dropsy having a hemorrhage for its cause guided me to the selection of China, which was repeated at proper intervals in 77m; while she was going down rapidly she began immediately to improve. No other medicine has been given and she is as well as anybody in the Home. As she had been so near the *angels* she has the liberty of the house and is a general pet; running three long stairs, visiting all the rooms and chatting and joking everybody. Old people recover when given the right remedy in suitable potency in a surprising manner. Some years ago I supposed that when an old person became dropsical his or her time had come. At present, I do not declare an unfavorable prognosis because of old age, but when the disease causing the dropsy. is one hard to manage regardless of age.

PART IV.

APHORISMS AND PRECEPTS

FROM

EXTEMPORANEOUS
LECTURES

It is no proof of man's undertaking to be able to confirm what he pleases; but to be able to discern that what is true is true, and what is false is false, this is the mark and charcter of intelligence.

— EMANUEL SWEDENBORG

KENT'S APHORISMS AND PRECEPTS

Truth, on every plane, is a sword, that wounds deeply; and blood flows freely.

The more idols a man has the less able is he to receive truth. He is sick.

You cannot divorce Medicine and Theology. Man exists all the way down, from his innermost Spiritual, to his outermost Natural.

A truth, on any plane, presented to different men, is accepted or rejected by each according to the good or evil of his mind.

The external man is but an outward expression of the internal; so the results of disease (symptoms) are but the outward expression of the internal sickness.

Everything is harmoniously working in the well man. Consider the man, heal the sick.

Hahnemann's was an unusual life. He was as circumspect as a woman, and that is saying a great deal. He had a duty to perform, and could do it. Clean, honorable, noble; a man of integrity to himself and his family.

The person who loves crime lives in it. It becomes a part of his nature and shows itself in the external man. The man who loves truth and humanity, lives in that idea, and it becomes a part of his nature, and can be seen in his looks and his life.

An immense amount of hardness of heart and lack of charity is engendered by trying to accumulate a large number of "Grand Operations" without asking, "Is this for the good of the patient?"

41

If you lose the attitude of mind which seeks the good of the patient you will lose your Homœopathy.

If Homœopathy does not cure sick people you are to despise it.

Those who say they have tested Homœopathy and it is a failure have only exposed their own ignorance.

So long as a man relies upon the senses to settle what is scientific and what is not, and does not use his understanding, so long will he be in confusion, and Sciences will oppose each other.

The Old School must know Pathology before they can treat disease, and they must have a *post mortem* before they can know pathology.

So long as man is capable of believing that Diabetes is disease, and that Bright's Disease is a disease, so long will man be insane in Medicine. His mind is only directed toward the results of disease.

It is not Homœopathic to say "Can you cure a cancer?" or "Can you cure Epilepsy?"

Technicalities are condemned in Homœopathy. Only frame in your mind that you have seen a species of Scarlet Fever, a species of Measles, or a species of Tuberculosis, or Diabetes, and speak of them as such; that the speech may be a true outward representation of the internal thought.

A physician's attitude in performing his duty to the sick, is different from that of any other person. He has a different sphere from that of the ordinary man. This is a thousand times amplified in Homœopathy. One who has entertained that peculiar "circumcision of the heart," always looking to the good of his patient, never thinking of the criticism of man, acquires an ability to say what is right to do. He establishes a garment of righteousness.

There is a state of insanity in the Sciences of the present day. They put all laws aside, in order to accept, for instance, the Molecular theory, because they want something that in its aggregate will be large enough to be felt with the fingers.

If there were no Idiosyncrasy there would be no Homœopathy. Every individual is susceptible to certain things; is susceptible to sickness, and equally susceptible to cure.

Cure rests in the degree of susceptibiliness.

Remedies operate as by contagion. He caught the disease, and catches the cure.

Dynamic wrongs are corrected from the interior by dynamic agencies.

Principle teaches you to avoid suppression. A Homœopath cannot temporize. Those sufferings are necessary sometimes to show forth sickness in order that a remedy may be found.

The affections make the man.

You must see and feel the internal nature of your patient as the artist sees and feels the picture he is painting. He feels it. Study to feel the economy, the life, the soul.

You cannot depend on lucky shots and guess work, everything depends on long study of each individual case.

This opens a field of tedious labor, and many failures,

but if once in awhile you succeed in curing one of these lost ones it is well.

Memorizers have no perception; they can only remember what they see, and they see only the surface.

Memory is not knowledge until it is comprehended and used; then grows the ability to perceive.

Understand the remedy first, the keynotes last.

Every ignorant man thinks that what he knows is the end of knowledge.

The physician who violates his conscience, destroys his ability to perceive.

What appears to be intuition comes from using that which is in the understanding.

It is the imperfect machine that causes death. The Vital Force is of the Soul, and cannot be destroyed or weakened. It can be disordered, but it is all there.

Man cannot be made sick or be cured except by some substance as etherial in quality as the Vital Force.

It is unthinkable to speak of Motion or Force without a simple, primitive substance. Force, or action of a nothing is unthinkable.

It is a serious matter to allow the mind to drift into thinking of anything but quality when speaking of force.

There is nothing in the world which does not exist by something prior to itself. With the grossest materialistic ideas man can demonstrate this.

There is at the present time, a continual discussion of

Force as an energy having nothing prior to it. This is confusion.

There is an Innermost to everything that is, or else the outermost could not be.

The Simple Substance is the substance of substances, and all things are from it. It is really first, in which rests all power.

Weight cannot be predicated of the Simple Substance, neither time, nor space.

No power known to man exists in the concrete substance, but all power exists in the Primitive Substance.

The Primitive Substance, or Radiant form of matter, is just as much matter as matter in its aggregate form.

The real holding together of the things in this world is by Simple Substance.

Every individual with whom you converse, has his own ideas and theories. When he questions you about Homœopathy, you hesitate because he has not the beginnings.

When he questions you about Homœopathic facts, if you tell him what your opinion about it is he will listen to you; but when you say it *is* so and so, he looks at you in wonder and doubt.

Your enemy on the ground of *common sense* can say so much more than you can that many individuals can be reasoned away from you.

Anything which looks away from exactitude is unscientific. The physician must be classical; everything must be methodical. Science ceases to be scientific when disorderly application of law is made.

Eternal Principles, themselves, are authority. The Law of Similars is a Divine Law. So soon as you have accepted the Law of Similars, so soon have you accepted Providence, which is law and order.

If you do not use your Homœopathy you will lose it. This is a responsibility so great that where one has gone into the Truth and does not make use of his knowledge, he will become like Egypt of old.

The sick are entitled to exact knowledge, not to guess work.

Leave names out when prescribing. They are only for the foolish and for the boards of health.

The disease is not to be named but to be perceived; not to be classified but to be viewed, that the very nature of it may be discovered.

Throw aside all theories, and matters of belief and opinion, and dwell in simple fact.

The human mind should not be burdened with technicalities. They destroy description, and close the understanding.

You must be able to recognize every ambassador of the internal man.

A profane man can have no more idea of the sentiments of a gentle, highly religious woman, than can a lobster.

The physician must see and feel, as the artist does his picture. He must perceive, by his knowledge of the human heart, that good woman's state whose religious melancholy he could not otherwise understand.

Every scientific man to-day is trying to find something he can claim as his own. Such a man cannot understand Homœopathy. He worships himself. Has dwelt on the externals so long that it is impossible for him to think rationally.

Whenever a man settles all things by his eyes, and fingers, pseudo-science and theories, he reasons from lasts to firsts; in other words, from himself, and is insane.

Man's unbelief and opinion do not effect truth. The experience which the Homœopath has, is experience under law and confirms the law and by this order is maintained.

What matters it what people think of a just man? His reputation will take care of itself.

A man, whose services are worth having, can starve in the gutter, in order that he may do good, for the love of his neighbor; and he will acquire this power, this perception. Such a physician may realize what it is to have a duty to perform.

Materia Medica never inspires perception. The physician must have the love of its use, and he becomes wise in proportion as he loves his use, and in proportion as he lives uprightly with his patients; that is, desires to heal them; beautify their souls. Can the physician, who does not love his neighbor as himself, get into this position?

One can never look from the toxic, to see what is in harmony with the dynamic, but may look from the dynamic to see what is in harmony with the toxic.

Toxicology shows the ability, or the extent of the effects of a drug.

All human beings have like possibilities of degredation; so we cannot look down on any member of the human

648 APHORISMS AND PRECEPTS

race. We sometimes find the lowest, characteristics that are the noblest.

You cannot meditate on even the extreme of the human race. It becomes your solemn duty to heal the good, bad, and indifferent.

Does any one know what Chemical Affinity is, except that certain substances seek to take a liking to each other?

If it were not for the Simple Substance, such states as antipathy, sympathy, or affinity, could not be. It is the sphere of Homœopathy to deal with these things; to glean what is the real *Esse* and existence.

There are two worlds; the world of thought, or immaterial substance, and the world of matter or material substance.

What reason has man to say that Energy or Force is first? Energy is not energy *per se*, but a powerful substance. The very *Esse* of God is a scientific study.

Bodies are not drawn together by means of their bodies, but by means of their Primitive Substance.

The Simple Substance is the means of identification in nature. The mineral, the oak, the wheat, are all identified by their Primitive Substance, and exist, only, because of their Primitive Substance, which makes them what they are.

Name everything that is, or moves; it is sustained from, and by power of this Primitive Substance. We do not argue that it is first power, but this is first substance.

Susceptibility is only a name for a state that underlies all possible sickness and all possible cure.

Now when a person becomes sick, he becomes susceptible to a certain remedy, which will affect him in its highest potency; while upon a healthy person it will have no effect.

When the dose is too large to cure, man receives it as a sickness.

Susceptibility exists in the Vital Force, and not in the tissues.

Measles and Smallpox are not on the outside. Man is protected on the outside, and is attacked from the inside when there is susceptibility.

There are degrees in susceptibility. The Old School calls a certain kind of susceptibility "Idiosyncrasy," though they have failed to find out what this is.

Think how susceptible a man is to sickness, when the Rhus vine will poison him when he is on the windward side, half a mile away.

An individual may be susceptible to nothing else; gross, coarse, vigorous in constitution; yet there is one thing he is susceptible to, and that is what he needs.

The signs are visible, but the *Esse* is invisible.

The tendency of the human mind to run after things visible, that can be felt with the fingers, leads one to adopt foolish theories like the Bacteria doctrine and the Molecular theory.

A physician above all men if not innocent should be anything else but a doctor. A bad man has only coarse, vicious ideas of the human heart.

When a man thinks from the microscope, and his neighbor's opinion, he thinks falsely. Nothing good can come from this. Evil must take place, and changes, which are the ultimates of his internal thought, will take place in the body.

The time may come when Homœopathy of the purer kind will be popular, but it is a very long time ahead.

Some have been confused by primary and secondary effects of medicine. You need not worry over this. You only need to know that certain symptoms follow each other. Primary and secondary action reverse themselves in different individuals.

The sharper the edge of the tool you fool with the more harm you can do; so it is with high potencies in unskilled hands.

A remedy is not known simply because it has been used upon the sick. That is a confirmation only, and gives more ripened knowledge.

The rational mind can go far beyond the idea of a molecule.

The Homœopathic physician who thinks in quantities only, has such a crude mind that he cannot realize true Homœopathy.

The old Philosophers were engaged in constant controversy, here converging, there diverging. If they had only known something of Simple Substance, as does the Homœopath, they would have had confirmation.

In chemistry one color obliterates another. This is an illustration of the outermost changes. The causes of such change lie in the primitive substance and not in the external form; so it is with the causes of cure.

Homœopaths have a consciousness of what life is, what the life force is, what the nature of disease is, and can apply to all theories of the world our measure and test them. They can realize the philosophies.

There is nothing in the outer world but what is representative.

The song that is within the heart is a million times more intense, more beautiful, than can be produced by the larynx. Everything that is, or appears as real before the eyes, or to the ear in sound, is only representation of the real world; because everything of this character is perishable.

All Art has its Internal and External. If music is in the soul it will give the outward reflected image of the delight which is song.

The world to-day accepts things perfectly incongruous and calls them science. Modern science accepts nothing which cannot be heard, felt, or seen.

Take a body of scientific men: after a lengthy discussion the conclusion is, that "we have concluded so and so," by the majority, after a general average is taken, and the conclusion is Science.

The microscopist has failed to show that there is no Vital Force, no Simple Substance, no Dynamis in drugs seen, and how can we expect him to foretell when the substance cannot be seen?

The different Philosophies do not agree about the Simple Substance, upon which they all touch in theory. They have no confirmation which could be had in the Homœopathic potencies, and in their action upon the sick.

The personal stamp is upon every disease and upon every proving, and the individual must be permitted to stamp himself upon the disease as well as upon the proving.

There are no two things alike in the universe. This is so of diseases and of sick people, of thousands of crystals of the same salt. No two stars are alike. When this thought presents itself to the mind of the physician, he can see that no remedy can be substituted for another.

A disease may be suppressed by a medicine as well as by a stronger dissimilar disease.

In Epilepsy, so long as Bromides suppress, nature is paying more attention to the disease of Bromides than to the disease of Epilepsy.

Epilepsy is not a disease; you cannot prescribe for Epilepsy. The symptoms which represent the nature of the sickness are not in the fit, but those which the patient has had in infancy up to the time of the fit.

The Homœopathic remedy only becomes Homoeopathic when it has established its curative relation; the relation between two dynamic influences.

Homœopathicity is the relation between the symptoms of the patient and the remedy which will cure.

Homœopathy is an applied science not a theory.

It is an injustice to Science to practice without exact knowledge and reasons for what you do. The whole world is but a swirl of this round-about inheritance instead of knowledge.

If we could accept opinion we should have to go back to Allopathy, because we find there only a record of man's experiments; a mass of heterogeneous opinions.

Experience teaches the Allopath to give Muriatic acid in Germany for Typhoid Fever, Nitric acid in England, cold bathing in Paris for the same. This is the doctrine of the Old School by "experience."

It is an injustice to one's self to remain in bigotry, intolerence and hatred.

When you have discovered that this Life Force resides in a simple substance you see at once that death is not an entity. The body has no life of its own and therefore it cannot die.

Therefore there is no death, but we do observe and perceive that there is a separation, of one that is alive from another that never was alive; a disjunction of that which lives from that which never lived.

That changes in the body correspond to wrong thinking is true. The fault of the world to-day, is reasoning from externals. Man elected in the early part of his history to think from lasts to firsts, and thereby lost his ability to know.

One sick man is to be treated, not the disease.

Man must be studied as he is, as he was, everything of man and of the human race in general in order to understand disease.

In proportion as man thinks against everything, his country, his God, his neighbor, he wills in favor of himself. Therefore this forms man into the nature of his affections.

Thus man wills against everything but himself. In proportion as he does this he becomes a form of hatred, or a form of self love; he is that. Allow this to proceed and ultimates are inevitable.

Thus man is what he wills. As his love is, so is his

life. When man thinks about the neighbor, he wills one of two things—he wills good to his neighbor or the opposite.

Psora is the evolution of the state of man's will, the ultimate of his sin.

This outgrowth, which has come upon man from living a life of evil willing, is Psora—is the life of Psora.

Now in proportion as a man falsifies truth or mixes or perverts truth; in proportion as he mixes willing well with willing evil, so does he adulterate his interiors until that state is present.

When Psora had become a *complete* ultimation of causes, it became contagious.

Everything that is a thing, has its aura or atmosphere. So as a race or class, the entire human race has its atmosphere or aura also. Each individual has his aura, or atmosphere.

This aura becomes intensified with the growth of evil in the interior of man.

Thinking, willing, and doing, are the three things in life from which finally proceed the chronic miasms.

The whole Miasm in a chronic disease, does not come out in an individual, but in the human race.

The human race exists as a changed *Esse*.

The Homœopathic principles, when known, are plain, simple and easily comprehended. They are in harmony with all things known to be true.

It is not a matter of theory, or belief, or opinion; we must have something more substantial. Homœopathy must rest upon facts.

When a microscopist can examine a grain of wheat, and tell whether it will grow if planted in favorable soil, he may be of use to Homœopathy. When he can examine a smallpox crust and tell whether it is still contagious, or whether its power has been destroyed by heat, then he may be of use. When he can examine the Aconite root and tell how it will affect man, we can do away with provings, but we have to enter by a different door.

One cannot afford to be liberal with principle.

When you make failures you may be sure that they are within yourself. If you think the failure is in Homœopathy you will begin your corrections on the wrong side of the ledger.

All quick prescribing depends upon the ability to grasp comparatively the symptoms.

If you do not know sickness you are apt to think all things strange and unique.

Sharp prescribing is attended with immediate results. If you do sharp work you will see frequent aggravations of the remedy. When you do poor work you never see them.

True pathology is entirely unknown to the medical profession outside of Homœopathy. It is morbid anatomy alone that is known.

If you love Homœopathy it will love you; such is natural charity.

One who is vicious in his real life, may preserve a placid exterior for a time, but will be shunned by good people ere long.

We owe no obedience to man, not even to our parents,

after we are old enough to think for ourselves. We owe obedience only to Truth.

When old symptoms return, there is hope. That is the road to cure and there is none other.

The physician spoils his case when he prescribes for the local symptoms and neglects the patient.

It is an entirely different business to comfort from what it is to cure.

What is man? Is he a body? If so we are justified in thinking of his parts, his liver, and lungs and skin, and extremities, and his body as a whole. But we are to consider man as from the life to the body.

Man is made up of what he is. The very *is*, or being, or *Esse* of man is his will. The difference between two human beings would scarcely be more than the will.

The will is expressed in the face; hence the difference of countenance of people. Has the murderer and evid-doer a placid face.

What a man wills to do is his life and character.

Proceeding from the will is man's understanding. If the will is good to obey the commandments, he selects his very education in accordance with it.

Memory is the gateway to man. The outermost envelope of this *Esse* is formed to be a receptacle for the will, the understanding, and the memory.

The upright man whose desires are good, wants the truth. His perceptions are intensified.

A prejudiced mind, decides without wisdom the way he wants to have it.

Every man has his affections, his pet theory to subdue.

These things enter into the symptomatology. **Hence** know the human heart.

Man, to-day, is destroyed as to his interiors· so that truth looks as black as smoke, and false philosophy as bright as the sun.

The outer world is the world of results. The inner world not discoverable by the senses, but by the understanding.

When we conceive that innumerable causes may give rise to the same pathological conditions we see that the pathological condition in itself, cannot furnish us with the slightest idea of the remedy.

Under Homœopathic treatment progress of chronic disease the highest degree of susceptibility must be present. until a cure sometimes becomes possible.

When you look at morbid anatomy from the symptomatology you are looking at it from the interior. Morbid anatomy must not be studied as a basis for prescription making.

Irregular action expressed in signs and symptoms is the disease. The disturbance in the Vital Substance has no other means by which it can make itself known to the intelligent physician. This is in accordance with law. This leaves morbid anatomy out of the question.

You need not expect great things when you have only pathological symptoms.

When pathological changes have gone on extensively the symptoms withdraw, seemingly discouraged that there

42

is no physician. So soon as a patient falls into the hands of a real physician the symptoms become orderly.

Unit of action in health, unit of action in sickness, unit of action in cure, all are one.

The Old School materia medica is known only to the Homœopath. To the Allopath it is really unknown.

It would seem as if the Old School would have asked long ago "What are the effects of drugs upon healthy people?" Their experiments on animals do not answer this.

"This remedy has proved useful in such and such conditions·" they say. Homœopaths know that such medicine has produced such and such effects on provers·

Man is more susceptible to drugs than to a disease, because their action may be forced upon the economy. In disease the highest degree of susceptibility must be presnt.

One who is not acute in observation, goes through life, seeing only indifferent similarity. Most men only know the toxic power of a drug.

Man is susceptible to all things capable of producing similar symptoms to those which he already has.

The record of symptoms derived from cases of poisoning, is the poorest kind of evidence for the Homœopathic materia medica. They are useful only as collateral evidence.

Individualization is blocked by this inability to distinguish between the finer featurs of sickness, and of medicines.

With the true physician, discrimination is not with the eye alone; the consciousness of discrimination seems to occupy his entire economy.

No two remedies are absolutely equal in their similitude.

The whole aim of Homœopathy is to cure.

He who sees not in Bright's Disease the deep miasm back of it, sees not the whole disease, but only the finishing of a long course of symptoms which have been developing for years.

The law of sickness, is the law of sickness, whether produced by drug or disease. It is the law of influx.

It is inconsistent and irrational to think that there are several active diseases in the body at the same time.

Take the simplest form of substance known to have life. If we subject it to physical and chemical forces it is killed; it no longer moves, feeds, propagates, or can be killed. There is then, something that can be withdrawn by physical force. Can we not perceive that 'tis a something added to these forces that makes it alive? It is not merely a motion of this substance, for move as you will, it is dead. Something is withdrawn, which can only come within the perception of the understanding.

These simple substances are the primitive powers of the earth. Gravitation must be something or we could not predicate anything of it.

Only quality can be predicated of the Simple Substance.

What things can we predicate of the Simple Substance? It cannot be found by Chemistry, nor seen with the eye, nor felt with the fingers. It must have a medium of operation, in order that it may become manifest to the sensorium.

For example, Electricity and the machine. Electricity is a simple substance, and needs the conductor to make it manifest. Until Electricity was discovered through a medium, it was unknown.

Cohesion is a primitive substance, and will obey all the laws that govern primitive substance; so also is the Vital Force.

Light also is a simple substance and will obey all the laws laid down for Vital Force.

This Primitive Substance abides in everything that grows, or has individuality or identity. It is the Vicegerent of the Soul.

If the Primitive Substance is normal, that which it creates is normal. Disease, which flows into the body, comes from within by influx through this Primitive Substance.

All motion, harmony and order, are due to Simple Substance. It not only operates all things, but is the cause of operation of all substances that are material. The very sounds of the forest have harmony and co-operation.

All matter is capable of reduction to its "radiant or primitive form.

Contagion does not come by quantity but by quality.

The quality of contagion is similar in its nature to the cure.

The symptoms, themselves, point to the thing which the individual is sensitive to, and every one is susceptible in just this way to the remedy that will cure. That which he most wants, is that which Nature has provided him with the means of reaching out after by the symptoms.

A patient may be poisoned by a crude drug, when the substance potentized would have cured him. The individual comes in contact with too much of something he is sensitive to· and gets sick.

If a man were in perfect health he would not be susceptible.

The same susceptibility is necessary to prove a drug, as to take a disease. That is the Homœopathic relation. Hence we see what contagion is.

We now see that we have something substantial; that something is disturbed by something as invisible and substantial, as itself. These two, coming together, disturb each other under fixed laws relating to Primitive Substance.

That which we call disease, is but a change in the Vital Force expressed by the totality of the symptoms·

Never amuse the patient with things that will injure him.

All prescriptions that change the image of a case cause suppression.

It is just as dangerous to suppress symptoms by drugs, as it is to remove them with the knife.

It is better to do nothing at all than to do something useless; it is better to watch and wait than to do wrong.

The idea that you must relieve a patient of his chills at all hazards, that you must give him Quinine, and Arsenic afterwards, if that does not work, is all wrong. You will be tempted to do these things, unless you have grown up within yourself a new conscience, and realize that it is criminal.

Diseases, themselves, cannot be suppressed, but symptoms can. The totality of the symptoms must disappear in an orderly manner in order to constitute a cure.

All physicians recognize that suppressing an acute rash is dangerous, but all are not far-sighted enough to see that such is the case with chronic eruptions, excepting that the resulting symptoms come more slowly.

The value of the service is nothing, your use is first, and so long as you have this in mind, you will grow.

Man must continue in his uses in order to continue to understand.

The physician who ceases to study a case before he sees what the patient needs, is neglecting that case. He falls into a habit and it becomes second nature to prescribe without reflection.

You see Homœopathy in a superficial way only when you see the similarity of the symptoms to the remedy, the mere outward manifestation. You must see that the interiors are related to each other.

When the materia medica is fully learned you see at a glance the image of the remedy. It looms up before you. You know it as a physician of experience knows measles or scarlet fever.

Only a few drugs will be similar enough to cure, and there will be only *one* similimum.

We cannot educate a patient until after he is cured. We have to let him think about it in his own way. But steal in and cure him. Do him good. This is the all important thing.

A memorizer applies the exact sentence of the proving to the exact sentence of the patient and Homœopathy never becomes alive in him.

Man must keep on plodding as long as he lives. He

must be patient and toil on; candid, kind, and gentle as a lamb, ready and willing.

Perception comes with use.

There is plenty of room for lazy doctors the other side of the gulf of knowledge. They can render a night's sleep and open the bowels.

The quiet, silent manner of perception is to be cultivated.

The physician must be sober, candid and able to receive.

The more ignorant the physician the more he will do.

Most doctors have gone crazy over the "vicious microbe" as being the cause of disease, and think the little fellows are exceedingly dangerous.

As a matter of fact, the microbes are scavengers. I wonder if scientists reflect when they make statements about bacteria. Naturally they would say that the more bacteria the more danger, but this is not so. It is well known that shortly after death a prick from a scalpel is a serious matter. This is due to ptomaines of the corpse; but when the cadaver has become green and filled with bacteria it is comparatively harmless.

The microbe is not the cause of disease. We should not be carried away by these idle Allopathic dreams and vain imaginations but should correct the Vital Force.

Save the life of the patient first and don't worry about the bacteria. They are useless things.

The Bacterium is an innocent feller, and if he carries disease he carries the Simple Substance which causes disease, just as an elephant would.

It would seem that with only the occasional cures from Bromine, and Secale, and Hellebore, that the Old School might have long since discovered the Law. But their books say "No Law." All their books say "No Principle, only Experience." Therefore their students are debarred from looking for law or expecting law.

It is easy enough to find something different, but one may look a long time to find a similar. It is more natural to suppose that the curative remedy would be found in the similar which is so rare and requires so much labor to find.

That man may enter and look from within upon all things in the physical world is possible. He can then account for laws and perceive the operation of laws.

The record of symptoms on the healthy human family then, is the first thing to be known. We store up our Materia Medica in this way. On the other hand the Old School physician stores up his diagnosis of diseases. It is out of comparing these great storehouses with each other that we may ascertain whether there is such a thing as law.

It is a law that if man does not think from firsts to lasts, he becomes disposed to sickness by doing evil through thinking wrong. This state precedes susceptibility.

Susceptibility is prior to all contagion. If an individual is not susceptible to Smallpox he cannot take it, and will not receive it though he goes near the worse cases, or eats a smallpox crust.

A piano tuner has restored harmony to a piano; has added nothing and taken nothing from it, yet has restored it to harmony. A change that is unknown to one who does not think is visible to the internal eye.

If man has no chronic miasm he would not have acute disease. It is because he is susceptible to these outside influences.

All diseases exist in a Simple Substance, which can penetrate when resistance is lost. This lack of resistance constitutes susceptibility.

When an individual is made sick by the crude substance, and even by the lower forms of Simple Substance, as in Rhus poisoning, it shows that he needs that substance on some plane. The dose has been yet too large to cure.

Much belongs to man and the outer world which the microscope has not yet revealed.

The Outermost has all within in to the Infinite in degree.

This Primitive Substance abides in everything that forms, grows, feeds, or has individuality, or identity. It is that which ultimates an exterior form suitable to its own existence. That causes the Aconite plant to be Aconite, and nothing else to the end of the world.

Simple Substance is continuously endowed with intelligence from first to last, mineral, plant, and animal kingdom.

Radiate substances have degrees within degrees, in series too numerous for the finite mind to grasp.

Arsenic, for example, is capable of identification from its Outermost to its Innermost. In the external form the degrees are limited. When it has passed to simple substance, the Radiant form of matter, it has infinite degrees.

To express the degrees from the Outermost to the Innermost, we might say a grain of Silica is the Outermost; the Innermost is the Creator.

It is from this primitive Substance that man is created his intellect made, his body formed. It is subject to all the laws of influx.

How describe a condition of affinity? When you see the attracting correspondence between spheres by which they are drawn together, you wonder. What a world it is in which we don't live or only partly live!

Every body has its atmosphere, just as the earth has its atmosphere. It is not the Smallpox crust that is so dangerous, it is the Aura which emanates from it.

Aura is a means by which warning is given between spheres; between plants and objects, between animals and persons. Objects are related to each other and give out. We find affinity and repulsion by this aura.

The aura of crude substances increases in intensity and breadth by the elimination from the lower to the higher. This is the order of things in relation to auras, that is, Simple Substance.

If you have an idea of the nature of sickness, you will know about the action of remedies.

Everywhere this Simple Substance is a bond of order. The Vital Force, like Electricity, is a bond of order. It builds in accordance with its necessities because of that which was prior to it.

Disease comes from within through this Primitive Substance. It is subject to disturbance, and creates a form corresponding to its own sick self.

Antipathic medicine produces opposite effect, singles out the region. It is in this way, in a general sense, with similars, and would, if given in small doses, be Homœopathic.

Bromides in minute potencies are capable of relieving conjestion to the brain in a most wonderful manner, but in using them in doses large enough to force contraction of blood vessels, the Allopath shows that he is only in a shadow of the truth.

Mongrel cures are by this method, and their cures are not permanent. It is antipathy and suppresses all symptoms that disappear.

The old definition used to say that anything capable of extinguishing the Vital Force was a poison. This cannot be denied to-day, but we may say now, that anything capable of engrafting itself upon the economy so as to produce incurable injury, is a poison. The tincture or third potency of China, if Homœopathically indicated, may establish another disease very quickly in a strong constitution.

The man who thinks it rests in the size of the dose does not know Homœopathy. One who lives in his sensorium thinks that way from without inward. He operates because he has seen others do so.

The physician will never grow stronger and wiser, so long as he thinks there can be a substitute for the remedy.

In regard to alternation, if the remedy is found which is similar to the condition, you do not need two remedies, and if neither are similar of course you do not.

When two remedies antidote each other, it cannot be said that one is more powerful than the other. It is like an alkali neutralizing an acid, the one added last seems more powerful, but this is only in appearance.

Power, then, is due to degrees in similitude. It is true that as it is more similar the remedy is more powerful and *vice versa*. Nature never cures except by similars. Year by year you will gain respect for this similar.

Every accidental cure that has ever occurred is founded on this law.

The Homœopathicity cannot be increased by increasing the dose. If it is right at all, you increase its Homœopathicity by elevating its quality toward its interior nature so that it corresponds more perfectly to the Vital Force.

We do not take disease through our bodies but through the Vital Force.

When a man takes a remedy in too large a dose, *he* feels worse and his symptoms are worse; with a higher potency *he* feels *better*, though his symptoms may be aggravated.

It is all important to see the remedy in its nature as a sick being.

Disease is a proving of the morbific substance. It is not true that there is one law for disease and another for drug effects, but the degree of susceptibility governs.

Whatever man is susceptible to, such he is, such is his quality.

One who thinks from the material, thinks disease is drawn in from without, but it is drawn out from within.

When a child takes Scarlet Fever it doesn't get the dose exactly adapted to it, so it has the disease.

The one who has had Smallpox is no different so far as his character would reveal, or the microscope, yet he has no susceptibility. It has been satisfied in that particular direction.

When we think of susceptibility we think of a state of the Vital Force in which it can be easily made sick by certain other simple substances.

Now, when a person susceptible to Rhus gets a whiff of air from a vine, he at once has the disease fastened upon him, and is not subject to further poisoning though he lie under the tree from which he was poisoned until he recovers.

It is the same with Scarlatina. If he were not fortified against the poison· at the instant he took it then it would continue to affect his system, and poison him more and more until it killed him.

If you think names you will think remedies, you cannot help it.

Any physician with pathological notions in his head, if he find no organic disease, is apt to think his patient is sick only in the imagination.

The prejudiced mind is not content to write down simple facts and symptoms but says "I will examine the organs and parts, and see if congested or inflamed, and then I shall know what to do."

All causes are external which flow from exterior to interior.

Organic changes constitute the same as external causes, because it is the external man. It is like the influence of the atmosphere, or like a splinter in the tissues.

The results of disease never form the image of the nature of the disease, the symptoms alone do this.

We must think what makes the patient sick; not what causes changes in his liver, his kidneys and his other organs.

When the ignorant reason about pathology, they should correct pathology by the patient instead of trying to correct the patient from a pathological standpoint.

There is no cell or tissue so small that it does not keep its soul and life force in it.

Would you think of curing a tumor? If you would you misunderstand this grand philosophy. You may administer a medicine which cures that which is wrong with the patient, and as a result the tumor disappears.

The physician is not called upon to cure the results of disease, but the disease itself. All pathological changes must be regarded as the results of disease since all disease is dynamic.

Homœopathy causes aggravations; it touches the very secret. It relates to the patient. All disease causes exist in this realm.

Note the difference between the aggravation of the disease, and that belonging to the remedy. Large doses really aggravate the disease, high potencies aggravate the symptoms of the disease.

Avoid unnecessary aggravation of symptoms by adjusting the potency to the patient.

The action of the remedy is mild. The medicine does not act violently, but the reaction of the economy in

rowing off the disease may be violent. As soon as order
is restored a tumultuous action may begin.

Crude drugs aggravate the disease, while high potencies aggravate the symptoms of the disease, and do not
engraft upon the economy a drug disease, provided the
remedy is not repeated.

We have in the image of the disease an exact representation of the image of a remedy. Do all things come
by chance? Can man meditate and become an Atheist?
A man who cannot believe in God cannot become a Homœopath.

We cannot even see all the symptoms in disease. We
can see the expression of the face but cannot know what
that represents. There is nothing in the outer man that
does not have its beginning in the inner man.

Don't change the slightest symptom, observe everything. Receive the message undisturbed and get it
on paper, there is no other way for a physician to perform
his function and do his duty.

How dare you meddle with that image? How dare
you meddle with those symptoms? There is an intelligence
at the other end of the wire.

The questions of palliation will annoy you, especially
in early years. You will be pressed upon all sides by
women who wring their hands and by men who hear the
cries of women. But what authority have you to hush the
cries of the patient, if by palliating you do away with the
ability to heal him.

When symptoms are removed by the reaction of the
economy they are more likely to stay away than when

removed by the action of drugs. Crude drugs given on theory only suppress symptoms.

If a remedy whose superficial symptoms agree with the superficial symptoms of a disease, but whose nature is different be given, it will cause a suppression if it acts at all.

An inappropriate prescription may be the stepping-stone to breaking down.

It is the same if the physician prescribes for this and that group of symptoms. Avoid this, for it is not healing the sick.

The more violence you see, and the more necessity for haste, and the more severe and the greater suffering of the patient, the more harm you can do by a false and foolish prescription.

A man who prescribes from a keynote for everything mixes the case up, and has to wait a long time to see the sickness as it really is.

When you give a remedy be sure that the nature of the remedy and the nature of the disease (as well as the symptoms) agree.

Can you not see that it is not another disease simply because this or that organ is affected.

An inflamed liver is not the disease. The liver is not the cause of itself.. It is under the control of the Vital Force, and it is what the Vital Force makes it.

We can never be good Homœopaths if we think of tissue changes as diseases. They are but the results of disease. We must think from within outward.

A cure is not a cure unless it destroys the internal or dynamic cause of disease. A tumor, if removed, does not cure the patient because its cause still continues to exist.

Irregular sensations are the evidence of disease. The Vital Force undisturbed gives natural sensations. Only a sick Simple Substance (Vital Force) can give abnormal sensations.

Power comes in the direction of similitude, not of intensity, and gains power only in proportion as it is similar.

It does not take any enormous quantity to cure people any more than to make them sick.

It is only by sustaining the sharpest kind of work that you will keep up your reputation, and be able to cure sick people.

How is it that bread and meat nourish the human body? We cannot say. How the Homœopathic remedy cures the disease will never be known, but the direction in which life flows into the body and the direction of cure can be known.

If the quality in the medicine is changed into quantity this is not a similar. It is antipathic and becomes dissimilar in its nature. The dose may be too large to cure, yet large enough to produce an effect.

When crude drugs are used for proving on those not susceptible to potentized doses, one or another organ is affected. These are fragmentary provings; are not true provings. They do not give the image of the remedy. Do not touch the man himself, or if you get the whole image it must be from hundreds of such provers.

43

The Soul, which is the most interior of man, cannot be affected by drugs. This can only be affected by man's own will.

When the third potency cures there is something higher in it. No substance permeates the Vital Force when it is coarse enough to be seen.

You cannot demonstrate any vital problem by the microscope.

Drug effects when carried to pathological conditions are too much alike. It is the same with disease.

So far as there is morbid anatomy to account for symptoms, so far is it unimportant as a symptom, for if no other symptoms are present you can find no remedy.

The dynamic plane is more interior or above the nutritive plane; it presides over it and commands it. This is the plane of provings.

The lower potency corresponds to a series of outer degrees, less fine and less interior than the higher.

The word disease really means the signs or symptoms before organic disease has taken place.

If you go at it like a common tinker you may cure acute sickness but, on your life do not tamper with these chronic diseases.

In the infant we see the father's history; in old age the history of youth. This enables us to look into the future to see whether a patient will recover, or die, or be palliated.

Sickness exists on varying planes. Acute diseases occupy an outer plane and do not take so great a hold upon the life. The chronic diseases reach what we may call the innermost potency of man.

The Acarus, then, is the ultimate of an internal condition, and indicates that the conditions are such in the economy as are suitable to ultimate an Acarus.

In acute miasms the whole disease is found in one individual, in chronic miasms this is not so.

How is it that the allopaths can cauterize the chancre and sore throat and send the manifestations of the disease to the internal organs? There is a vital ulcer ten times greater than the external one. Just so sure as ulcers are removed from the throat, will the Vital Force suffer, and the ultimates come in the form of organic changes.

The physician must penetrate the inner recesses of symptomatology. The very life of the patient must be opened. Learn the fears, instincts, desires, and the aversions of the patient. The remedy often crops out through the affections.

If you can get your patient to talking you can find out how he is sick. It requires a good deal of experience to keep a patient talking to the line.

It is not an easy matter to keep your mouth shut and let the patient tell his own story. It has to be acquired.

This flopping about, and not waiting for the remedy to cure is abominable. There are periods of improvement and periods of failure. Let the Life Force go on as long as it can, and repeat only when the original symptoms come back to stay.

We do not have to go into a plane called the other world to find a place where spirits dwell. Spirits are no longer unthinkable.

The consciousness between two substances is that atmosphere by which they know each other; a correspondence of spheres. They are in harmony, or antagonistic.

Every person and animal has an atmosphere.

You may potentize tubercles so high that there is not a shred of a microbe left in the liquid, yet if given to a susceptible person it will produce its own disease because of its Simple Substance.

You must see that the Vital Force may take on, or permit to flow with it, another Simple Substance (disease cause, or remedy that will cure). This occurs when electricity and sound are conveyed at the same time over a wire as in the telephone.

All disease causes are in Simple Substance. We must enter the realm of causes in order to see the nature of disease.

We potentize so as to render the remedy simple enough to be drawn in by influx by the Vital Force.

The direction in which sickness flows is from the within to the without.

Homœopathy exists as law and doctrine, and operates in the world of its causes. If this were not so it could not exist in the world of ultimates.

As soon as the vital powers are turned into confusion there is no order; confusion reigns as in a mob. In Old School treatment the confusion is made worse.

Low potencies can cure acute diseases because acute diseases act upon the outermost degree of the Simple Substance and the body. In chronic disease the trouble is deeper seated, and the degrees are finer, hence the remedy must be reduced to finer or higher degrees so as to be similar to the degrees of chronic disease.

The Vital Force dominates, rules and co-ordinates the human body.

The Simple Substance is again dominated by still another higher substance which is the Soul.

The Clairvoyant has an intensity in her nature she is highly electrical, sensitive to spheres, is annoyed by everything. This is sickness. These things show the nature of susceptibility and sympathy.

It is not enough to say that people have lost equilibrium, this is a technical way of expressing it. Individuals who are too sensitive are sick, repulsed by every one they meet. This is due to a deeper sickness than the one from the exciting cause.

Never look for a cause within the thing itself. It must be prior, or within the organism.

These chronic skin troubles are not local diseases. It is contrary to all science and logic (except in Allopathic medicine) to say that anything that exists is itself a cause of itself, or that it is capable of working changes in itself.

The Vital Force holds all in harmony, keeps everything in order when in health; just as Electricity in its own natural state is a bond of order.

The idea that an organ like the liver which is under the control of the Vital Force and whose action the Vital Force governs is able to set up a disease itself and thereby make the patient sick, is preposterous.

As soon as the Vital Force is sick or deranged it acts upon the liver in a different manner from what it does in health, consequently the liver (its action being governed by the Vital Force) must act in a sick or deranged manner.

As long as the Vital Force is acting harmoniously the organ (being governed by it) cannot act in any way other than a harmonious manner.

Cure is brought about by changing the diseased or sick Vital Force back to its normal (health) condition.

Hahnemann was always in a state of humility, he never attributed anything to himself.

Every sensation has its correspondence to something that is within.

Work must be done from within out, in order to be permanent.

Two sick people are more unlike than two well ones.

It would be difficult for the Old School to define what their system is. "We are regular," they say. When they relieve pain by anodynes, and constipation by laxitives, they do not know that there is a reaction. When the Vital Force is sick it is disorderly and they attempt to imitate this disorder. A perfect imitation would end in Homœopathy.

Here we have on the one hand the action of disease upon the healthy, and there the action of drugs upon the healthy. We find one a duplicate of the other. Is this not peculiar?

Every action in Homœopathy must be based on a positive principle.

Belief has no place in the study of Homœopathy. The inductive method of Hahnemann is the only way.

It requires expert judgment to make few blunders. The less you know about the sphere of sickness the more blunders.

The one who understands best the nature of his remedies will remember most about their peculiarities.

Ten years of practice will be a revelation to you, so that you will understand people and their minds. You will almost know what they are thinking, and will often take in a patient's constitution at first glance.

Now you should never think of Measles or Scarlet Fever as a fixed form of disease which you have sometimes treated thus and so, and expect to treat again in the same way. You must keep your mind from getting into ruts.

Anything that exhausts makes manifestations internal.

Vital Force and Soul are in the cell as well as in the body. The same thing rules the remedy and, stripped of its grossness and placed upon the tongue, it will be taken into the economy instantly. I went a thousand miles once to place a dose of Zincum on the tongue of a paralyzed woman who felt its effects in less than sixty seconds and in six weeks her paralysis left her.

There is not one law for contagion and another one for proving. They are both one.

The remedy pervades the economy silently and completely with its prodromal period; then comes the evolution of the disease which runs its course.

If morbid anatomy has taken the place of symptoms there is not much chance of cure. When organs are destroyed little guiding symptoms seem to pass into the shade and the prehistoric (before the pathological changes) symptoms are forgotten. The guide has disappeared. There is no other way of making it known.

If the Vital Force has not that extra susceptibility that allows a breath of the similar remedy to cure, repeated doses may suppress the symptoms but will not cure; you are getting only the primary action, the curative action is not at work. The reactive energy of the Vital Force is not brought into play.

You know that the infant at the mother's breast becomes as thoroughly medicated as the mother. Do not think, however, that if not indicated in the mother, it will reach the infant. It is not done through a funnel. The mother must be susceptible to it and thus vitalize it.

It is inconsistent to say "I gave a Homœopathic remedy and it did not cure." The administration of Homœopathic remedies is an applied Science.

Simple Substances combine and help each other to flow in the direction of the least resistance as much in things invisible as in things visible.

If we were to undertake to study with the microscope what susceptibility is or what affinity is, we would not succeed.

The microscope, then, only furnishes us a field of results, and, beautiful as they are· the cause is not visible, we see only the results.

There is a plane of nutrition and a plane of dynamis. Common salt is appropriated by the normal individual who receives it on the plane of nutrition, but the sick one who needs it eats it constantly and it does not make him well because he needs it on a higher plane.

Now when man reasoned falsely he created such a change in himself, in his Primitive Substance, that the body became changed, then he became susceptible to outer influences.

The body became corrupt because man's interior will was corrupt.

To-day no eruption is allowed to show its head. Everything is hushed as soon as it gives evidence of being. If this goes on long enough the human race will be swept from the earth.

Confusion comes from losing one's head, prescribing on few indications and giving medicine when no medicine should be given.

The increase of conditions shows increase of sickness; the increase of symptoms often shows diminution of disease.

When Hahnemann speaks of disease it would seem to be limited to disease activities.

It is worse than useless to give a second dose until the effects of the first dose have ceased.

Do not apply externally the indicated remedy. If it does no good there is no use in using it. If it cures it does so by healing up the external disease before the internal one is cured and thereby leaving no opportunity for the internal disease to come out.

Never, under any circumstances, make use of local applications for an internal derangement. It is the highest order of medical profanity!

The most natural thing to do is to remove external

obstruction, but anything that comes from within must be treated from within.

It is a very superficial view to take of Homœopathy to see that the symptoms correspond.

There are general, common, and peculiar symptoms. The general is used in the sense of the general of an army, and the generals command all other symptoms and really control the patient.

The modern provers note down only the common symptoms and the morbid anatomy which the remedy produces· and have left out the generals and peculiar symptoms.

Often you may think a patient has all the symptoms in the Materia Medica when in reality there is not a general or guiding symptom on which to prescribe. Such lack of symptoms is due to feeble vitality.

If you see that a patient must go in twenty-four to forty-eight hours, and suffering, it is a delightful part of Homœopathy to administer Euthanasia to arouse vital action suddenly and permit the patient to go.

If you can feel in your old age that the well proved remedies are all your friends, you should feel a state of humility that you are an instrument of such service.

There is much more to be learned about disease from the medicines, because disease is more obscured by the culminations.

The limit of drug action is symptomatology.

It is only after a careful and complete study of the finer provings of drug and the same of the finer features of disease that a law can be demonstrated.

The finest degrees of sensation are to be perceived for these changes constitute the nature of the disease. If drugs could not produce these changes they could not cure. This is the foundation. If you would discover whether the law of similar is the law of cure you would need to draw upon this store of finer symptoms.

Pathology has no place in an effort to select a medicine for the sick.

The microscope is only suitable to demonstrate the most concrete of matter. When the third potency of Gold cures it is because some portions of it are finer.

There never was a genuine Homœopath who discouraged the real genuine study of anatomy and physiology.

As soon as you begin to prescribe on peculiar symptoms you prescribe on keynotes, and will not do good work. When you have three symptoms—keynotes—it is true you may possibly get the right remedy, but what do you know of your *patient*, or of the image? You will never have the case in hand, or grasp the true nature of the case in this way.

When a remedy has benefited a patient satisfactorily, never on your life, change your remedy, but repeat that remedy so long as you can benefit the patient. Do not regard the symptoms that have come up.

The remedy has actually led to a change. Don't reason that if you had given a certain remedy in the beginning you could have cured your patient. The masked symptoms come out as a result of the remedy.

The more you cultivate Homœopathic methods, and the finer you discriminate, the better you see and the more you can understand.

Positive principles should govern every physician when he goes to the bedside of the sick. The sick have a right to this if it can be had.

The most villianous doctors are always hunting for something strange and peculiar. Those out of the way symptoms and strange pains are not what we prescribe on and will seldom serve you. The generals are the ruling symptoms and are what *the patient says*, the individual himself.

Never prescribe for a chronic case when you are in a hurry; take time. Never give a dose of medicine until you have duly considered the whole case.

You cannot count twenty-five decent provings since Hahnemann. They leave out what they call imagination and put in morbid anatomy.

Just so sure as you prescribe a one-sided remedy for an Hysterical case, just so sure will she leave you after a while because you do not cure.

The physician must be possessed of a knowledge of the human desires, must be a reader of human nature, not only as it relates to the sick room but in health.

If you place your trust in the Vital Force you will not hammer away with remedies. You must have confidence enough in the economy so that when you have started a commotion you can rest. There is a very quiet change going on.

A keynote prescriber is but a memory prescriber; he has memorized only and has not made it a part of his understanding. Such prescribers are almost useless and it is among them that we find "falling from grace."

The Psoric condition will result, in one, in brain disease, in another in organic liver disease, or structural change in the kidneys. The symptoms which present themselves after organic changes have occurred are far less important though not to be ignored.

When we recognize the fact of the long years of existence of chronic cases, also that they are often inherited for several generations, if a cure is made in the course of two or three years it is indeed a speedy cure. It takes from two to five years to cure chronic diseases.

We must remember that Vital Force is Simple Substance, and that which cures must be Simple Substance.

The greatest comfort on earth to man in incurable diseases is Homœopathy.

In incurable cases where there are extensive structural changes, use short acting remedies and such antipsorics as do not relate to the case as it was in the beginning. The remedy that fits the previous condition will tear the case down.

In old incurable cases when we give a remedy that fits the whole condition, the result is one of three things: first, aggravation of the symptoms with advance of the disease; second, no action, and third, Euthanasia.

Unless the inner nature of the remedy corresponds with the inner nature of the disease the remedy will not cure the disease but simply remove the symptoms which it covers; that is, suppress them.

Such antipsorics as do not relate to the constitutional condition of the patient are comforting and palliative and act as short acting remedies.

In advanced Phthisis with pathological symptoms, if

you prescribe for the old symptoms which should have prescribed for some years before, you kill your patient.

A Sycotic is never cured unless a discharge is brought back.

All things that change the aspect of a case should be avoided.

When a case comes back in a few days with all the symptoms changed, unless they are old symptoms, the prescription was inaccurate and unfortunate.

We are told that the afterbirth must be removed, and scraped off if necessary; these are insane acts and jeopardize life.

The body is covered on the outside and inside by a membrane that protects it from all noxious influences except violence. It is the same with the parturient, so long as you do not denude the uterus with officious interfering, there is no danger of blood poisoning. But if the placenta does not come away by gentle traction and abdominal pressure let it alone. Treat the cause and not the effects of disease.

There are degrees of fineness of the Vital Force. We may think of internal man as possessing infinite degrees and of external man as possessing finite degrees.

We see the difference between short and long acting remedies from this. Short acting remedies are only capable of corresponding to the outermost degree of man.

It is known that old fashioned medicine of all sorts fails to recognize that there are principles of plain and intelligible governing the practice of medicine. They regard it as a mere matter of "experience."

In vaccination when a new disease comes on the former is suspended during the time, and comes on again even though the crust had not formed. This is related as most wonderful, but this the Homœopath understands. Syphilis makes symptoms of Scrofula to disappear in the same way and after Mercury subdues the Syphilis, then the Scrofula comes back. One occupies some hidden precinct in the economy while the other is active.

The knowledge of complementary remedies is necessary of the nearest remedy in its nature and not in a few symptoms. Thus in a series of complementary remedies, the conditions must be there as well as the symptoms.

Keep in a series of complementary remedies. We can never cure if we select a remedy for a part of the symptoms, and as others come up, give a remedy that is not the complement.

In regard to nosodes, when prescribed upon the symptoms which they produce upon the healthy, they will cure the same as other remedies. But to use these things indiscriminately is an outrage.

Structural changes are not the basis for a prescription, but the symptoms which existed before the structural changes appeared.

The mind symptoms, if you can know them, are the most important. If the pathological symptoms seem to contra-indicate a remedy, and the mental symptoms to indicate it, these are to be taken.

In cases without symptoms, the patient must be kept on Sac. Lac. until you can discern some general, such as aggravation of symptoms in the morning, or at midnight. If the patient is only "tired," without guiding symptoms, you may know that it is liable to terminate in some grave disorder—Consumption, Bright's Disease, Cancer, or the like.

A copious discharge protects many an individual from changes in organs.

When derangement localizes itself upon one particular place it is for the purpose of tearing that organ all to pieces. If it sets up a discharge, that is a sort of safety valve and the other organs are protected.

Hahnemann did not mean simply Scabies when he said Itch, but all skin diseases as a class.

No applications which are capable of doing anything can be used without injury. If so simple that they do not change the symptoms they are of course useless.

The healthier the patient becomes the more likelihood there is for an eruption upon the skin. The vital energies must be sufficient for this. A cure progresses from within outward.

All susceptible provers will bring out the image of the remedy. The prover catches the drug disease from one or two doses just as people do the Scarlet Fever or the Grippe.

There are degress within degress to infinity. All may be made sensitive or become so to certain things and with differing degress of susceptibility; hence what folly to lay down the rule for a fixed dose beyond which the result would be fatal, and beyond which if a physician should go he would be responsible in case of death.

The expressions by which we know that he has been sick for a long time we know by our study of pathology and anatomy. These are the results of disease, but the primitive disease is evidenced by the symptoms, the morbid sensations.

Never leave a remedy until you have tested it in a higher potency if it has benefited the patient.

Higher means interior in quality.

The interior man is superior to the external man. Through this outer instrument everything is reflected or rather conducted.

The physician cultivates his eye for everything that it is possible to pass judgment upon and must write down everything that is unnatural, everything that is expressive of illness.

One remedy must be more similar than the other. It is true that one not conversant with the subject will be unable to see the finer shades of difference. Some are color blind, yet others can pick out colors.

The Homœopathic physician must continue to study in the science and in the art before he can become expert. This will grow in him until he becomes increasingly astute and he will grow stronger and wiser in his selections for sick people.

The wisest will make mistakes in perception, but the aim must ever be to find the most similar of any medicines proved, and to recognize that there is one most similar of all.

INDEX

PART I.—KENT'S NEW REMEDIES

PART II.—LESSER WRITINGS, 197

LESSER WRITINGS.—Continued

PART III.—CLINICAL CASES

CLINICAL CASES.— Continued